"The Drs. Petersen have cracked open a [...] one that causes untold suffering for millions. The Gluten [...] remarkable window into the innumerable ways in which gluten— that sticky little molecule found in our staff of life, bread, and hidden in so many other places—can cause everything from autism to dementia, from depression to psoriasis and so much more. If you have nagging symptoms that just don't go away, and you have no idea where they come from, you may be suffering from the gluten effect. This book can save your life!"

—Mark Hyman, MD, *New York Times* best-selling author of
UltraMetabolism, The UltraSimple Diet and *The UltraMind Solution*

"Gluten intolerance is an increasing issue in our health today, yet it takes the average person nine years to be diagnosed. Gluten intolerance and celiac disease wear many faces yet most people are treated for their depression, their arthritis, their lack of energy and their digestive issues separately. Drs. Vikki and Richard Petersen have done a great job translating the current scientific research into usable information about the ONE underlying cause of illness for many people who seem to have so many health ailments: gluten intolerance. Reading this book can be transformative for many people who are suffering needlessly."

—Liz Lipski, PhD, CCN, CHN; author of *Digestive Wellness*,
Digestive Wellness for Children and *Leaky Gut Syndrome*;
director of doctoral studies at Hawthorn University

The Petersens have brought to light a phenomenon observed in my practice and in those of many clinicians that when addressed, can change the health of those affected. Food allergies, gluten being one of the more common, have long gone undiagnosed and even scoffed at as an important cause of chronic illness. Pharmacists are involved in helping patients every day with all sorts of allergies. It is my hope they will expand their approach to health to include gluten and other food allergies as basic education for their patients.

—Lisa Everett, RPh, CCN, FACA

"In *The Gluten Effect* the Drs. Petersen take the neglected and often misunderstood subject of gluten sensitivity and make it understandable to the layperson.

Previous reading material on the subject of gluten intolerance has literally put me to sleep. This is not the case with *The Gluten Effect*. Knowledge is power and this book delivers the knowledge in a way that is not only easy to understand but interesting.

I was personally diagnosed with gluten intolerance fifteen years ago. I eliminated gluten from my diet and as a result of my improved health have embraced the gluten-free lifestyle. I host a gluten-free blog and am currently writing a gluten-free cookbook, and yet it wasn't until reading *The Gluten Effect* that I fully understood all the far-reaching implications gluten has on the body.

Prior to visiting HealthNOW Medical Center and working with Dr. Petersen I had suffered from migraine headaches since the age of thirteen. I was exhausted by the age of twenty-six and despite outward appearances of good health my body was beginning to betray me. At thirty I was starting to feel like an old woman. What an amazing discovery it was to find that I could reverse these effects on my body with what I ate.

The Drs. Petersen give us the power to improve our health and change our lives in *The Gluten Effect*."

—Carol Kicinski, author of www.simplygluten-free.blogspot.com

"The story this book tells of how gluten ravages the body and the HealthNOW Method, which counters this by enabling the body to repair the damage naturally to restore vibrant health, is a breakthrough. Although the chemistry in our bodies is extremely complex and the story is not simple, the Drs. Petersen take the reader clearly and accessibly through the labyrinthine processes and destructive roles gluten plays in nearly every system of those with gluten sensitivities. Since we are what we eat, gluten's reach extends far beyond the digestive system. The central nervous system, the glands (which regulate hormone production and balance), our organs—none escape its havoc.

I write this from experience. Although leading a generally healthy lifestyle, my health started to seriously fail in my late forties. By fifty-five I had a constellation of the very serious problems described in this book. Naturally, being Italian-American, pasta and bread were central to me and I was quite skeptical, to say the least, that gluten had anything to do with any of my problems! But all else had failed and I was deteriorating. So, at my wife's urging, I went to the HealthNOW office six years ago. That visit transformed my life at every level and I am healthier than I have been in over ten years. I have since referred many family and friends with "mysterious" symptoms that evade mainstream medicine to HealthNOW, and they have had similarly positive results. I will always be grateful for the Petersens' help."

—Louis Allamandola, PhD; fellow of the American Physical Society and the American Association for the Advancement of Science; winner of the Presidential Rank Award for Meritorious Senior Professional; senior scientist, NASA

"This book fills an important place in consumer literature by supplying a practical, step-by-step program of recognizing gluten sensitivity and then removing it from your life. As Drs. Vikki and Richard Petersen point out, gluten sensitivity can often be an underrecognized cause of a host of difficult-to-diagnosis symptoms. Food sensitivity, and gluten sensitivity in particular, is often called the 'great masquerader' because it can be the underlying source of a host of symptoms, ranging from fatigue to migraines, joint pain, autoimmune thyroiditis, osteoarthritis, eczema and depression. The Petersens have made a clear case for the importance of assessing whether you are likely to have gluten sensitivity by presenting a thorough evaluation of the subject and a plethora of convincing case studies of patients they've helped. They then make the practical application of removing gluten doable. While it can be challenging to remove this very common food ingredient from one's diet, it can be worthwhile and life-changing. In sum, this book can be a roadmap for individuals who have had chronic health problems and have yet to find an answer."

—Dan Lukaczer, ND, associate director of medical education
at the Institute for Functional Medicine

The Gluten Effect

How "Innocent" Wheat Is Ruining Your Health

Drs. Vikki and Richard Petersen, DC, CCN

True Health Publishing

For more information, please visit www.healthnowmedical.com
or email DrVikki@healthnowmedical.com

Book design by Arbor Books, Inc.
www.arborbooks.com

Author photo on cover by Jeffrey Hosier

Printed in the United States of America

The Gluten Effect: How "Innocent" Wheat Is Ruining Your Health
Drs. Vikki and Richard Petersen, DC, CCN

1. Title   2. Author   3. Health/Diet

Library of Congress Control Number: 2008911364

ISBN 10: 0-9822711-0-7
ISBN 13: 978-0-9822711-0-0

We dedicate this book to each other and to all our patients, both past and present. Their desire to improve their health and our ability to assist them has been a most rewarding team effort.

We also dedicate this book to our three children, who probably know more about the human body and nutrition than most adults due to hearing about it incessantly throughout their lives. Our greatest wish for them is that they find passions in their lives that they love as much as we love being doctors.

And, finally, we dedicate this book to those caring men and women who are committed to what they do and who try to make this world a better place. Those special people who are not afraid to buck the system and do what they know is right despite opposition are the true heroes of this world, and we salute them.

Table of Contents

SECTION FOUR
Other Gluten-related Disorders Including Depression, Weight Gain,
Fibromyalgia and Memory Loss

SECTION FIVE
Finding and Eliminating the Cause

Acknowledgements

Being a health practitioner is a journey that brings many gifts: the great joy of helping one's fellow man, the meeting of great men and women who are similarly devoted to improving the lives of others, and the knowledge that there is always more to learn and discover.

We have been very thankful to cross paths with some special people who have dedicated their lives to helping others and wish to acknowledge them here. They have impacted us in positive ways both personally and professionally, and this world is a better place for having them in it.

While we hope to include everyone, we apologize in advance for anyone we forget.

Dr. William Timmins, Dr. Jeffrey Bland, Dr. Mark Hyman, Dr. Terry Franks, Dr. Alan Beardall, Dr. William Kelley, Dr. Diana Schwarzbein, Liz Lipski, PhD, Ann Louise Gittleman, PhD, Dr. Tom O'Bryan, Dr. Dan Lukaczer, Dr. David S. Jones, Dr. David Singer, Dr. Barry Sears, Cindy Feshbach, Rick Manning, Judith Saldariagga, Ruth Valko, Darlene Eggen, Jackson Bain, the staff of HealthNOW Medical Center and L. Ron Hubbard.

Tips on How Best to Read This Book

This book is written for the layperson. A glossary is supplied at the back of the book so that you can look up terms you don't understand. Often, readers put down books because they run into words they don't fully understand, which results in their losing interest. We want you to get as much out of this book as possible, so please use the glossary whenever you need to in order to enhance your understanding.

Each chapter is heavily referenced so that you can show your doctor the scientific references that support the statements that are made.

Unfortunately, many doctors are not aware of the information contained in this book because when they were initially trained, it was not known. While awareness of gluten sensitivity has increased dramatically in recent years in the scientific community, the medical field has not yet caught up—a problem that we hope to remedy with this book.

We recommend that you start at the beginning of the book and read through to at least chapter seven. After that, sections III and IV contain chapters that give information about specific diseases and symptoms, and you may wish to turn to those that cover the subjects in which you have the most interest. Section V contains the last three chapters, which we encourage you to read as they sum up the entire book.

To your good health,
Doctors Vikki and Richard Petersen, D.C., C.C.N.

Introduction

Why We're Writing This Book

If you're picking up this book in the hope of finding an answer to your health problems, you have the right frame of mind. This book is about gluten sensitivity and its underappreciated ability to have far-reaching, negative effects upon your health. The decision to write a book about gluten came as a result of our many years of practicing a method of medicine identifying the root cause of people's health problems. We call this method the HealthNOW Method. Again and again we had patients describing how significantly their lives changed after discovering that they were gluten sensitive. This book aims to inspire you to seek out the root cause of your health problem and help you discover if the root cause is gluten sensitivity.

Why Do So Many Patients Suffer Undiagnosed?

It has now been more than fifteen years since we became interested in the effects of gluten on the health of our patients. In years past, the most commonly known form of gluten sensitivity, celiac disease, was a rare diagnosis. What is even more startling is that celiac disease is diagnosed in only a small fraction of affected individuals, even today. Why is this? The biggest reason lies in how standard medicine approaches health in general. Patients with gluten sensitivity, we have found, demonstrate many different symptoms. Likewise, the symptoms are usually nonspecific, which means that they could manifest from many different health conditions. As a result, more common conditions are investigated first and sometimes the underappreciated disorders, such as gluten sensitivity, go unnoticed.

Dr Vikki's Mother Started Our Gluten Adventure

Vikki's mother's case was an example of this. In addition to having many medical problems, including an adrenal gland dysfunction, she had long suffered from chronic headaches, fatigue, low blood sugar, constipation and a host of other complaints. She had undergone many tests and examinations, but none of these had given her an answer. Medicines were prescribed and treatments recommended, but in the end, the symptoms stayed the same.

We had just begun investigating gluten sensitivity in our office when we tested Vikki's mother for anti-gliadin antibodies. This is a test to see if the body's immune system is reacting to gluten in a negative way. Well, to our surprise, she had elevated levels of these antibodies. Even more intriguing was the fact that she responded dramatically well to a gluten-free diet. Her headaches, low blood sugar and constipation resolved after having suffered for well over fifty years of her life. Today she is a vibrant, healthy eighty-five-year-old who takes no medication and, by her own statement, considers that she is in "the best health of her entire life."

Our Youngest Daughter Proves the Genetic Link

To drive home the point even further, fifteen years ago our newly born daughter had been having persistent problems with projectile vomiting. When this is an ongoing problem, believe us when we say that you try to find an answer as quickly as possible. Not only is it painful to see your child suffer, but the mess is not much fun either.

After Vikki's mother was found to react poorly to gluten, and knowing that this can run in families, we tested our daughter. Sure enough, she likewise demonstrated gluten sensitivity and responded very nicely to the elimination of gluten in her diet. This started our crusade to evaluate the effects of gluten on people's health.

Why Is Gluten a Problem?

But what is gluten? You have possibly heard of it in recent years, with gluten-free foods being sold at health stores and the rash of gluten-free recipe books in bookstores. But what is it? And what is gluten sensitivity? Gluten is essentially the major protein component of wheat, rye and barley. As it is metabolized or broken down, it can give some people tremendous problems. In short, the body's immune system can see it as a toxin and therefore launch an attack against it. Varied and multiple symptoms are created depending on what tissues of the body are attacked.

Take the Gluten Sensitivity Self-Test
Check off the symptoms that apply to you:

Digestive
- ☐ Bloating and/or gas
- ☐ Constipation and/or diarrhea
- ☐ Nausea
- ☐ Weight trouble
- ☐ Iron-deficiency anemia

Hormonal
- ☐ Fatigue
- ☐ Sleep problems
- ☐ Depression, anxiety and/or mood swings
- ☐ Menstrual problems
- ☐ Infertility
- ☐ Thyroid problems
- ☐ Osteoporosis or osteopenia

Neurological
- ☐ Headaches and/or Migraines
- ☐ Memory problems
- ☐ Joint pains or aches
- ☐ Fibromyalgia
- ☐ Brain Fog

Immune System
- ☐ Get infections easily
- ☐ Arthritis, any type, you or family
- ☐ Cancer history, you or family
- ☐ Autoimmune disease, you or family
- ☐ Celiac disease, you or family

If you checked 1 to 3 boxes gluten sensitivity may be playing a role in your health problems.
If you checked 4 to 7 boxes there is a definite possibility that you are suffering from gluten sensitivity.
If you checked 8 or more boxes the likelihood is strong that gluten sensitivity is having a negative effect upon your health.

Let's Improve Your Health

Are you ready to consider a fresh approach to your health? Are you interested in finding what the underlying cause is rather than merely masking your symptoms? So are we. If you suffer from cramping, nausea, chronic bowel problems or stomach pains, the information in this book about gluten could be what you have been seeking. If you have chronic fatigue, sleep difficulties, depression, memory difficulty or anxiety, you will want to hear about how gluten affects the nervous system. If you have joint pains, rashes, chronic pain, weight issues or menstrual problems, don't rule gluten out as a potential base cause to your symptoms. If you are constantly getting infections or have other immune or autoimmune disorders, investigating gluten certainly is worth your time. While all of these complaints are varied in nature, their occurrences reflect how gluten may "stress" your health.

It wasn't until the 1970s that clinicians even appreciated how "bad" cholesterol and fats in our diet cause heart disease and stroke. Since that time, attention to these dietary components has significantly decreased these diseases. Likewise, we are just now understanding the effects that simple sugars have on our bodies' ability to produce insulin and regulate glucose in relationship to diabetes and glucose intolerance.

What You Eat Does Matter

Diet has always been a major influence on our health, and truly, we are what we eat. New vitamins, minerals and herbal nutrients continue to be discovered decade after decade. This is such a virgin field in this modern era of medicine, even though it would seem to be so basic. It is no wonder, then, that we are only now embracing how gluten can affect our bodies. This protein in wheat, rye and barley has been around for thousands of years. But its evolution, and its growing appearance in our diets, has finally caught our attention. For many of you, it indeed may be the root cause to your symptoms.

We have written this book because of experiences with our patients.

We love helping people get healthier so that they can live life to the fullest. Illness and symptoms keep a person from fully experiencing life and fully participating in life's pleasures. Our source of continued inspiration is our patients. Below is a letter that a patient wrote to us when asked how her life had changed after discovering that she was gluten sensitive.

Rachel's Incredible Story

It's very strange to think back and remember the years that I suffered because I didn't know I had gluten sensitivity. There is a very clear line of separation between my old life with gluten and my new life without it. It almost feels like I'd been living another life for so many years, like I was a different person. My story is relatively heavy on my symptoms, because I'd had my old life for almost twenty-seven years, and my new life is only six months old. I'm confident I'll be adding many more years to my new life...and many chapters to my story.

I'd had allergy-like symptoms year-round since I was six or seven, and I'd had the skin test for allergies when I was fourteen. I didn't react to any of the allergens, so my diagnosis was non-allergy rhinitis. My allergy-like symptoms persisted for another ten years, but since they had no distinct cause, I had no real treatment options and never experienced relief.

I started to have problems with acne before I was ten. I tried Proactiv and many other acne products, but none of them kept my acne under control. I even tried removing chocolate from my diet, since everyone seemed to blame chocolate for their blemishes, but that had no effect. Even in my mid-twenties, I still had the complexion I'd had as a teenager: oily and blemished. I eventually was convinced that I would never have clear skin.

My hair was always thin when I was young, but by the time I was twelve, it was quite obvious that my hair was thinning. My hair continued to thin all the way through college and beyond. I could see my entire scalp through my hair when I looked in the mirror. I felt there was no point in styling it anymore, because even the hairdressers I went to didn't know what they could do with my hair, besides fluffing it up with mousse and hairspray. My hair was simply falling out and not growing back.

By sixteen, I had started feeling overly fatigued. I no longer had the energy to stay up late. Every day, I would come home from school and take a nap until dinnertime. My memory started to suffer, and I was experiencing the notorious "brain fog" effect. I had always been at the top of my class and somewhat of an overachiever scholastically, but slowly, I was losing the ability to grasp new concepts, and homework assignments that normally would have taken a short time would drag on for hours. I would often lose control of my eye movements while reading, which only added to my frustration and multiplied the time and effort I would spend on my studies.

I seemed to catch every cold and flu that made its way to my school. I could count on having bronchitis twice a year, usually coupled with tonsillitis or a sinus infection. I would have random skin infections that resulted in hospital visits once or twice a year. It just seemed like my immune system couldn't keep up.

I often wondered how the other students in my classes could finish all of their homework AND play sports AND participate in after-school activities and clubs... It just didn't seem possible to me. I would complain about spending three hours on my calculus homework the night before, and my classmates would stare at me like I was crazy and say they only spent an hour on the same assignment. Still, I managed to keep my grades up, but at a tremendous cost mentally and physically.

I slowly realized over the years that I would have to give up my dream job. I had wanted to be a geneticist, but I knew I wouldn't survive such demanding college coursework if I could barely keep afloat in high school. I settled for a subject that would be less demanding on my mind and body, but that I still had interest in.

By then, the pain had started to set in. The pain started in my back and eventually moved through my torso and into my limbs. It was a deep, aching pain, unlike a sore muscle or a vertebra out of place, and always seemed to radiate from my back. My pain levels would fluctuate on a daily basis, but I normally found hugs to be especially painful, and feeling the pressure of my back against any piece of furniture would worsen the pain considerably. Ibuprofen would usually dull the pain, but pain was my constant reminder that something was awry.

I didn't really have the energy to drive, but when I finally got a car and started providing my own transportation, one very serious problem presented itself. Every time I would have to drive for longer than ten minutes at a time, there was a one-hundred-percent chance that I would fall asleep at the wheel. It was never the result of a gradual sleepiness; it was always abrupt, like my brain switched itself off. I would usually wake up a few moments later, also abruptly, and I would spend the rest of my drive battling sleep. If my drive to work took twenty-five minutes, it wasn't unusual for me to fall asleep fifteen or more times. I sometimes resorted to punching myself in the leg to try to keep myself awake, but I would often fall asleep anyway and awaken to find myself still punching my leg. In all those years, I actually never had any wrecks as a result of my sleepiness, and I only ran off the road once... I knew I was VERY lucky, but I also knew that someday my luck would eventually run out.

I fell into deep depression after college. I knew my body wouldn't hold up long enough for me to go somewhere, socialize and go home, so I didn't really have a social life or a network of friends for a few years. I felt old and worn out and very much in pain. Many times in my life, I just wanted a hug of encouragement, but I knew that a hug would only cause me more physical pain; constantly having to weigh emotional comfort against physical pain ultimately made me feel even worse about myself. I felt so alienated from my old friends, and several of my relationships ended because I wanted to spend most of my time resting at home instead of going out and having fun. My life was going nowhere.

My daytime sleepiness worsened to the point that I would fall asleep while sitting at my desk at work. I would sometimes crawl under my desk to sleep, because I was too exhausted to walk to my car and take a nap there. It was almost as if I could feel a command to sleep, like something in my brain would switch off and I had no choice but to obey. I no longer felt rested at all, no matter how many hours I allowed for sleep. I hated sleeping, I hated being awake, and I hated the grey area in between.

My digestion was suffering also. I felt bloated all the time and was usually constipated. I tried a diet very high in fiber, which is, of course, what is recommended, but my digestion never improved. It didn't seem to matter what I ate; I just couldn't process the food and move it out of my system.

I was in my early twenties and at the time, dressed like a skater girl. Some of my doctors constantly asked me if I used recreational drugs, because they couldn't come up with any other medical reason why I should be having so many seemingly unrelated symptoms, and I guess my looks were deceiving. Of course, I didn't use drugs, and I know the doctors were just trying to rule out all the possibilities, but I encountered the same questions from the same doctors, visit after visit. It was like they didn't believe me, or didn't want to believe me. I think one of my doctors eventually wrote me off as a hypochondriac, but I don't have his notes, so I'm not certain. I was very reluctant to seek help for my problems for a while afterward.

But I needed help so I continued to try to find it. However, the doctors throughout the years didn't know how to treat me. My symptoms were all over the map. There was a routine I came to expect. I would visit a new doctor and explain some of my worst symptoms, and they would respond with a smile and say, "Ah... I bet I know what's going on..." The usual suspects were fibromyalgia and multiple sclerosis. The doctors would have blood drawn and run all kinds of tests, sometimes series of MRIs and MRAs, but in the end, no doctor felt comfortable declaring any diagnosis. For years, all I wanted was a diagnosis...any diagnosis...so I could receive some kind of treatment. Instead, I usually received the generic "diet and exercise" response.

I decided to give the "diet and exercise" plan another try. I didn't have the energy to go to a gym, so I bought a dance mat for my PlayStation and played Dance Dance Revolution for my aerobic exercise. At least three times a week, I danced until the game said I had burned 200 calories—usually about twenty minutes. I would then collapse from complete exhaustion. I tried warming up and cooling down, drinking more water, eating a healthy snack beforehand to give me energy, and reducing my goal to 100 calories, but the result was always the same. I hated exercise, and I didn't understand how anyone could think exercise would improve their energy levels. I could only force myself to exercise at night, after I didn't have anything else I needed to accomplish that day.

I was eventually referred to a sleep specialist, who suspected I had narcolepsy or some other sleep disorder and had me do an overnight sleep study at her clinic. She studied my results and could not offer a solid explanation for my sleepiness. I had some, but not all, of the symptoms of classic narcolepsy, but she prescribed Provigil anyway to see if it would help, and I saw incredible improvement. I still didn't have the energy to do too much more physical activity, but my daytime sleepiness waned. I was, however, very dependent on Provigil, and I would start falling asleep again if I missed a dose.

I was very near the point of giving up when a friend referred me to the doctors at HealthNOW Medical Center. I truly felt the doctors there actually listened to my problems and wanted to help me, so when I was ordered to go on a modified elimination diet, I hated the idea, but I decided to make the effort and try the diet. No other doctor had given me such a radical piece of advice, and it sounded crazy enough to work.

After just a few days on the diet, I experienced heavy withdrawal symptoms. My body was craving *something*...craving it badly...but I didn't know what or why. I was especially moody, impatient and unpleasant, and none of the food I ate would comfort me. Not long afterward, the doctors at HealthNOW told me that my saliva test confirmed that I did indeed have gluten sensitivity. So...I was having gluten withdrawal. The concept blew my mind. I hated to admit it, but I knew they were right. They had started me on the right path, and I had a diagnosis I could work with.

My body's first noticeable, positive reaction to my gluten-free diet was completely unexpected. I woke up one morning and realized that my bed sheets felt "different." My clothes also felt "different." It was almost as if everything I touched had a more pronounced texture. I put on my sandals to go to work and noticed that the straps were no longer tight enough to keep my feet from slipping out. Apparently, my body's reaction to gluten had caused quite a bit of swelling, especially in my feet, that I had never noticed.

The pain, my old constant companion, began to subside. I could finally sit in my expensive, ergonomic desk chair at work for longer periods of time without worrying about my back hurting just from the pressure.

After a few weeks on a gluten-free diet, my acne cleared up considerably, and after a few more weeks, blemishes became more and more of a rarity. My hair slowly started to thicken until

I could no longer see so much of my scalp through my hair. My coworkers noticed my clearer skin and thicker hair before I did.

During the last cold and flu season, I only caught one cold from a coworker. That's a record low for me. Most of my allergy-like symptoms have subsided, so I no longer feel I have to carry a box of tissues everywhere. My immune system seems much more efficient and much less stressed.

My digestive system has also started to work more efficiently, and I rarely encounter the digestive issues I'd dealt with in the past. I quickly lost about eight pounds during the first few weeks of the diet, and my weight is still much more manageable.

I have even survived a few days without Provigil. When I miss a dose, I still feel sleepy, but I don't battle to stay awake anymore. I am hopeful that I will progress to the point that I no longer have to rely on that medication at all.

I feel so much less pain.... It's incredible (but still slightly strange) to be able to enjoy hugs again. The radiating pain is mostly gone now. I usually only feel pain when I've earned it with an injury.

It's still very difficult sometimes, knowing that I won't be able to go out to eat with friends at most restaurants without bringing my own food. I still have so many food options, so I try to focus on what I *can* eat instead of what I *can't* eat. I'm slowly becoming a better cook, and I am more comfortable eating my own culinary creations because I know exactly which ingredients went into the food.

I know I am the same person I was before I kicked gluten to the curb, but the difference in my quality of life is staggering. I'm just so much healthier, and life is so much more vibrant than it was before. I still occasionally deal with brain fog and fatigue, but certainly not to the extent that my symptoms impact my life so greatly anymore.

Hope is a wonderful thing.

—*Rachel F.*

We Want You to Have a "Health Miracle"!

Such "miracles" are almost daily occurrences in our practice. Is that rewarding? Absolutely! Do we only want such benefits for the patients that are within driving distance of our clinic? Absolutely not. If reading this book doesn't improve your health, it is very likely that it will improve the health of someone you know. Gluten intolerance is that pervasive and, at the same time, that unrecognized. We are committed, through our endeavors, to increase people's awareness of it.

SECTION ONE

Why All the Sudden Interest in Gluten?

One

Introduction to Gluten Sensitivity

Angelita's Story

Angelita could not believe it. For the first time in almost fifteen years, she felt "normal." No cramping, no bloating, no fatigue. These and so many other symptoms that she had suffered from over the years had gradually dissipated, almost miraculously, in just a few weeks.

What had made the difference? Angelita had been diagnosed as having gluten sensitivity, a dietary intolerance to a protein called gluten. Since she had eliminated gluten from her diet, all of her complaints had resolved. The days of missing work due to the unpredictable nature of her bowels were over. She was no longer at the mercy of her body. Angelita was now in control. The frustration and irritation of her chronic symptoms were now replaced with a sense of relief.

But at the same time, Angelita could not help but feel a bit resentful of the delay in finding the root cause of her problems.

In the prime of her life, she had been forced to adapt to the constraints of her bodily handicap. In what was supposed to be the age of modern medicine, why had this diagnosis escaped the slew of physicians she had been seeing since she was a child?

Doctors "Miss" Gluten Sensitivity When Diagnosing Patients

Such case studies are all too typical. What complicates the picture even further is that most clinicians have yet to distinguish gluten sensitivity from celiac disease. As an overview, celiac disease is a type of gluten intolerance that specifically damages the digestive tract. Celiac disease represents the most well-known gluten-related disorder, but it is by no means the most common one. Thousands of people suffer from non-celiac gluten sensitivity, as will be explained in this book, and it is our goal to increase awareness of the entire spectrum of gluten health disorders. Celiac disease simply represents one variety of gluten intolerance, as you will learn.

It Takes, on Average, Eleven Years to Get Diagnosed

On average, there has been a delay of eleven years between the time of symptom onset and a diagnosis of celiac disease for those who have actually been diagnosed. Since celiac disease is the most commonly recognized gluten-related disorder, the delay in diagnosing gluten sensitivity is presumably much longer. Opinions support the idea that the less than twenty-five percent of our population who is suffering with gluten intolerance has been accurately diagnosed.[1] Today, there are many diagnostic tests that aid the diagnosis, and it appears that one in every 250 people of American and European descent has celiac disease,[2] but this represents a small fraction of all gluten-sensitive individuals. And while celiac disease is the major known form of gluten sensitivity, how many other people have the lesser-known gluten intolerance, which results in many serious and variable symptoms?

Although described by Aretaeus of Cappadocia in 250 AD, celiac disease was originally described scientifically in 1888 by an astute clinician named Gee.[3] A century later the majority of the cases are still unidentified.

Doctors Don't Look for the Root Cause

In today's era, no different from centuries past, there exists a large number of people who suffer from a multitude of symptoms for which traditional medicine has yet to identify the cause. This has occurred despite tremendous advances in genetic research, diagnostic abilities and knowledge of the body's physiologic and pathologic processes. These symptoms range from fatigue, depression and stress to chronic pain, joint aches and many, many more. So, like Angelita, who endured test after test that continued to show normal results, modern medicine seeks to comfort the symptoms and wait for the cause to declare itself, or for better diagnostics to evolve.

Masking the Symptom Is Not the Answer

How many people now take a pain reliever or a sleep aid on a daily basis? Certainly these medications can have beneficial, though temporary, effects for many people. But it is not reaching the root cause of their problem. If a symptom exists should we just mask it with a drug or should our goal be to detect the underlying, root cause that created that symptom? We feel that it is self-evident that the answer is the latter, and we call our approach and philosophy the HealthNOW Method.

For years, Angelita had tolerated her stomach bloating, painful, intermittent cramping and loose movements. She had been told to try fiber, then a series of medications, to relieve the cramping and diarrhea. While sometimes things appeared to be improving, the symptoms would always return sooner or later. She had seen multiple specialists and undergone many blood tests and probing diagnostics, none of which gave a clue as to the cause of her condition. She had essentially resolved to accept that she indeed had irritable bowel syndrome, and that relief was unattainable.

Angelita Found Her Solution—So Can You!

Eventually, Angelita came to our clinic and began the HealthNOW Method. She was found to have a dramatic response to eliminating gluten in her diet, and her blood testing did show borderline abnormalities, suggesting gluten sensitivity. All of her stomach and intestinal complaints resolved. Like so many others, what was thought to be irritable bowel syndrome turned out to be gluten sensitivity. The solution was simply a change in diet and not an array of medications or other treatments.

Labeling a Disease Is Not the Same as Curing It

Irritable bowel syndrome is a diagnostic label that many gluten-sensitive patients carry prior to their eventual diagnosis. It is a disorder assigned to patients who complain of abdominal cramping and alternating bouts of constipation and diarrhea (and negative diagnostic exams). In theory, this disorder represents a defective ability of the intestines to move digested material along the digestive tract. If it is too fast, cramping and diarrhea occur. If too slow, constipation develops.

A cause of this disorder is not well-defined, and it's likely that many people carry this label even though their root cause may be gluten sensitivity. Several diagnostic labels such as this exist in medicine. They provide patients with a name for their group of symptoms and can help organize research, but at the same time may deter individuals from continuing to look for the real cause.

What Do You Do When Lab Tests Are Normal, But You Still Feel Sick?

With conditions like migraines, chronic fatigue syndrome, fibromyalgia and insomnia, it is evident that diagnostic medicine has significant limitations. All of these represent similar labels to irritable bowel syndrome. Tests and exams are repeatedly normal, and patients are left without any clear understanding of their conditions' causes. Theories about a genetic flaw or a relationship to stress are often given as explanations, and a medication is prescribed to hopefully alleviate the symptoms. The patient then leaves feeling hopeless and perplexed.

Such is the case for those with gluten sensitivity. Their symptoms continue despite medication Band-aids that seek to appease their woes temporarily. Fortunately, there is a growing interest not only in preventative health and lifestyle, but also in diet, nutrition and the environment. This is helping to accelerate our understanding of health in a much broader sense and expand our scope for other potential causes of poor health.

Is the "Art" of Diagnosis No Longer Practiced?

Interestingly, traditional medicine used to handle patient care differently. Prior to all the high-tech radiology procedures, the advanced blood tests and the vast arsenal of prescription drugs, patients' symptoms and physical exam findings were the bases for treatment. Likewise, therapies that were anecdotally effective were introduced long before research evidence validated their benefit. With the advance of diagnostic testing and medication treatment, medicine has adopted stricter rules before implementing therapies. This has not necessarily been a bad thing, especially when it can prevent an unknown side effect of a new drug. But what has developed concurrently has been a shift in the approach to the patient. Clinicians have begun to rely more heavily on test results and less so on symptoms, behavior and lifestyle.

In other words, the creative art of medicine has lost some of its creativity.

A Fresh Approach to Patient Care

In trying to approach health from a fresh perspective, it is important to evaluate all the potential causes of a patient's symptoms. This not only includes family history, medications and known allergies but also diet, nutrition and lifestyle. Symptoms are the body's way of indicating that something is wrong with its normal ability to function. They may be minor, or they could be major and noteworthy. Regardless, they are warning signals that something is affecting the body's health and normal functioning.

Symptoms Can Take Years to Develop

What is not always intuitive is that the cause of these symptoms may have been days, months or even years in the making. For instance, plaque from high cholesterol doesn't develop during the few years before a heart attack; instead, as studies support, arteries develop plaque formation decades earlier. The effects of poor diet, poor exercise and genetics actually begin insidiously before the actual disease (the heart attack) is realized.

Likewise, for someone with multiple sclerosis, a disorder affecting the brain and spinal cord, symptoms of numbness and dizziness can appear years before the diagnosis is made by standard medical testing. Therefore, time association can be quite poor when trying to manage health problems.

The Body Often Responds Quickly to the Correct Therapy

Once Angelita eliminated gluten from her diet, it took about a few weeks to feel significantly better, and within a few months, all of her abdominal complaints resolved. This delay between the cause and the effect was what made it impossible for her to figure out that her condition was a dietary problem. Once gluten is removed, the inflammation that is already present in the small intestines must heal, and this takes some time.

Some Patients Revert to Bad Habits

Many patients make the mistake, months or years later, of adding gluten back into their diets. Usually, within days, weeks or months, symptoms recur. If it takes a long period of time, sometimes patients don't realize that it was the reintroduction of gluten that created their problems. All too often patients mistakenly believe that negative dietary changes will result in a rapid onset of symptoms. When this isn't experienced, they assume that the food is not a problem.

Many disorders of our health are not realized for long periods of time after the inciting causes are introduced. Unless a clinician can continue to probe into all the areas of a patient's health and continue to focus on what systems of the body are creating the symptoms, it can be a challenge to find the true underlying, root cause. Foods and toxins in the environment likely pose the biggest challenges since their effects are difficult to measure within the body, and symptoms can develop very insidiously over time.

Gluten Affects Many Systems of the Body

There is also evidence that gluten intolerance can cause many symptoms outside of the digestive system.[4] Inability to break down this protein fully in the intestines can result in effects in other areas of the body including the nervous system, the immune system and the hormonal regulatory systems. For most of those affected, there are no digestive-related symptoms at all. This fact has certainly contributed to gluten sensitivity as an overlooked diagnosis, as most consider that food reactions will create digestive symptoms.

Gluten intolerance has been implicated in symptoms such as headaches, joint pains, infertility, menstrual irregularities, depression, fatigue, sleep difficulties and many others. All of these will be discussed in detail in later chapters, but suffice it to say that intolerance to gluten in our diets is much more common than appreciated.

Gluten Acts Like a Toxin in Your Body

For a patient with gluten sensitivity, gluten is unable to be broken down well in the upper intestine and absorbed. Instead, it combines with digestive enzymes and triggers the body's own immune system to actively inflame the intestinal wall. The immune system sees the gluten-enzyme complex as foreign and launches an inflammatory assault to rid this foreigner from the body. Unfortunately, the battlefield is your small intestine, and it becomes inflamed and damaged in the process. This results in intestinal symptoms in many, but also affects the intestine's ability to absorb other nutrients. As a result, poor nutrition, vitamin and mineral deficiencies, and exhaustion of the body's immune system can occur, creating many other problems. This is a common mechanism by which gluten intolerance can be the root of so many different complaints.

Gluten Enters the Bloodstream and Creates Havoc in Other Organs

In addition, if gluten (a protein) is digested or even partially digested and reaches the bloodstream, there is ample evidence that this protein complex can have detrimental effects on other organ systems. This also occurs through immune system processes.[5] For instance, children with autism routinely have improvement in behavioral abilities when gluten is eliminated from their diets. Antibodies (substances your immune system makes to identify and neutralize foreign objects) directed against gluten have also been implicated in seizures through effects on the brain in patients.[6]

Gluten Affects the Brain

While, again, diagnostic testing lags behind any objective evidence of cause and effect, gluten, through immune reactions, negatively interacts with certain brain receptors, causing these symptoms. This indicates that gluten can affect one's health in other ways besides its direct effects on the intestinal wall and digestive system. Case reports support evidence that there is much more to gluten's health effects than is currently accepted in traditional medicine.

Wendell's Depression and Fatigue

Wendell is an interesting example of this type of situation. Wendell had complained of fatigue and sleepiness for years. Sleep disorders had been considered, but a cause for his lack of sleep, as well as treatments directed toward insomnia, had provided no relief. He tried to exercise to see if this would help, but, honestly, his lack of energy was a huge deterrent.

Diagnoses of chronic fatigue syndrome and depression had been suggested by different clinicians over the years. After trying several medications to treat his symptoms, all of which had minimal benefit, he decided to come to our clinic. At the time he was taking several medications for sleep and depression, but was very dissatisfied.

Through our HealthNOW Method, he demonstrated positive blood tests for gluten sensitivity and had an improvement, in only one and a half weeks, to a gluten-free diet. Wendell's energy and level of alertness improved significantly, and he has progressively been able to stop taking all the medications previously prescribed.

Though the many prior medical tests and examinations had failed to show a root cause, eventually, Wendell was able to identify gluten as the culprit. What is most interesting in Wendell's case is that he had suffered no digestive symptoms. If a clinician only associates gluten with celiac disease and not the vast number of other health disorders, an accurate diagnosis is unlikely to be found.

Is Gluten a Toxin That Is Creating Your Symptoms?

Just as nutrition can help provide our bodies with the necessary tools to maintain our health, our diets can also introduce substances or toxins that can cause detriment.[7] For many people, gluten falls into this category. It represents not a food but, rather, a toxin that creates adverse effects when it interacts with various body systems.

Detecting food intolerances can, of course, be very difficult, especially when the reaction is insidious and subtle. This is where the challenge lies when trying to truly find the problem's root. The lack of an "evidence trail" by standard diagnostic means imposes a significant roadblock to many physicians. What is required is a symptom-based approach with special attention to the body's systems. Incorporating this into a more global picture of health will lead to better chances of establishing the true cause. The HealthNOW Method contrasts dramatically from the current pervasive method of masking symptoms with drugs creating a false and temporary illusion of health.

What Parts of Your Body Are Affected by Gluten?

So what systems are important when trying to find the root cause of one's symptoms? As mentioned above, the digestive system and immune system are usually the primary systems involved for the gluten-sensitive patient, but secondarily, other systems can be affected as well. Nutritional deficiencies can affect the nervous system, the skin, blood cells and several other body systems. Often joint and muscle systems are symptomatic, as are hormonal balances.

Identifying symptoms and then aligning them with the affected systems of the body can give clues as to the root cause. When standard examinations and tests fail to reveal the problem, a search for other causes must be explored. Details of diet, activity, environment, travel, relationships and chronology can be helpful in narrowing the search for the cause. In essence, this infuses the art of medicine back into the evaluation process. Today's practitioner is too quick, in our opinion, to send a patient on his or her way on the sole criteria of negative laboratory tests, which are mostly looking for disease or pathology. If a patient is suffering, it is our job to isolate the root cause. There always is one.

Angelita and Wendell—Different Symptoms, Same Root Cause

In comparing Angelita's symptoms to Wendell's complaints, one would never think that gluten was the problem for both individuals. However, both had persistent symptoms that escaped accurate diagnosis by standard medicine techniques. In retrospect, there are some similarities that may have been helpful in facilitating earlier diagnosis of gluten sensitivity. Both individuals had chronic symptoms that were not responding to treatments. Also, both had no obvious causes to their complaints based on common tests and diagnostics. Their persistent symptoms and lack of response to treatments should have extended the search for a root cause, and this should have then included a more detailed investigation into their diets and lifestyles. Throughout this book you will see how important these two health factors are in getting to the cause of people's symptoms.

You Can Be Sensitive to Gluten and Have No Digestive Complaints

Certainly, with a digestive system disorder, diet and food groups are very important to evaluate. This likely would have led to a diagnosis of gluten intolerance earlier for Angelita. For Wendell, dietary causes may not have been as apparent since no intestinal complaints were present, but diet affects all of our body's functions. Fatigue and sleep difficulties certainly can be the result of dietary substances. When obvious solutions failed to work in Wendell's situation, examination of dietary toxins should have been explored.

Gluten can definitely be one of those toxins for many people.

Approaching patients with a primary focus on their symptoms allows for a greater awareness of potential causes to their problems. Appreciating that cause and effect can be separated over long spans of time helps keep diagnostic considerations more open.

How Does Gluten Exert Such a Wide Variety of Negative Effects?

In exploring all the effects that gluten can have on our health, a detailed description of what gluten is, how it is broken down and how it can cause physiological effects within our bodies will be discussed. One of the important questions is, why does it seem as though gluten only recently became a health issue? Several factors have evolved that likely provide reasons for this.

Overall, gluten can have widespread effects and symptoms in a person who is intolerant to its digestion and metabolites (a substance produced by metabolism or breakdown). While this creates a daunting task for a diagnostician, it is no different than a variety of other nutritional disorders that have diffuse effects on many cellular functions throughout the body. Vitamin B12 deficiency is a good example of this as it can cause symptoms ranging from fatigue to numbness to memory loss to imbalance. Gluten intolerance, therefore, is no different in its variable manifestations of symptomatology.

What Percentage of the Population is Gluten Sensitive—Thirty Percent, Forty Percent?

Fortunately for Angelita and Wendell, they were able to eventually identify gluten intolerance as the root cause of their health conditions and subsequently improve their quality of life. In examining other case reports and literature, gluten's effects constitute a major cause in many patients' symptoms that have yet to be diagnosed, and as high as thirty percent of the entire population may have gluten sensitivity.[8] This is an amazing figure! And the range of these symptoms can be quite broad.

Don't Give Up—Gluten May Be Causing Your Symptoms

By understanding how gluten ingestion can result in physical problems, patients can help clinicians investigate this as a possible cause of their complaints. Some may have become frustrated with a lack of an answer and decided simply to accept their symptoms. Others continue to struggle along from test to test, hoping that eventually that elusive diagnosis will surface.

The human body is indeed amazing and complex. Paying attention to diet, nutrition, environment and lifestyle can assist the body's own healing mechanisms. And in the case of someone who is gluten-intolerant, it can make all the difference in the world when this offending protein is avoided.

Two

Wheat and Mankind— A Healthy Partnership or a Dangerous Liaison?

Why Is Gluten Suddenly a Problem?

You may wonder why wheat and other grain products are becoming the focus of health attention as of late. Let's face it: Since you have been alive, wheat products, cereals and breads have been a staple in your diet. So why now? Fiber and whole wheat are supposed to lower your cholesterol and lower your risk of colon cancer, so how can they also be potentially harmful?

Gluten's Effects on Your Body Can Develop Slowly

All of these are good questions that highlight the ambiguity around gluten and its effect on our health. The answer lies within how gluten interacts with our bodies and through which mechanisms it affects our well-being. The effects of grains on our health are often indirect and delayed.

There was a program on the National Geographic TV network that demonstrated how the Rocky Mountains had been formed geologically. In short, two very large land masses, called "plates," had pushed toward each other until they'd collided. As they'd continued to push against each other, wrinkles in the land surface had occurred, forming mountains.

This was not some big collision in which the land masses crashed together like an explosion. Instead, it was a gradual process that developed over hundreds of thousands of years, and the end result was the magnificent and majestic Rockies of today. The important point is that small changes over long periods of time can result in enormous results. This is one way to think of the effects that gluten can impose on our health.

How Long Have Wheat and Grains Been in Our Diets?

Did you know that grains have only been in our diets for about 10,000 years?[9] Now, this seems like a long time, but our ancestors have populated the earth for more than one million years. In the scheme of things, the time that grains have been in our diets is less than one percent of all the time the human diet has been around. Therefore, given its relatively short presence, wheat and other grains are just now being identified as having negative health effects.

Imagine a group of our ancient, cave-dwelling ancestors sitting around a fire. Some were hunters and some were gatherers, but it is unlikely that they had a need for grains as a dietary source. Grains were dry, hard and difficult to digest. Techniques to make them more palatable were not available and honestly, there was likely no need for them since other foods were more accessible.

Were Our Ancestors Gluten-Free and Healthier?

What is noteworthy is that our ancestors' stature and height were greater than ours are today, and their bone health appeared to be better, based on archeological studies.[10] While other factors may have accounted for this as well, dietary influences are undoubtedly a major influence.

What did our ancestors eat prior to 10,000 years ago? Interestingly, most of their diets were made up of animal and plant foods. Nutrition during the days of the caveman came from both lean and fatty animal meat and an abundance of vegetables and fruits. Wheat and grains were absent.

Grains Are Relatively New in Our Diets

Grains are naturally difficult to digest, which is why they require refinement, even now, before being used in our diets. It was not until the Agricultural Revolution, about ten to twelve thousand years ago, that these began to appear in everyday meals. Even then, it took some time before wheat became a common dietary adjunct. Milling techniques still had a long way to go, and grinding wheat and other grains into a digestible form was not easy or efficient.[11]

There may have been a few reasons why wheat and other grains appeared in the diet at that time. First, knowledge of agricultural farming improved and facilitated larger crop production and greater harvests. Grains could be stored for long periods of time, whereas meats could not. This provided an incentive to cultivate grains as a component of the diet.

Secondly, there gradually began to be a reduction in the larger animals to be hunted. Large animals with higher fat content declined, and leaner meats from smaller game became more common as a meat source. The reduction in fats was subsequently replaced with carbohydrates from grains so that daily calories could be maintained.

We Begin to Crave Grains

As grains began to be eaten more routinely, people became somewhat dependent on their presence in their diet.[12] Many grains, including wheat, are metabolized to substances that exert effects on our brains that stimulate cravings. Therefore, once wheat became part of our diet, there was a natural tendency to maintain its presence through dietary cravings.

Carbohydrate Addiction Is Born!

The addictive nature of foods is an interesting subject. It is well-known that simple sugars and carbohydrates can give a "quick fix." What essentially happens is that the sugar, or glucose, from these meals causes the blood sugar to rapidly rise. This, in turn, causes insulin to be released from cells within the body so that the glucose can be utilized by the cells. Subsequently, because glucose is so efficiently utilized by our cells in the presence of insulin, the glucose level drops abruptly. The body's natural response is to then seek more sugar to replace the sudden drop. This is just one facet of how our own bodies' metabolisms stimulate cravings.

In the movie *Supersize Me*, it demonstrates that this addictive tendency can be used to encourage a good customer base. McDonald's restaurants add sugar to just about all their products including sandwiches, fries, desserts, breaded chicken, etc. Not only does it enhance the immediate taste, but it also provides a sugar stimulus that leads to craving more of these foods once metabolized.

Drug-Like Effects Associated With Wheat Consumption

What you may not realize is that the wheat products in their breads likewise carry some stimuli for cravings. In the case of wheat, metabolites (breakdown products) called gluteomorphins have effects on morphine-like receptors in our brains.[13] Now, this is not the same as taking heroine or morphine, but there is a very mild, positive effect that leads to emotional cravings. As with glucose, there are believed to be other physiological cravings that develop when wheat becomes a regular component of our diet.

Evidence that grains were becoming a part of the human diet can be traced back several thousands of years, but they may not have been a significant component until more recently. There is evidence that the Egyptians used wheat and other grains to make breads and beer approximately 1,600 years ago. Recent bone research on ancient Egyptian mummies has shown tetracycline within the bones. Tetracycline is usually derived from grain molds, thus allowing us to verify that the Egyptians indeed used grains in their diet routinely.

Grains offered a more stable supply of nutrition in areas where vegetation was scant and animals scarce. It could also be stored for use later, during times of famine.[14] These features also made the use of wheat grains more popular in certain climates and regions.

Grains Have Worsened Our Health Status

You may wonder why the Egyptians or earlier cultures didn't demonstrate poor health effects from grains, if grains were so unhealthy for them. That's a fair question. But, maybe, they actually did. In comparison to our Paleolithic ancestors from thousands of years ago, humankind has shown a decline in many health areas since the time grains were introduced into our diets. Overall, average stature has become reduced, bone and tooth decay have become more prevalent, infections and cancers have been more common, and anemia has become a common finding. Even lifespan has reduced in comparison.[15] Across the board, consistent findings show changes in bone and dental health as well as overall changes in our nutritional status since grains were incorporated into our diets.

Linking Gluten to Our Health Problems

What is the basis to link these as cause and effect? Were there not other factors that could be accounting for this? While this may well be the case, there is strong, clinical research that supports gluten and wheat as being strong culprits.

Interestingly, even patients today with gluten sensitivities show changes in bone health, dental health and multi-system dysfunction. Children diagnosed with celiac disease are known to have poor bone maturation and short stature. Anemia is a common manifestation as well. Also, grains contain phytates, which can hinder the absorption of other nutrients. This, in turn, can result in poor mineral absorption, poor vitamin absorption and malnutrition. Normal blood cell function, bone health and an effective immune system all rely on proper nutrition. Therefore, the association between these physical findings and the introduction of grains has been a consistent finding. This makes for a rational cause-and-effect relationship.

What Happens When Grains Are Introduced to Primitive Cultures

But additional evidence even furthers this hypothesis. Researchers in the early twentieth century actually studied primitive cultures that did not have grains as a part of their diets and compared them to other grain-consuming cultures from around the world. In addition, the health effects over time were assessed within those primitive cultures once grains were introduced. In each case, it appeared that within twenty years of introducing a grain-based diet, ill health effects began to develop.

The Rule of Twenty Years

Thomas Cleave was one such researcher. He found that after refined flours were introduced, heart disease, hypertension, diabetes, gall bladder disease and colitis all began to appear. He coined the phrase "the rule of twenty years" due to the consistent findings he discovered.[16]

When assessing the benefits and detriments of a particular diet, effects are often delayed. It therefore can be very difficult to establish a scientific, cause-and-effect relationship unless patterns are consistent and large numbers of people are investigated.

There is now good evidence that wheat and other grains result in digestive stress to our bodies.[17] In turn, this causes negative effects on our health that previously were not present when our diets consisted of animal and plant foods. While grains provide protein and carbohydrate nutrition, they appear to be at the expense of other important nutrients and to cause ill health effects.

Why Gluten Creates More Health Problems Today Than in the Past

More recent history sheds some light on why gluten and wheat are more problematic today. In the late 1800s, the Industrial Revolution brought steel roller mills to societies around the world. This allowed wheat and grains to be refined quickly and inexpensively. As a result, flours became more available in Europe, America and a few other locations where importation was prevalent. What was once available only to the wealthy now became accessible to the masses.[18] In this regard, the use of wheat flour on a large scale has only been present for about 150 years.

Refining Process = More Gluten

As stone mills were replaced with refineries, the flour became more "pure" and white. The impurities, which consisted mostly of wheat bran and wheat germ, were incompletely processed with stone milling and therefore gave the flour a browner appearance. As a result, white flour had a higher protein content per pound and was superior for baking purposes. Higher protein content also meant higher gluten content.

Science was evolving in the wheat industry as well. Better wheat seed was developed to allow crops to be grown in areas with short seasons. These "harder" wheats had a higher protein and gluten percentage as well.[19] So, wheat and other grains became more accessible, and the concentration of gluten and protein in the wheat gradually increased as technologies improved.

Grains Are Cheap Food

As the industrialized world began to produce and import refined flours to a greater extent, innovative entrepreneurs like Kellogg and Post, around the turn of the twentieth century, expanded the presence of grains through the production of breakfast cereals. Hot and cold cereals increased utilization, and, according to USDA reports, wheat usage peaked between 1875 and 1900. Refined grains were able to be manu-factured at low cost, provided an inexpensive food source for many people, and could be stored for long periods of time.[20] As a result, wheat became a strong part of the daily diet.

Through the twentieth century, wheat production and usage fluc-tuated up and down. As groceries began to diversify their products more with fruits and vegetables, grains made up a smaller percentage of the American diet. This was the result of better importation and a better transportation infrastructure. Products that were locally unavailable or out of season could now be shipped in from other areas by boat or railway. American diets became more varied as a result.

Gluten Becomes an Integral Part of Our Diets

You might expect the incidence of gluten sensitivity to decline during this time, but actually, the reduction in wheat in the diet was not profound. Wheat and other gluten-containing grains were still a strong part of the daily dietary consumption. In addition, even though we were beginning to understand more about the immune system and how it reacted to various proteins, it was still a budding, new field. Recogni-tion of gluten's effects on the body was still very poor, and there were no really good diagnostic means to assess its effects in a clinical setting.

In the late part of the twentieth century, there were two significant developments that again increased the use of wheat in our diets. First, the data from the Framingham study demonstrated that fiber diets reduced cholesterol and heart disease. This, almost overnight, resulted in a tremendous increase in whole wheat products and high-fiber diets in the marketplace.

Fast Food Means Gluten

And while this was dramatic, the second development had a larger impact. We were now part of the "fast food revolution." Women entering the workforce, higher numbers of single-member households, and compression of time all resulted in the need for quick meals on the go.[21]

These meals utilized many bread products including sandwiches and breaded chicken, which also increased the amount of wheat grains in our diets.

Gluten continues to be a stable part of most people's diets in breads, pastas, breaded foods, etc. Fast food still has a secure part of the dining market, and eating out at restaurants has continued to increase as our society has become more affluent.

Technology to Diagnose Gluten Sensitivity Is Available but Not Used

Within the last ten years, the medical community has become more aware of gluten's effects on health and of people with gluten sensitivities. But even today, the number of individuals accurately recognized as being gluten-sensitive is a small fraction of the effected population. For every one celiac disease patient, there are eight who have asymptomatic gluten sensitivity.[22] It is estimated that between thirty-five and fifty percent of our population has some form of gluten sensitivity.[23]

Gluten Is in Hiding

We understand more about our immune system now, and we have many blood tests and other procedures that help us "see" how gluten affects some people. But we are just scratching the surface. It is not a surprise that a protein in our diets that has been causing bone, dental and nutritional changes for centuries still is not fully understood in its full scope of effects. Gluten has stealthily hidden itself from obvious view and continues to do so for much of the traditional medical community (a mistake we hope to correct with this book).

Gluten—Anatomy of a Grain

Now would actually be a good time to talk about what exactly gluten is in terms of wheat anatomy and why the body has such a hard time with its digestion. You may now appreciate the fact that wheat is present in the diet more commonly, and that its gluten content has increased, but why does gluten give the body so much difficulty? The body metabolizes many other proteins without significant strife, so why is there such an issue with gluten?

Gluten Is a Protein

Gluten itself is the main protein in wheat, representing eighty-five percent of all the wheat proteins present. The others that make up the remaining fifteen percent are of little significance. Once wheat is refined into flour, the end-product contains protein (almost all gluten) and carbohydrates (wheat starch). Gluten itself is made up of two proteins, which are gliadin and glutenin. These are present in equal, fifty-fifty portions for the most part. Gliadin gives wheat its ability to be stretched, known as extensibility. Glutenin gives wheat its ability to return to its shape when stretched, known as elasticity.[24] Both are needed to make good breads.

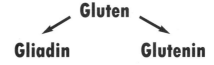

The Protein Gliadin Creates Digestive Problems

Of the two proteins that make up gluten, gliadin poses a greater problem when it comes to digestion. Like all proteins, it is made up of smaller components called amino acids. These are like Lego building blocks that snap together to make a bigger structure. In this case, that bigger structure would be a protein. Gliadin contains two problematic amino acids, proline and glutamine, that cause the body a problem during digestion.

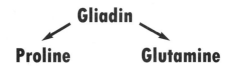

While the details of why these are a problem will be covered a little later, suffice it to say that their structure can trigger an immune reaction in some people. This immune response is what then causes many of our health problems related to gluten.

Gluten Also Creates Neurological and Immunity Problems

So about this time, you are afraid you enrolled in Chemistry Class 201. Unfortunately, in order to comprehend the relationship between gluten and our health, some science has to be described, but we promise to make it painless. Part of the reason why gluten's effects have been disguised for so long is that it triggers indirect effects through our body's own immune system. Therefore, difficulty with balance may not be thought of as a gluten problem, but evidence clearly now shows that gluten can cause neurologic disease that results in this symptom.[25] The same can apply to disorders of the thyroid, the skin, the heart, the reproductive system and many others. Immune system disorders have markedly increased in this century alone.

Gluten, Your Gut and Your Immune System— A Dangerous Triad

Celiac disease itself, while it may have been around for hundreds of years, was first scientifically described as an illness in 1880 by Gee.[26] Was it because medicine had evolved enough to begin to describe more occult illnesses? Or maybe the marked increase in dietary wheat increased the prevalence of the disorder enough to make it more noticeable. Either way, it is noteworthy that wheat and grain usage peaked in the U.S. at the same time that gluten sensitivity was identified in the medical arena.[27] This is a coincidence that again supports a cause-and-effect relationship. As noted before, when diet is the cause of delayed health effects, it is hard to identify unless large numbers of individuals are evaluated. The marked increase in wheat and grain usage in the last century has facilitated this.

Gluten Creates Problems via a Complex Route

What we have learned about gluten in the last few decades has been substantial. There have been tremendous gains made in detailing how gluten is digested and metabolized, and how it interacts with our immune system. And, as you might expect, it is not a simplistic mechanism by which gluten causes various health disorders. It appears to be quite intricate and complex. But, then again, if it were easy and straightforward, the effects of gluten would have likely been obvious hundreds of years earlier.

In order to understand how gluten can cause health problems, let's first look at its normal digestion as we eat that whole wheat bagel. By comparison, it will then be easier to understand changes that lead to eventual problems with our bodies' functions.

How Is Gluten Digested Normally?

What we now understand about a normal digestive process is that the gluten ingested in our diet dissolves into the proteins gliadin, glutenin and an array of other less-important nutrients. After the gliadin passes from the stomach into the small intestine, the lining of the intestine, or mucosa, has lining cells that absorb the gliadin from the bowels. They are the cells that begin its metabolism. Along the sides of these lining cells, there is little to no space for the gliadin to "sneak" across the intestinal wall. This is due to sections called "tight junctions" that hold the cells together on their sides. That means that the only way for the gliadin to go from the intestine into our bloodstream is through the cells' digestive processes.

As the gliadin is absorbed into the lining cell, a special enzyme, called tissue transglutaminase (tTG), begins breaking down some of the amino acids on the gliadin. The end product is now called "deaminated" gliadin, and this digested protein then proceeds to other cells for further digestion and metabolism.[28] (See Diagram 1.) In normal individuals who do not have gluten sensitivity, there are no problems, and the process proceeds smoothly without any harm to their health. But there is an important reason why gliadin is not seen as a danger in these people.

NORMAL GLUTEN DIGESTION

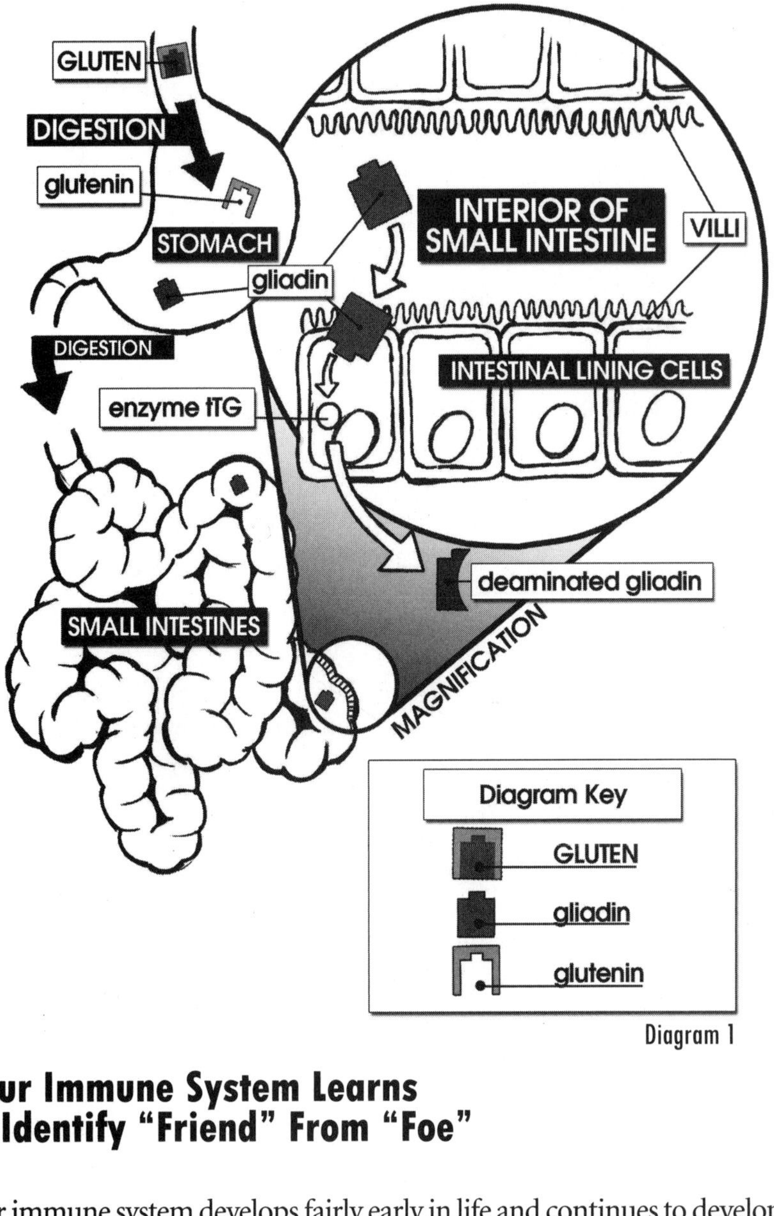

GLUTEN

DIGESTION

glutenin

STOMACH

gliadin

INTERIOR OF SMALL INTESTINE

VILLI

DIGESTION

enzyme tTG

INTESTINAL LINING CELLS

deaminated gliadin

SMALL INTESTINES

MAGNIFICATION

Diagram Key	
GLUTEN	
gliadin	
glutenin	

Diagram 1

Your Immune System Learns to Identify "Friend" From "Foe"

Our immune system develops fairly early in life and continues to develop further as we age. However, during the immune system's development in a fetus, and during the first year of life, it must identify tissues and proteins that are part of the normal body and diet. If it didn't, our immune system would constantly be attacking all of our organs and tissues, as well as everything we ate.

For instance, if our immune system had no way to identify our heart muscle as our own, it would detect it as a foreigner and fight it like it would an infection. Therefore, it is crucial that our own bodies' tissues, and normal foods in our diet, be recognized as "safe" so that the immune system will work effectively, only fighting legitimate foreigners like bacteria and viruses.

The Principle of Oral Tolerance

Normally, as infants and children are gradually exposed to foods, including wheat and gluten, the immune system catalogs these as "safe" and normal. In this way, when the gluten and gliadin process through our digestive system, there is no immune attack triggered. Because the immune system learned early in life that this is beneficial to our nutrition and causes no harm to our health, it tolerates these substances. This is the principle of oral tolerance.[29] Interestingly, it also applies to the normal bacteria that live in our intestinal tract. These "good" bacteria are needed to fight off "bad" bacteria, and provide some vitamins and digestion for our bodies as well. The immune system, by way of oral tolerance, is able to view these bacteria as "safe," which, in the long run, promotes our overall health.

Gluten and Your DNA—It's All in the Genes

So, what happens when someone is gluten-sensitive? This is where we have come a long way in our understanding of gluten sensitivity. It has been medically proven that individuals with certain genetics are more prone to developing gluten disorders.[30] In our genetic DNA profile, there is a group of genes that carry the blueprint for the cells of the immune system. Specifically, these are referred to as HLA genes. In people who are gluten-sensitive, a group of specific blueprints keep surfacing on these HLA genes. These have been labeled HLA-DQ2 and HLA-DQ8. In addition, there are some others that are currently being researched, but these are the most common. In short, our immune cells that carry these DNA patterns affect our ability to see gluten as a "safe" dietary protein. The result is that the immune system begins attacking the gluten molecules.

Environmental Triggers Cause Genes and Diseases to Express Themselves

There are many disorders that show similar effects of genetic risk. In other words, a person's DNA carries a pattern that, only if exposed to something in the environment, will develop into a health disorder. Some examples of these disorders include high blood pressure, diabetes, cancers and others. It is not until an infection, a food, an injury or some other trigger stimulates the expression of this gene to develop into a health disorder. In this way, gluten and gliadin expose the genetic risk of a gluten-sensitive person to develop a subsequent medical condition such as thyroid disease or cancer.

Childhood Illnesses Can Increase the Risk of Gluten Sensitivity

Additionally, there are other factors that affect the development of gluten sensitivity. One of the major factors can be concurrent infections, especially early in life. A common virus, rotavirus, has been identified as a risk for developing gluten sensitivity. This virus, and possibly some other infections to which we are exposed, causes the intestinal lining to become "leaky." This means that the tight junctions between the lining cells become disrupted due to inflammation, and gliadin particles can directly bypass the lining cells and gain access directly to the bloodstream.

How You Develop a "Leaky Gut"

For sensitive individuals, the gliadin can result in an immune reaction if they have the DNA blueprint that places them at risk. Other stresses can also result in "leaky" tight junctions and allow gliadin to cross through without proper digestion. (See Diagram 2.) These can include alcohol, aspirin and even extreme, vigorous exercise.[31]

HOW A LEAKY GUT DEVELOPS

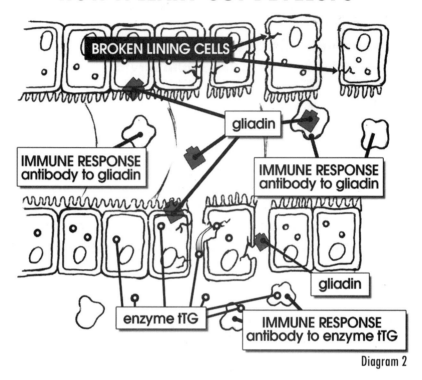

BROKEN LINING CELLS

gliadin

IMMUNE RESPONSE
antibody to gliadin

IMMUNE RESPONSE
antibody to gliadin

gliadin

enzyme tTG

IMMUNE RESPONSE
antibody to enzyme tTG

Diagram 2

These types of factors that cause changes in the intestinal mucosa fall
under the category of "stress." Stresses can be chemical, like medications,
toxins or foods. Stresses can also be physical, like extreme heat, extreme
cold, vigorous exercise and trauma. Emotional stress also falls under this
category. It has not been clearly defined which of these stresses play roles
in developing gluten sensitivity except for the ones mentioned, but it is
likely that other stresses are important.

So, suppose you are someone who carries these specific HLA genes.
You have a normal childhood and have normal health up until you are
twenty-one years old. You then develop a flu-like illness, but it resolves
after a couple of weeks and things are back to normal.

But, over the next year or so, you begin to develop fatigue, weight
gain and just an overall bad feeling. After several tests, you eventually
find out that you have Hashimoto's disease. This is a thyroid disorder

wherein the immune system has "attacked" your thyroid gland and resulted in low hormone levels. You begin replacement and many of your symptoms improve, but not completely. Why would anyone ever suspect that gluten in your diet may be the root cause?

Gluten Can Trigger an Autoimmune Disease to Develop

What has been found is that gluten can trigger other immune disorders of many other organ systems, including the thyroid.[32] These will be detailed later in the book, but gluten has proven to be the root cause of many disorders. In the above scenario, the viral infection may have resulted in a leaky intestinal lining that allowed gliadin to come across into the blood stream. Because you have the HLA genetic risk for being gluten-sensitive, your immune system sees the gliadin as foreign and begins an immune attack.

Proteins Within Your Body Resemble Gluten and Are Attacked by Your Immune System

In many gluten-related disorders, however, the immune attack is sloppy and fails to simply go after the gliadin. Instead, it also focuses on other, similar proteins in different organ systems, thereby causing disorders. Because the attack is against your own tissue, these disorders are called "autoimmune "disorders. Diseases such as arthritis, cancer, diabetes and others are known to have an autoimmune component.

Viruses Can "Mimic" Gluten to Your Immune System

Maybe the infection you had was the rotavirus. Rotavirus, in particular, also carries proteins within it that look very similar to the gliadin or deaminated gliadin particles. In this way, not only does it cause a disrupted intestinal lining, but it can also directly trigger the same immune attack as gliadin. It is as if the rotavirus is an imposter for gliadin, and the immune system fails to recognize the difference. So, it proceeds the same way, as if gliadin was present.

Putting It All Together

So what exactly causes one to be gluten-sensitive? First, you need to have a genetic profile that makes your immune system susceptible to developing an intolerance to gluten. Secondly, you must, at some point, eat gluten, which can trigger this sensitivity. These are the two requirements, but additionally, there is another. Either due to some type of environmental stress that results in a "leaky" intestinal lining or due to a failure of your immune system's oral tolerance to develop correctly, your immune system reacts abnormally to what should be a normal dietary food.

Gluten sensitivity develops to varying degrees in susceptible people according to their ability to tolerate these stresses and according to what extent their oral tolerance developed.[33] This is why some people with "risky" HLA genes may never develop gluten sensitivity. Their ability to tolerate environmental stresses is high, or they developed good oral tolerance that protects them from reactivity to gluten.

What's Your Risk? About a Flip of a Coin

So, how many people have the HLA DQ2 and/or DQ8 genes that never develop gluten sensitivity? Important question. It appears that between twenty and fifty percent of the population has at least one of these genes.[34] The exact number of the entire population with gluten sensitivity is not known because a large number of gluten-sensitive individuals have not been diagnosed.

Celiac disease, the most well-known form of gluten sensitivity, exists in about two to four percent of the population, and reports show that as high as ninety-five percent of celiac patients have the HLA genes.[35] Based on progressive evidence of how many other ways gluten can affect our bodies, it is likely that many people that carry the genes indeed have undiagnosed gluten sensitivity; and as a result, are suffering from the ill effects that gluten can silently create on their health.

It Is Imperative to Discover if Gluten Is the Root Cause

This is why it is imperative to search for gluten as the root cause of many disorders beyond celiac disease. Testing for genetic risk and gluten sensitivity in many others with various disorders will eventually help us have a more accurate figure of those who are at risk and have gluten sensitivity.

As will be detailed in later sections with specific body systems, evidence will show how many medical disorders can be caused by gluten sensitivity. We have just begun to identify how this wheat protein can cause such widespread health effects and how it acts through our body's immune system in doing so.

Gluten Damages Your Small Intestine

Likewise, there are significant, nutritional effects that occur with gluten as a result of its damage to the intestinal tract. The amount of scientific literature and research that has become available continues to direct us toward further evidence of gluten's role in many people's daily symptoms. And while it is important that we accurately identify gluten as the culprit, it is also imperative that we look at how to promote better oral tolerance early in life in susceptible individuals, and to help protect the integrity of their digestive system.

Even though grains have been around for many centuries, wheat has become increasingly present in our diets, and its gluten content, likewise, more concentrated. Because of the means by which gluten causes illness, it is no wonder that the association between it and disease has been difficult.

Understanding gluten's relationship to our immune system's development, gluten's effect on our overall nutrition, and, specifically, how the immune system operates in autoimmune disorders will lay the necessary groundwork to better grasp the scope of gluten sensitivity today. In the next chapter, these and many other details will enlighten you even further about gluten's hidden effects within our bodies.

Three

How Your Immune System Works and Why It Reacts to Gluten

You have now been indoctrinated into a bit of the science behind the body's immune system and how gluten interacts with it. It is important to again state that through the immune system, gluten exerts most, if not all, of its negative effects on our health. In people who have a genetic pattern that puts them at risk, gluten can trigger their immune system to affect a number of organs within their body. While the digestive system is the most common, many other areas of the body can be affected. In each case, it appears as though the immune system acts as its messenger in carrying out an inflammatory process. This inflammation then, eventually, leads to symptoms and disease.

Gluten Sensitivity and Immune Disorders— A Strong Link

Did you know that of all patients with gluten sensitivity, more than twenty percent have other immune disorders?[36] This figure is likely much higher because testing is limited in detecting all immune system dysfunctions. At what age does this start? For many, gluten can start this process immediately after birth. By examining the development of your immune system from conception forward, you will be able to better understand how gluten plays a role. Not only will this help shed light on gluten's part, but it also can give some guidance how to minimize its negative effects.

Your Immune System and Oral Tolerance— Or How You Successfully Fight Off Bad Guys

While you are still snug and cozy in the womb, your immune system is already hard at work. And for good reason. The task at hand is to make sure that the immune system is ready to fight off infections and other "foreign" attackers, yet avoid any damage to the body's own tissues.

Your Immune System Knows Self From Foreigner...Most of the Time

So, how does your immune system detect what is "foreign" and what is "self"? You certainly don't want your immune system attacking your own liver. Early in the development of your body, cells of the immune system (called T cells and B cells) begin to seek and destroy other cells that would normally attack your own body. The first wave of this is called central tolerance.[37]

The reason it is called "central" is because it occurs within the central portions of your body's immune centers. One center is called the thymus gland (which is where T cells are found, mostly) and the other center is the bone marrow (where B cells predominate). Pretty clever to name them according to the first letter of the area in which they reside, huh? Each "center" selects immune cells that would normally recognize your own "self" tissues as invaders and eliminates them. This leaves only those cells that would then accurately attack foreign bacteria or other particles.

If central tolerance did not occur, this would be a major problem. Essentially, every function of your body would be affected as the immune system would be attacking them while they tried to do their jobs. While some autoimmune disorders result from central tolerance being defective, this is not the case with gluten. The immune dysfunction with gluten is elsewhere.

When Healthy, Your Body's Immune System "Suppresses" Itself From Attacking You

The next phase of the immune system's development occurs away from the thymus gland and bone marrow. It occurs in the tissues and bloodstream and is therefore called peripheral tolerance. In the "periphery," away from the immune centers of your body, there is still work to be done in fine-tuning the immune response. This operation is handled most by special T cells called regulatory T cells. Basically, they continue to identify immune cells that are targeting self tissues, but instead of deleting them, as is done in the thymus gland and bone marrow, they suppress them or make them inactive.

Regulatory T cells make these self cells incapable of attacking other cells or tissues by rendering them ineffective. This process starts while you are an embryo and continues throughout your life.[38] There is a constant monitoring process by these regulatory T cells, which watch out for autoimmune cells.

Acquired Tolerance—In a Perfect World No One Would React Badly to Food

The third phase of the immune system's development is acquired tolerance. This is the area that mostly pertains to gluten. Acquired tolerance develops in response to things that are truly outside the body yet are safe and needed for our health, like food. In this way, these "triggers" to the immune system are indeed foreign, but not harmful. Although these particles can gain access to our bodies through the air and through our bloodstream, most present to our bodies through our mouths and digestive tracts.[39] This particular category of acquired tolerance is termed oral tolerance.

Just imagine if everything you ate were identified as a foreign invader to your body. You would quickly become malnourished as your immune system would seek and destroy every morsel you ate. It is very important that oral tolerance develops so that necessary nutritional substances that your body requires can be absorbed and metabolized. In addition, it is also important that some bacteria that protect our intestinal tract be viewed as "safe" bacteria by your immune system. These bacteria prevent "bad" bacteria from harming you. All of this is accomplished by oral tolerance.

Recognizing Safe From Unsafe

Oral tolerance is essentially orchestrated in the same way as peripheral tolerance. Regulatory T cells, early in life, are able to categorize different foods and bacteria as safe and others as unsafe. Once they identify the safe proteins, and the good bacteria and foods, these regulatory T cells then suppress the immune cells that would normally attack these substances. For instance, with gluten, in a normal individual who is not genetically at risk for gluten sensitivity, gluten will be recognized as safe. The immune cells that would normally attack gluten are turned off, allowing gluten to be absorbed and metabolized unharmed.[40]

Your Digestive Tract Has a Strong Immune Defense Army

Our digestive system alone contains a very large number of immune cells, including regulatory T cells. The reason for this is that our intestinal lining is a major barrier between us and the outside world. As we ingest medications, food, bacteria, viruses and many other substances, the intestinal lining represents our front line in battle. It has the role of determining what is safe and what is not. And for things that are unsafe, it must launch an immune attack to destroy them. As you might imagine, it requires a great deal of activity to constantly be on-guard against potentially harmful particles. Therefore, the gastrointestinal system requires a full army of immune cells to be ready for battle.

Oral tolerance is most active immediately after birth and during the first year of life. It is also active throughout your life, but it gradually declines as you age. Therefore, the period of infancy is the most important period in which oral tolerance matures. This has significant meaning for those who may be sensitive to gluten.

Can You Lessen a Child's Risk of Developing Gluten Sensitivity?

If you are at-risk for gluten sensitivity, there are ways to encourage or discourage oral tolerance to this protein. The occurrence of gluten sensitivity is both time-dependent and dose-dependent.[41] Therefore, when you first are exposed to gluten and how much you are exposed to influence oral tolerance and intolerance.

When Should Gluten Cereals Be Introduced to a Child?

While it is true that the majority of people diagnosed with gluten sensitivity are adults, it is clear that the process of gluten intolerance begins in childhood. But exactly when does this start? At what point does your immune system become "triggered" by gluten to cause problems?

The answer to this is variable, but it is clear that oral tolerance plays a big role. As mentioned, oral tolerance is most active immediately after birth and through the first year of life. Of course, this is when foods are being first introduced into a baby's system. Therefore, it stands to reason that this period of time is important for children who are at risk for developing gluten sensitivity.

An Immature Immune System Can Result in Higher Reactivity to Gluten

There is now good evidence that timing plays a key role in the development of gluten sensitivity. In one study, 1,560 children with genetic risk for celiac disease were followed for about five years and categorized according to when wheat products were introduced into their diets. Interestingly, for those who first had gluten cereals between zero and four months, there was a five-fold increase of subsequent celiac disease/gluten intolerance compared to those infants who first had cereals between four and six months of age. This supports the idea that an immature immune system may result in higher reactivity to gluten if it is introduced early.[42] These infants with early exposure also had an increased risk for developing insulin-dependent diabetes.

Risk of Developing Diabetes Increases Five-Fold

Another study examined children of parents who had insulin-dependent diabetes. Insulin-dependent diabetes is an auto-immune disorder, and it was theorized that gluten may increase the risk for this autoimmune disorder if given early in life. In this case, infants who received gluten cereals between zero and three months had almost a six-fold increase of developing diabetes before the age of five years, compared to infants who only received breast milk during the same time. This finding was similarly supported by another diabetic study.[43]

As will be discussed shortly, gluten sensitivity is associated with many other immune disorders beside type I diabetes. These findings in children of diabetic parents indicate that the timing of gluten early in life influences the occurrence of autoimmune illnesses as well.

Breastfeeding Can Be Protective Against Gluten

From the above findings, it is encouraged to delay gluten cereals until at least four months of age for infants, especially if either parent has gluten sensitivity or an immune disorder. It also appears helpful if infants receive breast-fed nutrition. Breast milk has many immune antibodies from the mother that helps protect the early infant while his or her immune system is developing. In a large, Swedish review study, breast feeding protected infants from developing gluten sensitivity compared to those who were not breast-fed. In a German study looking at 143 children with celiac disease and 137 with normal health, breast feeding for greater than two months reduced the risk of gluten sensitivity by sixty-three percent.[44]

The bottom line is that if gluten is going to be given, you want to delay introducing gluten-containing grains until at least four months of age. If cereals are required for other reasons prior to this, choosing a rice-based cereal that does not contain gluten would be wise. In addition, breastfeeding during the first six months likely has protective effects in preventing gluten sensitivity from developing. During this time, the infant's immune system is developing and maturing, and oral tolerance is still adapting. Allowing these to become independently functional before challenging their digestive system is helpful.

Is Gluten Sensitivity Putting Your Child at Risk for Disease?

Given the fact that it generally takes five to ten years to accurately receive a diagnosis of celiac disease, and even longer for non-celiac gluten intolerance, the number of children with gluten sensitivity is significantly underestimated. On average it takes evaluations by five different physicians before the diagnosis is usually made.[45] Not very impressive statistics. We are just now beginning to dig below the surface and identify what seems obvious: Many children have gluten sensitivity.

Many "Adult" Diseases Actually Begin in Childhood

But if gluten sensitivity is diagnosed mostly in adulthood, how can it be a childhood disorder? You only have to look as far as other inflammatory conditions to get the answer. The number-one disease causing mortality for men and women remains vascular disease. And this disease clearly affects most people after the age of forty years. But what has been found in heart disease research is that atherosclerosis and changes in the heart and blood vessels actually begin in teenage and early adulthood years. In other words, there is a delay between the actual beginning of the disease and when symptoms first appear. To take it a step further, there is even a delay between its onset and when tests can detect its presence.

More Than Seventy-Five Percent of Gluten-Sensitive Patients Have No Digestive Complaints

The same is true for gluten sensitivity. The inflammation that begins as the immune system reacts to gluten develops many years (and sometimes decades) before symptoms occur. More than seventy-five percent of all gluten-sensitive patients never have digestive complaints.[46] The remainder falls into "silent" or "latent" categories because they do not yet have symptoms, despite having gluten reactivity occur within their bodies, or because the inflammation cannot yet be detected. By the time symptoms of osteoporosis, infertility, malnutrition or many other conditions develop, gluten has been causing hidden problems for years. This is a big reason to check for gluten sensitivity early if risk is suspected.

Early Detection Is Critical to Prevention of Disease

Another reason to check for gluten sensitivity in childhood is that early treatment intervention can make a huge impact. Because gluten triggers immune dysfunction in sensitive individuals, it is associated with many immune disorders. In a retrospective review, it was found that twenty-one percent of the celiac disease patients in one clinic had other immune disorders.[47] In another study that examined patients with thyroid disorders, having celiac disease resulted in a 140-percent increase in the presence of autoimmune thyroiditis.[48] Many other examples exist between the association of gluten sensitivity and the development of immune disorders. And these disorders can affect not only the digestive system but almost every bodily system. By making interventions earlier with treatment, these other disorders can be curbed and health can be restored.

Gluten Sensitivity Does Cause Autoimmune Disease

To drive this point home, research shows that if a child is diagnosed with celiac disease before the age of two years, the chance of developing another autoimmune disorder is about five percent. However, if the diagnosis is made between two years and ten years of age, the risk increases to seventeen percent and if delayed until after ten years, the risk is then more than twenty-three percent.[49] This highlights the point that earlier diagnosis makes a great impact on health, and that gluten is actively affecting your immune system long before symptoms appear.

If Gluten Sensitivity Is in Your Family Tree, Don't Delay Getting Screened

If a parent or sibling of a child has a known gluten sensitivity, or if a close relative or family member has an immune disorder, evaluating the child for gluten sensitivity should seriously be considered. Waiting for symptoms to dictate when testing should occur can be detrimental to the child's health and quality of life. Testing has improved greatly in its ability to detect gluten sensitivity, and it is very simple to complete.

Gluten Sensitivity Can Be Latent or Hidden

Gluten sensitivity, whether it is celiac disease or non-celiac gluten intolerance, can lie hidden from view while it is laying the groundwork for later problems. For children, having a high level of suspicion, understanding how gluten interacts within our bodies, and taking into account the family's health history is important. Gluten disorders are much more common than we appreciate.

Autoimmune Diseases Are Among the Top Ten Leading Causes of Death

If you harbor the genetic traits that predispose you to gluten sensitivity, then your immune system is primed not only for gluten intolerance or celiac disease, but also for a host of potential immune disorders. Gluten sensitivity has been associated with several non-celiac, autoimmune conditions such as autoimmune hepatitis, immune thyroid disorders, dermatitis herpetiformis (a severe skin condition), autoimmune cardiomyopathy (a form of heart disease), lymphoma (cancer of the blood), rheumatoid arthritis and insulin-dependent diabetes. There are more than forty defined autoimmune disorders and, in total, these are among the top ten leading cause of death.

To put it in perspective, collectively, autoimmune diseases affect approximately eight percent of the United States population—twenty-four million persons. Cancer affects nine million people and heart disease affects approximately twenty-two million. And while that is an impressive enough figure it is dwarfed by the fact that only one-third of those afflicted with autoimmune diseases are diagnosed. This does not even include other gluten-associated disorders that likely have immune causes such as dementia, epilepsy, infertility, osteoporosis, dental diseases and others.[50] Gluten exerts its effects on our bodies through the immune system.

The Intestine Is Your Front-Line Defense... When It Works Properly

Going back to the intestinal lining (our front line of defense against the world), immune cells along the lining are constantly making antibodies. These proteins are found in the blood and used by the immune system to identify and neutralize foreign particles, which include unwanted bacteria, toxins, viruses, etc. Ingesting gluten, for sensitive individuals, stimulates antibodies to be made against it and, ultimately, leads to negative effects in the intestine and/or other parts of the body.

Why Your Immune System Decides That Gluten Is a Toxin

But why does this happen? The immune cells that contain genetic markers HLA DQ2 or HLA DQ8, for reasons that are yet to be defined, are not properly regulated by regulatory T cells. As you recall, regulatory T cells identify immune cells that are targeting self tissues and suppress them or make them inactive.[51] In gluten-sensitive patients, they are not suppressed and made ineffective. Therefore, these cells begin making antibodies for substances that should be safe under oral tolerance or should be safe because they represent self tissues.

You have heard of factory recalls at manufacturing plants. Suppose there were a machine along the assembly line that was defective because of the way it was built. And during its portion of automobile assembly, it repeatedly installed safety belts incorrectly. As a result, injuries skyrocketed once the car made it to consumers. Well, immune cells with DQ2 and DQ8 markers are the same. They are defective in the way they are regulated and in how they produce antibodies. And their defective "processing" results in injuries to the body.

Gluten Causes Inflammation and Damage to the Intestine

In celiac disease and in non-celiac gluten intolerance, sensitive individuals are at risk for immune dysfunction. As gluten enters the small intestine, it is recognized as "unsafe." Immune cells in the intestine then make antibodies against gluten, and this begins the inflammatory process. The intestinal lining becomes irritated. As the inflammation progresses, not only is gluten attacked, but the intestinal lining also

INTESTINAL INFLAMMATION AND DAMAGE FROM GLUTEN

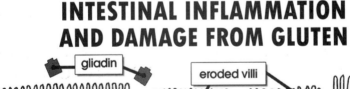

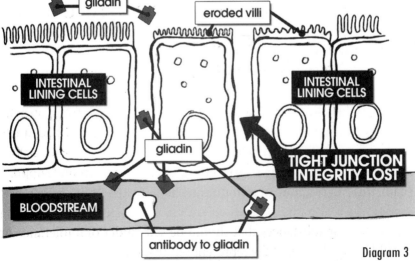

Diagram 3

becomes inflamed. In other words, the battleground is polluted as the invader is attacked. As the intestinal walls become inflamed, lining cells are disrupted and become "leaky." This means that these cells no longer form a solid front-line defense, but instead have pockets where invaders can sneak through the wall. And gluten is one of those invaders.

Some gluten makes it all the way through to the bloodstream without being touched by digestion; some of the gluten is broken down partially to gliadin, which then sneaks across the lining. Both of these proteins, once across the intestinal lining, trigger an immune response by defective DQ2 or DQ8 immune cells against them. This then leads to the formation of gluten-related antibodies that can circulate anywhere in the body. (See Diagram 3.)

The Attack on Gluten Spreads From the Intestine to the Bloodstream

So, the initial immune attack that started in the intestinal wall has now spread within the walls of the intestine and to the bloodstream.[52] This is how gluten causes effects far from the intestine. It stimulates an immune attack that can circulate to the brain, the heart, the joints and many other places.

Now, in addition, a couple of other problems arise. As the lining cells become "leaky," some of the proteins in the lining cells break apart and are released into the bloodstream and body. This does not happen in a normally functioning body. As a result, these lining cell proteins can also be seen as invaders and trigger autoimmune responses in many different systems of the body. Secondly, as gliadin crosses the leaky portion of the cell, it may attach to the enzyme responsible for its metabolism. This enzyme is called transglutaminase, or tTG. The combination of gliadin and tTG forms a new complex or compound. This new complex, likewise, can be seen as "unsafe" and as a potential invader. Again, this can result in an immune attack on tissues of the body.[53]

So, Let's Summarize

You have genes that make you sensitive to gluten. You eat gluten, and some of the defective immune cells attack gluten, thinking it is unsafe. The inflammation from the attack causes the intestinal lining to become leaky and inflamed. Gluten and gliadin then sneak across, into the bloodstream, triggering a further immune reaction throughout the body. Also, lining cell proteins and enzyme-gliadin (tTG-gliadin) complexes may trigger immune reactions. The end result is that auto-antibodies are made that can then injure or harm many other systems throughout the body by attack and inflammation, leading to autoimmune diseases. (See Diagram 4.)

Cellular Mimicry: How Gluten Triggers Disease Throughout the Body

One of the main ways these antibodies cause damage to other organs is through cellular mimicry. What is this? In essence, what it means is that some molecules of one tissue can look very similar to molecules of another. For instance, in heart research, it's been observed that the molecules of the tTG-gliadin complex look very similar in structure to molecules of some heart cells. Likewise, antibodies against tTG-gliadin complexes are seen to attack these heart cells. Even though the direct attack of the immune system is against gliadin and its enzyme, the final result is that it is unsuspectingly damaging the heart as well. The result is autoimmune myocarditis, an inflammation of the heart.[54] This phenomenon of mimicry is one way that gluten triggers immune disorders throughout the body.

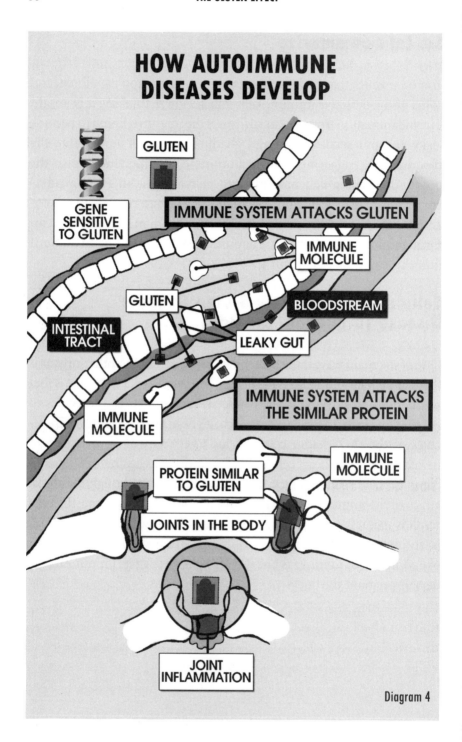

HOW AUTOIMMUNE DISEASES DEVELOP

GLUTEN

GENE SENSITIVE TO GLUTEN

IMMUNE SYSTEM ATTACKS GLUTEN

IMMUNE MOLECULE

GLUTEN

BLOODSTREAM

INTESTINAL TRACT

LEAKY GUT

IMMUNE SYSTEM ATTACKS THE SIMILAR PROTEIN

IMMUNE MOLECULE

IMMUNE MOLECULE

PROTEIN SIMILAR TO GLUTEN

JOINTS IN THE BODY

JOINT INFLAMMATION

Diagram 4

Inflammation Starting in Your Intestine Travels via Your Bloodstream to Trigger Diseases Elsewhere

These mechanisms will be described later in greater detail, as each individual disorder is described. For now, the point is that gluten initially starts inflammation in the intestinal area, but the eventual problem may be triggered elsewhere. It accomplishes this by way of the immune system and through the inflammation that follows.

Leaky Gut, Infections and Medications Can All Act As Triggers

There are some other factors that can also facilitate gluten's immune reactions. These include things that make the intestinal lining leaky even before gluten arrives. Infections, medications such as aspirin and anti-inflammatories, toxins such as alcohol, and even mechanical stress as in heavy exercise can cause disruption of the intestinal lining. These factors effectively weaken our defenses. Rotavirus, a common infancy and childhood diarrheal virus, contains proteins that can mimic gluten's structure and trigger a gluten-like immune reaction in some gluten-sensitive individuals.

You Can Prevent Further Damage From Occurring

Unfortunately, there is no way to re-teach your immune system that gluten is safe and not an invader. Gluten will remain a trigger for inflammation if you are sensitive. But reducing stress on your intestinal lining will help, and, of course, avoiding gluten completely will eliminate the trigger. These two measures keep the lining of the intestine from becoming leaky and prevent an autoimmune response. In this way, other serious autoimmune disorders can be prevented as well.

Can Gluten Stunt Your Child's Growth and Development?

As you are now aware, the inflammatory changes of the intestinal lining are the first site wherein gluten causes difficulties for gluten-sensitive people. Children are not any different. Additionally, because of their rapid growth and development, gluten's effects on the digestive system can be more profound.

Growth requires larger quantities of vitamins, minerals and nutrients per pound of body weight. If there is an absorption problem at the intestinal lining, this can lead to either specific or generalized malnutrition. In one study of seventy-five celiac children, there was an average nine-month delay in both weight and height by age seven years.[55] This may not be entirely due to nutrition, but, certainly, nutrition plays a role.

Years Can Pass Before Symptoms Develop

Another problem, as mentioned previously, is that gluten has a delayed presentation of symptoms. Under the surface, gluten-related inflammation is occurring but it may be years before symptoms or signs develop. Therefore, it is very common for children to have "silent" gluten sensitivity. It has been shown that for every one patient diagnosed with an autoimmune disorder, there are three more with pre-immune system disease.[56] This was determined by the appearance of circulating auto-antibodies in the bloodstream prior to the appearance of any complaints. Children are not only at greater risk because of more rapid growth, but also because they harbor symptomless problems even when gluten-sensitive.

Gluten Can Hinder Nutritional Health in Children

In relation to poor nutrition, some vitamins and minerals are used in greater amounts in childhood. For instance, bone growth utilizes greater amounts of vitamin D, calcium and phosphorus. Blood cell formation and growth require iron, vitamin B12 and vitamin K in higher quantities. Some vitamins that are poorly stored in the body (water-soluble vitamins) need to be supplied daily, like vitamin B6, vitamin C and vitamin B1. If absorption from the digestive system is reduced, greater consumption or supplements of these micronutrients may be needed. Gluten, therefore, can hinder nutritional health to a much greater degree in children for these reasons. They require these essential vitamins and minerals to successfully grow and remain healthy.

Uniformly, for gluten sensitivity, a gluten-free diet is the most effective treatment. Restricting gluten from the diet, at first glance, may imply further difficulties in keeping up with good nutrition. However, in actuality, this is not the case.

Gluten-Free Diets Are Healthy and Nutritious

Gluten-free diets are composed of greater amounts of natural vegetables and fruits, which are known to be loaded with vitamins and minerals. And, of course, broiled and roasted meats are better than batter-fried meats for several reasons. Replacing gluten-containing grains with others like rice, potatoes, and corn causes very little risk in terms of selective nutrition. Of the micronutrients that may be less available on a gluten-free diet, the main ones are thiamine, riboflavin, niacin, iron, chromium, magnesium, selenium, folate, phosphorus and molybdenum. While this may sound like a long list, a healthy diet, which consists of vegetables, fruits, eggs, meat and dairy products, will easily gain you all of these needed vitamins and minerals. We also recommend a daily, high-quality nutritional supplement (that is free of gluten, of course).

In addition to gluten, there are also other inflammation-provoking items in our diet that need to be monitored. A group called excitotoxins in today's prepackaged, preservative-enriched culinary environment can be particularly detrimental to the intestinal lining. These include artificial sweeteners, MSG and nitrites.[57] As with gluten, there also may be other food triggers that are poorly tolerated such as milk products, corn and soy. It simply depends on your genetic make-up and oral tolerance.

Lack of Symptoms Is Not an Accurate Yardstick by Which to Measure Gluten Sensitivity

The bottom line is that you should not be lulled into thinking that you or your child does not have gluten sensitivity just because symptoms are absent. If there is a predisposing family indicator, then have yourself and your child checked for gluten antibodies. Not only can the silent inflammation result in other illnesses, but it can also result in poor nutrition.

Likewise, diet is an incredibly important aspect of our health. If you never ate gluten, even though you were gluten-sensitive, you would never have a related problem. Pay attention to what foods and nutrients you eat. Diet is a powerful environmental factor that can reveal genetic risks that you may have.

What's Ahead

In the subsequent sections, we will delve into more details about specific symptoms that can occur as well as what systems of the body may be involved. Through the immune system's reaction to gluten in at-risk individuals, there can be multiple target areas for injury. Each system has different symptoms, and many people with gluten intolerance never have digestive complaints. This is what makes it very hard to define gluten as the underlying cause. But, armed with knowledge, you can raise your awareness and help detect gluten sensitivity sooner rather than later. You don't want to wait five to ten years to get your answer…for yourself or your child.

SECTION TWO

Is Gluten the Hidden Culprit Behind Your Symptoms?

Have you or someone you've known ever gone to a doctor because you had symptoms that were of great concern, but then was told that all of your tests were normal, and there was really nothing wrong?

Doctor, Please Listen to Me!

In American healthcare today, there is a tendency to focus solely on the objective. What do we mean by this? As a result of advancing diagnostic tests and demands for documentation by insurance companies, a positive test result, abnormal x-ray or observable examination finding receives more credence than a patient's symptoms. How many times has an insurance company failed to approve a medication or test because the findings on an exam or other test did not support it? Or, of greater relevance, how many times has someone with gluten sensitivity been ignored because all of their tests were negative?

The HealthNOW Method

This shift has been a gradual change over several decades, but in the process, the art of symptom assessment and recognition has fallen by the wayside.

We have coined the term "HealthNOW Method" to help distinguish the different type of healthcare we practice, and this should make our readers think about health in a new manner. We use this term throughout the book to show our thought process of evaluating a health problem.

The HealthNOW Method is distinguished from the common, allopathic view by addressing the root of the problem and not simply symptom relief. This topic, regarding a symptom-based approach, as well as the ensuing chapters that expand on this discussion, is a core component of the HealthNOW Method.

We have devoted this section of this book to the symptoms that occur in response to gluten sensitivity. Later, we will discuss the more well-known diseases or syndromes that are associated with gluten sensitivity symptoms.

Why You Should Listen to Your Symptoms

In our clinic, we recognize symptoms as the body's warning system. Symptoms are built-in survival mechanisms that indicate that a process within the body has resulted in some dysfunction. This may be mild and reversible, or it may be more serious. It may be a sudden development, or, like gluten sensitivity, may have been going on for years.

The bottom line is that symptoms are a guide to help identify the root cause. They point to certain systems of the body, which helps narrow down the location of the problem. Symptoms also may help distinguish what the actual cause may be in some cases.

Symptoms Don't Occur in Healthy Bodies

Symptoms do not occur in healthy tissues. It is only unhealthy tissues that will create a symptom. Again, the symptom is a protective mechanism built into our bodies to essentially inform us that something in the body is no longer functioning normally. It indicates a need to do something different from what we are currently doing in order to enhance the survival and health of the body.

Treating the Symptom or the Cause—Which Makes More Sense?

As an example, if a boulder has rolled onto the toes of your foot, the body gives you the symptom of pain, which would greatly inspire you to push the boulder off your foot to enhance its health and survival. If, instead of removing the boulder from your foot, you took a pain reliever so that you no longer felt the pain, would you consider that a good solution?

Well, taking a drug so that you no longer experience a symptom without doing anything to change what you are doing to your body does nothing to improve your actual health. It only makes the symptom less bothersome. With that said, there can be definite health benefits from taking certain drugs, as they may address serious problems. A blood pressure medication, for example, can lower the risk of stroke, but it still does nothing to improve the underlying reason why the person developed high blood pressure.

Even when standard lab tests fail to discover a problem, this does not indicate the absence of a problem if symptoms are present. Symptoms are still very important. This is why our focus has been to take a symptom-based approach to health and to use functional lab tests (which we will discuss later) to show us where and how the body is malfunctioning.

Gluten Has Widespread Effects

In this section, you will learn what symptoms are commonly assigned to different systems of the body, and how gluten influences the presence of these symptoms. Because gluten has such widespread effects in those who are sensitive, defining symptoms that can be caused by gluten helps increase our awareness. For instance, someone with headaches from gluten sensitivity may have no diarrhea or stomach symptoms. If you were unaware that gluten can be associated with headaches and migraines, you would never consider this as a potential cause. By knowing which symptoms gluten can cause, and why, you can begin to realize the scope of gluten sensitivity within our population. More importantly, you may identify gluten as the problem in your particular complaint.

Gluten Hides and Is Therefore Underdiagnosed

Some symptoms may be obvious in terms of where they originate, but others may not be. And it may be a surprise to find out how gluten can result in complaints completely unrelated to its effects on the small intestine. This is a big reason why gluten sensitivity is so underdiagnosed.

Don't feel alone. Many physicians do not appreciate the vast array of symptoms that can reflect gluten intolerance. A key factor in making an accurate diagnosis is the level of suspicion that a treating physician has for a condition.[58] If you never suspect gluten as a cause, you very well may never test for it or recommend a trial of a gluten-free diet. By increasing your awareness, you can assist your physician in raising his or her level of suspicion.

Four

Digestive Problems and Gluten: A Very Close Relationship

What Digestive Symptoms Can Gluten Cause?

Because gluten is a dietary protein, the immediate effects indeed involve our digestive system. This occurs both directly and indirectly, as will be explained. But what symptoms can you expect from a digestive tract problem? The answer is, quite a few. Our digestive system is responsible for many tasks. These include the breakdown and digestion of foods we eat, the absorption of nutrients into our body, the prevention of infectious organisms or toxins from gaining access to our body, and the maintenance of good fluid and electrolyte balance. As previously mentioned, it is a major interface wherein the outside world comes in contact with our body. Therefore, all of our digestive organs are important in providing good nutrition and fuel for normal health, yet preventing secondary problems like infection or toxin exposure.

In addition, symptoms from the digestive tract can be numerous because our digestive process encompasses many parts of our body. Think about it: Digestion begins the moment you put a bite of food into your mouth. Saliva begins to break down the food along with the action of chewing. Along the way, the stomach, small intestines and colon add

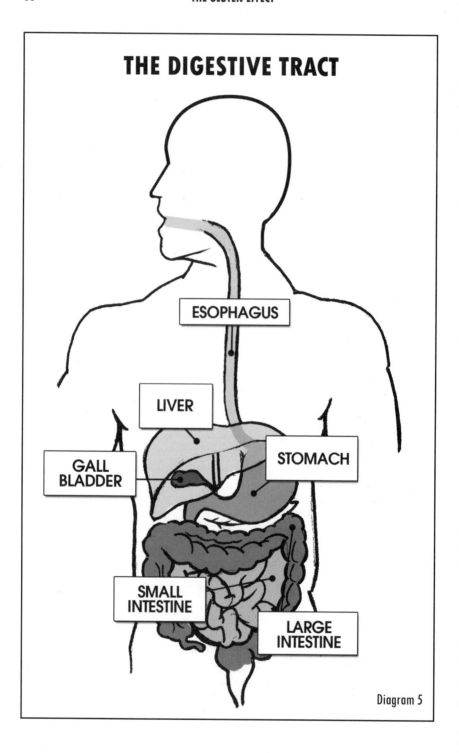

Diagram 5

to the process. In addition, other organs contribute including the liver, pancreas and gall bladder. Each one is needed for normal digestion to occur. Because of the length of the digestive system and the number of organs involved, symptoms can vary tremendously. But, even so, the constellation of complaints helps target the mainly affected area along the way. (See Diagram 5.)

Our Food Needs to Be Converted Into Good Fuel

Overall, it is quite simplistic. Our bodies require food and nutrition as fuel for normally functioning health. But this fuel has to be good fuel, not garbage. If you consistently put gasoline with high levels of contaminants into your car, parts of the engine will break down sooner and wear and tear will be accelerated. Our bodies are no different in this regard. If your fuel contains gluten, and you are sensitive to gluten, then it makes sense that your body will react negatively to it. Over time, it will cause wear and tear, and, eventually, symptoms will start to develop. It may be very difficult to "see" the damage by the current level of tests and exams that are available, but the symptoms are still there, signaling that something is awry. Is it so hard to believe that our diet can have this potential? Not really. It is common-sense medicine.

Food Can Act Like a Stressor Rather Than a Fuel

You recall, from the preceding section, that people have genetic risks for developing conditions, but only if exposed to certain environmental stresses. Diet represents one of the largest stresses in this regard. Other stresses can include infections, sleep patterns, toxin exposures, emotional stresses and exercise. All of these are important in trying to achieve a lifestyle that promotes good health. What you eat is a big factor, however, and there is still much to learn about how our bodies interact with what we eat.

Sixty-Nine Percent of All Americans Suffer From Digestive Problems

The small intestine is the site where most of the food we take into our bodies is absorbed. Approximately eighty-five percent of all foods are absorbed in the twenty-one feet of our small intestine. The surface area of the small intestine is enormous (it's equal to the surface area of a tennis court) so that it can accomplish this absorption.

Fifty Percent of All Symptomatic Individuals Are Gluten-Sensitive

In relationship to gluten, the most common complaints are related to our bodies' intestinal tracts. And, selectively, gluten tends to affect more commonly the small intestinal lining and, secondarily, our nutritional health. Overall, sixty-nine percent of all Americans suffer from some type of digestive difficulties.[59] Combining this piece of information with the finding that fifty percent of all symptomatic individuals have a form of gluten sensitivity[60] and it is no wonder that gluten in our diet is having a tremendous impact on our digestive health.

Common symptoms of gluten sensitivity include gas, bloating, diarrhea, constipation, abdominal pain, cramping, heartburn and nutritional deficiencies of vitamins and minerals. Symptomatic patients may have a few of these, though some may have all, and each helps indicate different potential problems. These will be detailed for you below.

Millions of Americans Needlessly Suffer From Digestive Problems

As you read this chapter, remember that having digestive symptoms are not required in order to have a diagnosis of gluten sensitivity. In studies, the number of confirmed celiac disease patients who had digestive symptoms was far less than the number who did not.[61] But there are many people, who have various digestive symptoms, who are still in search of a cause to their problems. All their examinations and tests have failed to document a cause, and medications have only provided limited relief over time. If you are in this group, this particular chapter may be quite enlightening.

Gurgling, Bubbling and Other Sound Symptoms

If these are your only symptoms, you may never have felt compelled to seek medical attention. You might live your life on over-the-counter medications for stomach symptoms. And you may have become used to the embarrassment of it all.

The symptoms are usually described as gurgling, churning, whistling or bubbling. Other terms include your stomach "making noises" or being "hungry." The basic cause of these stomach and intestinal symptoms is usually related to increased movement of the intestinal muscles, increased production of air and gas within the intestines, or both. Because of their cause, rarely are these symptoms in isolation if they are chronically present.

In gluten sensitivity, these symptoms occur for a couple of reasons. The main reason is inflammation caused by the gluten and your body's inability to tolerate it. As the intestinal wall becomes inflamed, muscles that line the intestines become irritated. And when muscles become irritated, they contract, which creates activity and movement within the intestines themselves.

Increased intestinal movement is one of the causes of these "noises" and sounds within your abdomen. Essentially, the lining cells of the intestine change in reaction to gluten when you are sensitive. Your immune system causes this reaction and it results in damage to the lining.[62] These lining cells change, the lining becomes more leaky, and the inflammation set in motion affects the entire intestinal wall. This includes the muscles that promote movement of food materials and the "churning" that you may hear.

Your Risk of Intestinal Infection Increases

The other cause of abnormal intestinal sounds includes the formation of air and gas within the digestive tract. It has been shown that gluten sensitivity increases the susceptibility to developing an infection.[63] The chronic effects on the immune system from attacking the gluten proteins eventually wear down your immune function. This is evidenced by low antibodies of IgA (the chief antibody found in the digestive tract) in many celiac patients.[64]

Because the immune system is not at optimal function, bacteria and parasites may gain access to the intestines that normally should not be there. Many of these organisms produce gaseous by-products as part of their normal metabolism, which then results in abnormal sounds.

This is probably starting to sound not too lovely. One of the key things we investigate in our clinics is secondary infections. By performing lab tests on stool samples, these infections can be identified and treatment can be started. While gluten is not the immediate cause, the effects it has on your immune system and the intestinal wall result in easier access of these infections to your body. And, sometimes, these infections result in just as many problems as the gluten itself.

Understanding this association helps you be aware that sometimes eliminating gluten from your diet may not be 100-percent effective in symptom relief. It may require treating secondary problems caused by gluten over time to achieve a full response.

Gas, Bloating and Other Pressure Symptoms

These symptoms may be more likely to grab your attention, but even so, many people simply tolerate them and self-medicate at their local pharmacy. Pressure symptoms commonly include gas, bloating and flatulence. These symptoms can be associated, of course, with increased intestinal noises (and often are), and therefore be quite embarrassing.

In addition, there exists a degree of mild discomfort with this that impacts your quality of life to a degree. Because of this, patients are more likely to mention these symptoms to their physicians, but only in the context of other complaints. The severity of these symptoms in isolation does not prompt many to seek attention for them.

Infections Can Be a Root Cause

So, what causes increased abdominal pressure? Is it really due to pressure, or can it be related to other things? With gluten sensitivity, these complaints develop probably in relation to a few processes. As with increased noises of the abdomen, pressure symptoms occur due to a secondary infection by organisms that produce air or gas during their metabolism. The mechanism is the same.

Infections gain access to the intestinal tract because gluten has worn down the immune system in sensitive individuals. Once they establish a residence in your bowels, gas by-products can cause symptoms of pressure. Why some people may experience bloating and pressure and others churning and gurgling is not clear. Many experience both simultaneously. Regardless, in some gluten-sensitive patients, secondary infections are a problem.

Debbie's Digestive Story

Debbie is one of our success stories (and there have been many related to gluten sensitivity!). She first saw us in the clinic, years back, with complaints of bloating as well as constipation. After her assessments were complete, not only was she found to be gluten-intolerant, but she also had a secondary bacterial infection called H. pylori. This is a common bacterium that has been found to cause ulcers within the stomach.

The gluten had caused inflammatory reactions in her bowel wall as well as triggered immune system reactions. As a result of this, over time, her immune system had become exhausted. This allowed her resistance to fall, and she developed an infection with H. pylori. These bacteria, of course, added insult to injury by infecting her digestive tract, where she was already having problems. Both the inflammation and the bacterial infection contributed to the bloating she was describing.

After she began a gluten-free diet and received antibiotics for the intestinal infection, all of her digestive complaints resolved.

Malabsorption of Nutrients

Another likely cause of gas and/or bloating is a reduced ability of the intestines to absorb nutrients from the diet. The inflammatory changes of the intestinal wall hinder nutrients from normally crossing the lining cells into the bloodstream. This delay causes more food substances to stay in the intestines. This then promotes a feeling of fullness and bloating.

What Is Causing My Big Belly?

Also, the inflammation itself, which, by definition, causes swelling, can result in pressure symptoms. As fluid and inflammatory cells enter into the intestinal walls, they enlarge, making you also feel bloated and full. It is not unusual for our gluten-sensitive patients to experience a major reduction in the size of their abdomens after removing gluten from their diets. The increased size of the abdomen was not from excess fat but from the physical swelling of the walls of the intestines.

Regardless of their cause, bloating and gas, as well as flatulence, indicate digestive symptoms. If gluten sensitivity is the cause, this could be the only complaint. Therefore, you should make a point to mention these symptoms to your physician, particularly if gluten sensitivity or autoimmune disorders are common in your family.

Symptoms uniformly improve on a diet if due to gluten intolerance.[65] And, if concurrent infections are present, these easily respond to antibiotic treatment followed by probiotic treatment. But, unless the symptoms are acknowledged and addressed, they can persist indefinitely while your health continues to suffer.

Abdominal and Digestive Pain

If you experience chronic or repeated bouts of abdominal pain, then you very well may seek medical attention. Pain in any fashion is the body's message to have something investigated more urgently.

With gluten sensitivity, pain usually comes in the fashion of cramping or colicky pain, and it is reflective of the inflammation ongoing within your digestive system. These are common symptoms in both celiac disease[66] and non-celiac gluten intolerance. Abdominal pain, however, can be difficult to localize. Pain mechanisms of the body within the digestive system do not localize pain the same way the skin does. Pain usually develops when intestinal wall muscles contract intensely, or when pressure causes a digestive structure to be overstretched. For many, there can be significant inflammation of the intestinal lining and yet no complaints at all.

If this were on the skin, pain would be significant. The nerve endings that signal pain from the skin respond quickly to heat, cold, cuts, scrapes, bruises, etc. They are very discrete and precise. The pain signals from the intestines are not. They are more generalized and respond more to pressure than to cuts and scrapes. As a result, pain occurs much later and differently when originating from the digestive tract.

Young Melissa's Story

One of our adolescent patients, Melissa, had suffered stomachaches for some time (in addition to cramps, bloating and a full, gaseous feeling). She had undergone the standard exams, but nothing had revealed a cause. Over the time of her symptoms, she had also become irritable and moody, with an overall sense of poor energy. Her parents found it difficult to deal with her moods, and her behavior was affecting everyone adversely. Melissa was not a happy young lady.

After our routine assessment, it was decided to try an elimination diet, and she was taken off gluten for a few weeks to see how she would respond. Amazingly, within that short time, all of her complaints improved. Currently, the only time she feels bloated is when she accidentally eats gluten-containing foods; plus, her energy level returned with a moderate degree of weight loss as well. The little "spare tire" she'd had around her belly was a thing of the past.

Gluten had been triggering her cramps and bloating as a result of intestinal wall inflammation, and it had also caused a lack of energy and irritability. Once Melissa decided to avoid gluten, the triggering cause was removed, and her symptoms abated.

Pain Can Result From Inflammation

Cramping and abdominal pain may also reflect underlying intestinal wall contractions. Just as described with gurgling and other noises, the muscles contract when inflamed by gluten, and if violent enough, can cause discomfort. Often, this will result in diarrhea, which is discussed next, and therefore cramping and diarrhea often go hand in hand.

Pain may also result from too much gaseous pressure causing the intestinal wall to swell and distend. Within the walls of the intestine are pressure sensors. If the walls expand too greatly, pain develops. This is what causes the ups and downs of colicky pain. As the walls expand in response to pressure within, the sharp pain hits, and then, as it subsides, the pain diminishes. In the case of gluten sensitivity, all of this is set in motion by inflammation as the immune system targets gluten for attack.

Heartburn and Indigestion Are Caused by Gluten Sensitivity

You probably realize how common heartburn and indigestion have become in our culture. Did you know that these are also common symptoms of gluten sensitivity in many patients? The sale of antacids and acid blockers over the counter and by prescription is a large money-maker for the pharmaceutical industries.

Gluten, through the body's immune system, can cause generalized stress to your body's health. Stress in all forms, likewise, increases the acid content of the stomach and leads to symptoms of heartburn.[67]

Once you remove the triggering agent (gluten), inflammation resolves, stress reduces and acid content returns to normal.

This is a more effective way of getting to the root cause, rather than putting a Band-aid on the symptom with medication. An antacid may neutralize the acid in your stomach for several hours, but the underlying stress and the reason for acid production increase have not been affected. You will be looking to medicate again once the antacid's effect dissipates.

Other Digestive Organs Can Be Affected

Other causes of abdominal pain related to gluten include conditions originating from the pancreas, liver and gallbladder. These are less-common sources of pain in gluten sensitivity but must be considered as gluten can provoke an autoimmune disorder in these organs. For liver and gallbladder symptoms, yellowish discoloration of the skin and eyes, called jaundice, can develop and light, tan-colored stools can be associated with bile disorders. Disorders of the pancreas may result in diabetic symptoms or back pain. Assessing these additional symptoms along with blood tests will help identify these less-common digestive disorders in gluten intolerance.

Don't Give Up—There Is a Root Cause of Pain

You are much more likely to seek help if pain develops, but it does not mean that biopsies or routine tests will reveal the cause. If these are negative, remember that gluten sensitivity may still be the cause. Sometimes, the only way to know is to eliminate gluten from your diet for a few weeks to evaluate the response. There are many causes of abdominal pain and cramping, and all of these need evaluation, but the key is not to overlook your diet, and specifically gluten, as a potential cause.

Diarrhea, Constipation and other Movement Symptoms

If you have these symptoms for any length of time, they tend to get your attention fairly quickly. Most patients will have sought some form of care if resolution has not been found in the local pharmacy, or if the symptoms did not resolve on their own within a few days.

If your intestinal wall contractions move things along too quickly, there is less time for nutrient and fluid absorption. Therefore, this results in diarrhea. If the contractions are slow, then the converse is true. There is greater time for fluid absorption to take place, and constipation develops. Both of these symptoms are very common with gluten sensitivity.

Diarrhea Can Cause Malnutrition

In the case of diarrhea, the inflammatory changes of the bowel wall stimulate the muscles to contract more violently and to speed the movement of food materials along the digestive tract. This occurs in gluten-sensitive patients because of inflammatory changes that irritate the bowel wall muscles. The more severe the inflammation, the worse the diarrhea can be for many people. With diarrhea, not only is cramping and pain often associated, but it also promotes malnutrition.[68]

Because food materials travel through the digestive system faster, there is less time for nutrient absorption. The gluten-induced inflammation has limited nutrient absorption already, so diarrhea only worsens the problem by speeding up the transit time.

The other reason diarrhea may develop is related to another phenomenon. It is called an osmotic process. Osmotic changes refer to the "drawing" effect of fluid toward solid material. In the digestive system, this describes solid food material inside the bowl actually pulling fluid into the bowel from the tissues around it. In a normal intestine that is functioning well, food is digested and absorbed efficiently and does not hang out in the bowel for very long. When gluten, however, causes villous atrophy (degradation of the lining of the small intestine) and inflammation, absorption is slowed and reduced. This causes food material to stay longer in the bowel and draw fluid into the bowel as well. This increase in bulk (food material and fluid) stimulates the intestinal muscles to push things forward more rapidly. This, then, causes diarrhea.

Jennifer's Thirty-Year Struggle

Jennifer had suffered cramping pains and diarrhea alternating with constipation for more than thirty years before coming into our clinic. She was also plagued with joint pains, headaches, asthma and dry, cracked skin. Heartburn "ran in the family," so she was convinced there was no hope for change in that area.

Once she began treatment with a gluten-free diet, she had resolution of her stomachaches and bowel movement problems over a fairly short period of time. In addition, her energy level returned to normal and her dry skin resolved as she started to absorb her nutrients. Her "familial" heartburn likewise resolved.

The only bad news was the fact that she had suffered unnecessarily for most of her life as a result of gluten sensitivity. The intestinal irritation and malabsorption caused by gluten had triggered the cramps and diarrhea and resulted in a decline in her daily energy. Once gluten was taken out of the picture, the intestinal lining was able to heal, and food digestion and absorption returned to normal. This allowed her diarrhea and other complaints to abate.

Marvin's Story

For other patients, constipation is a bigger problem. Marvin was one such patient. He had chronic constipation all the time, and always felt "clogged" and congested. Even after his constipation had resolved after being off gluten foods, he still noticed its immediate return when he accidentally ate gluten-containing items. He is still able to gauge the quality of his diet through his constipation.

In theory, constipation in gluten-sensitive people develops due to a lack of motility and movement of the intestines. Presumptively, because the villous atrophy of the bowel wall and inflammation reduces nutrient absorption, there is a greater amount of material remaining in the digestive tract. While this bulk often stimulates motility and possibly diarrhea, in other people, it actually delays movement. With greater time in the bowel, more fluid is re-absorbed and constipation occurs.

Gluten Directly Relates to IBS Symptoms

Whether it is diarrhea, constipation or, most commonly, alternating bouts of both, gluten can often cause these problems of bowel motility. A large portion of patients who have these symptoms get labeled with IBS (irritable bowel syndrome). Gluten may not be considered as a cause of IBS, and often, all other tests are negative. The important key, however, is that the symptoms remain, which indicates that something is wrong.

Of all IBS patients, more than half are found to have celiac disease.[69] In addition, many of the remaining percentage have non-celiac gluten intolerance. This demonstrates that when no other cause can be found in diarrhea and constipation complaints, gluten must be considered.

Gluten Causes Malabsorption of Vitamins and Minerals

An Eight-Year Tale of Woe

We diagnosed M. eight years ago with gluten sensitivity. Her initial list of symptoms was long and included sinus infections and bronchitis (which she got twice a year, every year), severe digestive problems including stomach pains, gas and lots of noises, swelling around her joints and fairly constant fatigue. In addition to being diagnosed with gluten sensitivity, we found a parasitic infection, Cryptosporidium, which is now resolved.

When she got off gluten, there was a 100-percent turn-around in her health. She was "mad as hell" at first because removing gluten from her diet was also eliminating many of her favorite foods. But, she now states categorically that it has been totally worth it considering how well she feels. She has learned what to eat and is happy with her choices.

M. realizes that she was malabsorbing nutrients most of her life as she still has some borderline anemia and some fatigue. In addition to anemia, her blood tests also showed low vitamin D levels. She wasn't diagnosed with gluten sensitivity until she was almost fifty, so she had done a lot of damage to her small intestine before getting the diagnosis. But, despite the chronicity of her situation, she doesn't get sinus infections or bronchitis anymore. The swelling around her joints has resolved. Her digestive complaints are a thing of the past, and while her fatigue is not perfect, it's much improved.

How Gluten Causes Malabsorption of Nutrients

While you may have a clear understanding of how gluten affects the digestive system and causes symptoms, you may be less aware of the symptoms it causes as a result of malabsorption. As gluten interacts with your immune system, an inflammatory attack occurs on the surface of the digestive lining. This lining is normally covered with finger-like projections, called villi, that serve to help nutrient absorption. These villi greatly increase the surface area of the intestines and allow a much wider area from which nutrients can enter our bodies for nutrition. However, when an individual who is sensitive to gluten digests wheat, rye or barley products, the ensuing immune reaction damages these villi. The end result is villous atrophy, or shrinkage of these structures, and this, in turn, hinders normal absorption of necessary nutrients.

Poor Absorption = Poor Health

Vitamins, as well as many minerals, are essential to your body's health, and when absorption declines, the lack of these micronutrients can cause all sorts of problems. As a general rule, there are two groups of vitamins. One group is water-soluble (meaning they dissolve in water) and the other group are fat-soluble (these can dissolve in fatty tissue). Fat-soluble vitamins can be stored more easily in the body than water soluble vitamins, so we must eat water-soluble vitamins almost daily to promote good health.

Regardless, both groups can become depleted when the villous atrophy and/or inflammation from gluten is severe enough. Even after treatment with gluten-free diets, half the celiac patients in one study were still depleted in vitamin B6, vitamin B12 and folate.[70] Therefore, nutritional needs must always be considered, even after gluten elimination.

In order to organize this section a little better, groups of common symptoms will be described that can be the result of selective vitamin or mineral deficiencies. But, sometimes, these symptoms can have other causes as well. Some of the other causes may even be related to gluten's effects on other organ systems besides the gastrointestinal system. If so, these will be covered in other sections. For now, it is important that you understand that our bodies need good fuel to operate optimally. This includes good nutrition and an ability to absorb it.

Fatigue, Lack of Energy, Easily Out of Breath

This doesn't sound like much fun, does it? Amazingly, these are common complaints for a number of different conditions, but malnutrition can be a reason.

In our bodies, all of our cells require oxygen to function well. Some tissues, like muscles, require it in much larger amounts. The way we obtain oxygen is through our lungs, as red blood cells, with the help of iron and hemoglobin, collect oxygen molecules and transport them to our tissues. In this process, there are four key vitamins and minerals that we must have. These include vitamin B12, iron, folate and vitamin K.

Gluten Sensitivity Can Cause Vitamin B12 Deficiency

Vitamin B12 is required to make red blood cells, and it is absorbed in the small intestines from our diet. Tuna, salmon, lean beef, liver, crab and oysters are some foods rich in this vitamin. What you may not know is that vitamin B12 requires a special enzyme in the lining of the digestive tract to allow it to be absorbed. And if gluten has induced deterioration of the lining, this crucial enzyme may be affected. As a result, no matter how much vitamin B12 you eat, it cannot be absorbed. While a loss of vitamin B12 results in many symptoms, anemia and fatigue are common ones.

Folate, which also helps build red blood cells, can be deficient with gluten sensitivity along with vitamin B12. It also is needed for the body to make red blood cells, and anemia can result from its deficiency. Allowing the lining to heal by becoming gluten-free will eventually allow replenishment of these vitamins through your diet.

Vitamin K is important because it assists in clotting. If you are suffering malabsorption of vitamin K because of gluten intolerance, it may result in a reduced ability to form clots. At least one case study reported severe intestinal bleeding in a celiac patient as a result of vitamin K deficiency induced by gluten intolerance combined with the use of anti-inflammatory meds. These medications are known to irritate the stomach and small intestine. And with a low vitamin K level, the irritation accelerated into bleeding.[71] Vitamin K is typically found in leafy green vegetables, as is folate.

Anemia Is a Common Symptom of Gluten Intolerance

Iron, of course, is needed to form hemoglobin, which binds the oxygen. If iron is low, red blood cells become reduced in number, and oxygen levels fall in the bloodstream. Increased bleeding demands more red blood cells to be formed, and this increases the need for even greater amounts of iron, folate and vitamin B12. If the intestinal lining is significantly inflamed, sometimes, low levels of bleeding can silently occur. Laboratory tests will identify this, but the underlying cause, if it is gluten sensitivity, may go unrecognized.

As red blood cells drop and oxygen levels are reduced, fatigue from hungry muscles develop, as does a lack of energy. If exertion occurs and your body has to utilize more oxygen, you then begin to breath more rapidly, to collect more air. The more air you ventilate, the more oxygen can be extracted for your red cells to use. But if they are limited in number, this will only help so much.

While lack of energy and fatigue may come from other gluten-related problems such as adrenal gland exhaustion, poor sleep, thyroid dysfunction and fibromyalgia, nutritional deficits can be an important cause as well. Correcting the nutritional depletion while eliminating gluten from the diet will improve these symptoms greatly within days to weeks in many patients.

Headaches

While gluten can cause headaches from other mechanisms, vitamin and mineral deficiencies from poor nutrition are definitely a cause. Specifically, B-complex vitamins can cause frequent, low-grade headaches when deficient, as can vitamin B12. B vitamins in general are needed for nerve cell function as well as muscle function. Either of these structures, when nutritionally depleted, could result in headaches.

In addition, headaches often accompany anemia, which was discussed above. Several of our patients had initial complaints of generalized, frequent headaches that resolved with treatment through a gluten-free diet. Whether this permitted healing of the digestive system to replenish nutrients or whether other mechanisms were involved is not precisely known. Regardless, gluten was at the root of the problem and their headaches resolved.

The Teen With Terrible Migraines

A. is a very bright, seventeen-year-old man in his final year of high school. Starting in seventh grade, he suffered from intermittent headaches and stomachaches. By tenth grade, they had become constant, and he was placed on medications—Elavil to start and Effexor, which he had been on for over a month when he came into the office.

His mother tried removing gluten and dairy from his diet, which seemed to help his stomach. Other foods seemed to bother his stomach as well, but nothing seemed to help the headaches. He was missing a lot of school despite scoring impressively high on his college entrance exams. However, if he wasn't able to spend more time in school, he would be in danger of not graduating.

His parents decided to wean him off the Effexor. This occurred during the first week as he also began the modified elimination diet. He didn't notice any change during the first week but halfway into the second week, he was feeling better and having less headaches. His lab test revealed a positive test to gluten sensitivity and a bacterial infection in his stomach.

Two months into the program, having successfully treated the stomach infection and removing gluten from his diet, his stomachaches were under control. His headaches were improved both in frequency and intensity and he resumed a normal school schedule. He noticed that dairy products created headaches as well, so he eliminated them from his diet also. As so frequently occurs, he occasionally stumbled into a little gluten. The results were intensely painful for him and a multi-day migraine would ensue.

Several months after he was back to normal health, his mother spoke to his pediatrician as she wanted to update him on the true source of her son's chronic stomachaches and headaches. Upon relating the entire story to the pediatrician, her doctor stated that the only way to know if A. had celiac disease was to put him back on gluten for a minimum of one to two months and then perform a biopsy of his intestine. A's mother was flabbergasted.

We realized, from the above case, how critical it was to alert everyone about the effects of gluten sensitivity and hopefully make the distinction between gluten sensitivity and celiac disease clear for doctors and patients alike. Needless suffering due to misunderstanding can be avoided with proper understanding and education. In this case, the root cause of the headaches and stomachaches could have been identified much earlier.

Muscle Difficulties—Aches, Pains and Fibromyalgia

Our muscles require a great deal of nutrients to function well. Our muscles utilize a tremendous amount of energy to move our limbs and joints, to pump our hearts, and to accomplish many internal activities such as digestion and swallowing. As a result, they consume large amounts of energy. Nutrients required for proper function of your muscles include calcium, magnesium, vitamin E, vitamin A and vitamin B12. And, unfortunately, all of these can be affected by malabsorption caused by gluten disorders.

Gluten-Free Diet Improves Fibromyalgia

You are likely aware that many diseases exist for which there are no known causes. For many of these, gluten is turning out to be a potential cause. Some muscle dystrophies and muscle conditions fall into this category. Fibromylagia, which is a disorder of fatigue, joint aches and muscle aches, is often present in patients with gluten intolerance. Fibromyalgia responds well to a gluten elimination diet for many patients, thereby supporting it as a major cause of this complaint. Low levels of vitamins E, A, C and B complex can trigger this condition as can low manganese, and these deficiencies can be associated with gluten intolerance.

Never underestimate how important your diet is for your health. Foods can be essential in providing key nutrients but can also, as in the case of gluten for many people, cause harm.

Evaluating Diet and Lifestyle Is Integral to a Proper Diagnosis

As you discuss your symptoms and complaints, try to localize with your physician the system within your body that is signaling a problem. Tests and exams that are performed are very important for detecting many illnesses and causes, but if these come up without an answer, it does not mean that it is time to sit back, wait and continue to suffer. Evaluating your diet and lifestyle can often uncover an answer.

If you have symptoms that relate to your digestion, be sure to consider gluten as a factor. People with digestive symptoms are twice as likely to have gluten sensitivity compared to the rest of the population.[72] And if gluten intolerance or celiac disease is detected, always consider nutritional malabsorption as contributing to the problem.

When You Can't Absorb What You Eat, Problems Ensue

Because our intestinal tract provides the pathway for fuel to reach your body, absorbing proper nutrition can be a problem when gluten affects the lining cells. Villi shrink, the lining becomes leaky and poor absorption is the result. Vitamins and minerals cannot be obtained for your body's needs, and this can affect many other areas of your health, as described. So, what begins as an intestinal problem evolves into a multi-system disorder.

Lastly, the stress from gluten on the body can lower its risk of infection. H. pylori, rotavirus, and proteus are some common infections of the digestive tract that occur more frequently in gluten-sensitive patients. When these are present, a gluten elimination diet may only partially resolve the complaints as the infection must be treated separately. Likewise, treating the infection only, and not identifying gluten as the root cause, will only result in temporary relief. Understanding how stressful gluten can be on both the intestinal lining and the immune system encourages consideration for secondary problems like these.

There's No Magic Pill

In looking ahead, some researchers are evaluating enzyme tablets that could be taken with gluten meals to aid stomach digestion. This way, gluten proteins may be digested well before they arrive at the intestinal wall. Whether this would be sufficient to reduce an immune attack is still under investigation, and we have our doubts.[73]

This therapy does not seem immediately around the corner, so for now, the best treatment is to avoid gluten if you are sensitive to it. If you do not know if you have a gluten sensitivity and have symptoms, get tested, because silent gluten disorders are common. If you have no symptoms yet have a strong family history of autoimmune disorders or gluten intolerance, also get tested. And, by all means, watch what you eat. Your diet determines a large part of your health.

Five

How Gluten Affects Your Brain and Nervous System

Gordon Just Looked Drunk

Gordon is a seventy-five-year-old gentleman who came in complaining of ataxia (trouble with balance), poor sleep, fatigue and high blood pressure for ten years. He was concerned because he knew that when he was walking, he looked drunk. He was concerned what people would think, but he was more concerned about his instability. He was at a loss of what to do and hadn't been receiving any help from his medical doctor.

Upon embarking on the HealthNOW Method, Gordon was found to be gluten sensitive by a positive saliva test. Furthermore, his stool test was positive for a bacterial infection.

After starting a modified elimination diet for three weeks, he began feeling better and his blood pressure reduced. After five weeks he was feeling stronger, and no longer had ataxia since being off the gluten. After six weeks he had no sleep apnea, his energy was much improved and his blood pressure continued to reduce. Gordon was a gentleman set in his ways, but he had to admit that he felt markedly different with the gluten-free diet and the other lifestyle changes he had implemented.

Is Your Nervous System Being Affected by Gluten?

You may be perplexed as to how a little protein in wheat can create problems in your nervous system. With the spotlight having been mainly on celiac disease and its relationship to gluten in creating digestive problems, few people have broadened their focus to look outside the digestive tract. What is now known about gluten sensitivity is that the number of celiac disease patients is much smaller than those who are gluten-intolerant. In essence, this figure is about eight to one.[74]

For this reason, it is extremely important to consider gluten sensitivity when dealing with many non-digestive symptoms. It is quite amazing how many other parts of your health can be actively affected by gluten without the presence of any digestive symptoms. Of all the other organ systems of your body, the nervous system is the area most commonly affected by gluten after the gastrointestinal system. And, because our nervous system handles so many important functions, symptoms related to the nervous system are quite varied.

Your nervous system incorporates central structures including your brain,, spinal cord,, peripheral structures that are made up of sensory nerves (which sense pain, hot, cold, etc.), motor nerves (allowing you to perform movements) and nerves that regulate your involuntary systems (such as your heart beating, breathing while you sleep, intestinal movements, etc.). In individuals who are predisposed to gluten intolerance, gluten triggers an immune reaction that can interfere with the function of these structures.

Is Your Brain "On Fire"?

There is an abundance of evidence that inflammatory changes occur in the brain and nerves that cause a variety of symptoms. These can range from clumsiness to headaches to numbness to mood disorders to memory problems. It has been reported that only thirteen percent of patients with neurologic symptoms from gluten sensitivity may have digestive symptoms,[75] and, often, neurological symptoms in gluten-sensitive patients precede digestive symptoms by months to years when they do occur.[76] For this reason, it is important to keep gluten in mind as a root cause when dealing with disorders of the nervous system.

In this chapter, categories of common symptoms that suggest neurological involvement will be described in detail. Remember, symptoms are the body's way of getting your attention and directing you toward the site of a problem. If standard tests and exams cannot reveal a cause, dietary factors, toxins, lifestyle issues and other stresses deserve your attention.

This is where gluten should be a strong consideration. Because gluten affects so many people silently, and because most of those symptoms are not related to the digestive tract, it needs to be an early consideration when addressing many health care problems. Examining the different way in which gluten affects your nervous system is an excellent way to appreciate the scope with which gluten results in a variety of symptoms. It also highlights the importance of your diet in relationship to your health.

Clumsiness, Imbalance and Coordination Problems

While this may not be the most common symptom of the nervous system related to gluten intolerance, it certainly is the most researched area. In medical circles, the term "ataxia" is used to describe poor coordination and balance. It can affect your walking, your ability to stand, or even your arms or legs in isolation. While many systems contribute to your balance (your inner ear, your vision, your sensations of your feet on the ground, etc.), your brain is the location that organizes all of this information and navigates your movements precisely. More specifically, the cerebellum, which is a part in the back of your brain, is the balance "control center."

Some examiners claim that ataxia is one of the most common disorders produced by gluten in relationship to the nervous system.[77] Poor coordination and clumsiness does occur with gluten intolerance and affects children as well as adults. But how does gluten cause the brain to function improperly and cause this imbalance? Evidence suggests that it is all due to the immune system's reaction to gluten itself.

Brain Cells That Help With Balance Are Destroyed

In your cerebellum (a part of the brain that plays an important role in the integration of sensation and control of movement), there are special cells called Purkinje cells. These cells are found in your cerebellum and are the main components of the balancing center. In patients with gluten sensitivity, it has been shown that there are antibodies against these Purkinje cells. The antibodies made against gluten (anti-gliadin antibodies) cross-react against these Purkinje cells.[78]

What this means is that in a person who is genetically at-risk for gluten sensitivity, gluten induces an immune attack against the protein gliadin, and this antibody not only attacks gliadin, but also attacks tissues far away from the intestines. In this case, through the bloodstream, these antibodies travel to the cerebellum and attack the Purkinje cells. As these cells become inflamed from the immune attack, the ability to coordinate all the balance information is impaired. Symptoms of poor balance and coordination then result.

Forty-One Percent of a Group With Ataxia Are Discovered to be Gluten-Sensitive

To further demonstrate this point, another study, out of Britain, examined 224 people with ataxia disorders. Some had inherited disorders of ataxia, some had ataxia combined with other neurologic symptoms, and some simply had ataxia without known causes. Of those who were without known cause, forty-one percent were found to have anti-gliadin antibodies supporting gluten sensitivity as a cause. Also, when looking at all patients in these groups who were positive for these antibodies, seventy-nine percent showed small cerebellums in MRI testing.[79] The gluten antibodies that had been generated from the immune system's reaction were not only directed against gluten proteins, but also against the cerebellum and its Purkinje cells. Over time, the size of the cerebellum had decreased.

Ninety Percent Show Beneficial Response to a Gluten-Free Diet

But the proof is always in the pudding. What happens if someone with poor balance is taken off gluten? In another study, ten patients with headaches and/or clumsiness were placed on a gluten-free diet. Over time, nine of the ten showed beneficial responses in all symptoms.[80]

The evidence is overwhelming. The presence of gluten antibodies, shrinkage of the cerebellum and the dramatic response to dietary change all support gluten as the cause. Yet, despite these obvious factors indicating gluten (a dietary component) as the root cause, the majority of the time, no digestive symptoms exist.

Brain Inflammation Can Occur Silently

In more than one study in patients with ataxia, other changes in the brain, revealed by MRI testing, have demonstrated inflammation and small areas of tissue damage.[81] These changes occurred silently, without anyone even knowing it until they grew large enough to create symptoms. But by the time symptoms occur, the inflammation has been evolving over a long time, for most people. For example, in individuals with small, silent strokes to the brain where symptoms are absent, eventually, enough tissue can be damaged to cause memory problems and dementia. By the time this is diagnosed, often, more than twenty percent of the brain is already damaged!

Poor coordination and clumsiness usually get your attention fairly early, and you are likely to seek medical care. But if testing fails to show a cause, strongly consider gluten as the culprit. Out of all the possible causes for unexplained ataxia, gluten intolerance is the most common cause.[82]

Numbness, Tingling and Pain

Think of your nervous system as an electrical circuit through which information flows to and from the brain and spinal cord. Thousands of nerves traverse your body, telling your muscles to move a certain way, and several sensors send information about touch, movement, pressure, temperature and pain back to your brain as well. When these nerves are unable to function well, false information can be sent back to the brain and cause many perceived symptoms. Of these, numbness, tingling and pain are the most common.

If you have ever slept on your arm incorrectly, you know how uncomfortable the symptoms of numbness and tingling can be. Imagine having this feeling all the time! If you slept in a poor position, as soon as you adjusted and moved, the compression on the nerve was released and the numbness faded away. In cases where the nerves are being damaged, however, changing your position does not help. This is called neuropathy.

Nerve Damage Related to Gluten

Neuropathy can be due to many causes, and diabetes is the most common known cause. Unfortunately, the majority of neuropathies are without a known cause. In addition to ataxia, neuropathy is fairly well studied in relationship to gluten and is a common neurologic manifestation of gluten intolerance.[83] The mechanism is related to the immune system.

Antibodies directed against gliadin or gluten can result in cross-reactions against proteins or fibers of the nerves, causing damage. Research supports that these antibodies have specific cross-reactivity with myelin (the insulating layer around nerves, composed of protein and fat) and neurofilaments (fibers that make up the nerve cell). Both of these are key components of nerves that relate to sensation and movement.[84]

Which portion and which set of nerves are affected will determine your symptoms. For instance, if nerves that sense temperature changes are attacked by gluten-related immune antibodies, then odd sensations of hot, cold or pain may develop. Or, if nerves that sense pressure and touch are involved, unusual pressure sensations or deep pain can result. While it may seem as though something that is hot, cold or painful is affecting an area of your body, there is really nothing there.

Are Your Nerves Short Circuiting?

But, your brain's perception is purely based on what the nerves tell it. So, if they are signaling "bad" information because they are inflamed or injured, you still feel the pain even though nothing painful is there. In this way, it is like a short circuit in a faulty monitor. The monitor's alarm is going off, signaling a problem, and everyone is hurrying to fix the problem, but no problem with the system is present. The problem is in the monitor, or, in this case, the nerve itself.

Studies Show Gluten to Be the Cause

How commonly does gluten cause these neuropathy problems? More often than you might think. In a study of twenty-seven children with celiac disease, eleven percent had some form of neurologic disorder. Neuropathy was the most common.[85] Another examined nine patients with confirmed celiac disease, and several different types of neuropathies were documented in this group, affecting many different sorts of nerves.[86]

When you consider how few patients with neuropathy carry a documented cause of their complaints, gluten may well account for a high number. Also, while diabetes accounts for the majority of neuropathy patients, the mechanism of how it causes neuropathy is still not clearly defined. Gluten, in these diabetic patients with neuropathy, may also be the primary cause. Gluten not only can cause an immunologic attack on the nerves through the immune system, but it also can cause diabetes through mechanisms of stress. Chronic stress results in adrenal exhaustion, which leads to insulin resistance and elevated glucose levels. In this way, gluten, directly and indirectly, can be the root cause of neuropathy complaints.

Again, the same rules apply. Symptoms of numbness, tingling and pain can indicate a neuropathy condition. Gluten has been well-documented to be a cause, and should be routinely assessed for a possible source of the problem.

Headaches and Migraines

Have you ever had a headache? Headaches are one of the most universal symptoms, and almost everyone has experienced a headache at some point. A migraine, which is as a specific type of headache, occurs regularly in as many as twenty-seven percent of the population.[87] So, when dealing with such a common condition, it may seem bold to claim that gluten, likewise, can cause headaches. Can we prove it? Let's take a look.

Migraines, and many other types of headaches, are influenced by stresses in our lives. This includes emotional stresses, but, in addition, encompasses diet, exercise, chemical exposure, etc. Migraines commonly are known to be triggered by these factors. As has been demonstrated repeatedly, gluten also is one of these triggers, and eliminating it from the diet in sensitive individuals can provide significant relief.

Headaches Show Favorable Response to Gluten-Free Diet

In a large study examining many patients with neurologic complaints, headaches were assessed along with a few other conditions. While all were gluten-sensitive patients, only some were celiac patients. More than half who did have celiac disease had neurologic disorders, and almost twenty percent had neurologic complaints but not celiac disease. The key finding was that, of all the neurologic symptoms assessed, headaches had the most favorable response to a gluten-free diet.[88]

A British researcher found similar results in the response of gluten-sensitive patients to a gluten-free diet. Ninety percent responded favorably to elimination of gluten in the diet.[89] Another researcher reported a case study of a woman who converted her intermittent, occasional migraines to chronic, daily headaches with the addition of wheat biscuits to her daily diet. Once these were stopped, her headaches reduced dramatically.[90]

The point is that gluten needs to be considered in people who suffer headaches. While it is true that migraine medications may be beneficial in alleviating headaches or adding some protective effects, how many times are we actually getting to the root of the problem? Why commit someone to the costs and inconveniences of taking a prescription medication when simple lifestyle or dietary adjustments may be the real solution?

Marsha's Battle With Migraines

Marsha had suffered from headaches and migraines her entire life. She had also suffered from cystic acne, which came on as an adult. She had been spending a lot of time and money on weekly face treatments, to try to treat it and to prevent scarring.

Marsha had no digestive complaints when she came to see us, so, therefore, was very surprised when we diagnosed her as gluten-sensitive. But, her surprise turned to delight when the acne disappeared while on a gluten-free diet. And the delight turned into downright joy when she ceased having migraines. We followed up with Marsha three years later; her migraines never returned unless she accidentally got into gluten.

She had been to many other clinicians and had tried many medications for her headaches, but in the end, she found the best relief by avoiding gluten.

The Correct Answer Is Often a Simple One

In our society, simplistic solutions and causes are often overlooked. Large pharmaceutical companies spend millions of dollars on the research and development of new drugs. And, there are powerful lobbyist groups for these businesses that benefit from investing in new medications rather than dietary changes.

Eliminating gluten from your diet does not require a prescription and does not support the cost it took to design the new migraine medication. This is a significant reason why dietary factors are ignored or overlooked. Yet, study after study supports a beneficial response to dietary changes in many conditions. If you are suffering from headaches, and traditional medical means have failed or only offered temporary results requiring you to ingest a medication, gluten may be an easy solution for you as well.

Memory, Brain Fog and Attention Difficulty

The way our brains process and retain information is extremely complex. The intricacies of how nerve cells interact with each other through a web of connections, and how different brain chemicals affect these connections, are a source of never-ending research. Because of this, many neurologic disorders that affect our ability to think, learn and remember escape a definition of cause.

Is Your Diet Putting You at Risk for Alzheimer's?

For instance, in Alzheimer's, many factors (including diet) have been shown to affect risks, but no single cause is evident. But, what has been demonstrated is that gluten does play a role in such cognitive disorders, in a percentage of people.

Losing your memory before the age of sixty years is considered very early. The term "dementia" actually means the premature loss of memory and other functions of cognition. In one recent study, patients under sixty years with dementia were assessed in their response to dietary changes. Of these, five were found to have celiac disease by biopsy. The notable finding was that treatment with a gluten-free diet showed improvement in dementia in four of these five individuals.[91] That is an eighty-percent response rate!

Gluten Can Damage Your Brain

But how does gluten affect memory as well as all the other symptoms described? The major mechanism is, again, through our immune system, but our memory and thinking are also affected by gluten in other ways as well.

In regard to the immune system, gluten invokes an immune reaction in persons genetically at-risk for gluten sensitivity. There is strong evidence that these immune reactions affect the brain tissue as well. CT scans of the head in dementia patients with gluten sensitivity have shown atrophy (also known as brain shrinkage),[92] and MRI studies of the brain have shown evidence of deep-tissue inflammation in gluten patients as well.[93]

It is suspected that this deep-tissue inflammation results from gluten-related antibodies attacking tiny blood vessels deep within the brain, causing inflammation and resultant tissue injury. Over time, this results in a reduced ability to pay attention and recall memories. In other words, the connections between the nerve cells are damaged and information cannot be processed or retrieved as well as before. If part of your computer's circuitry were damaged, the computer might seem to operate fairly well, but in the process, you may have lost some files. This is what occurs in gluten-sensitive people who suffer gluten-induced effects within their brains.

Gluten By-Products Have Morphine-Like Effects

The other mechanism by which gluten causes reduced attention and memory is chemical means. Gluten has by-products in its metabolism that form substances known as gluteomorphins. The "morphins" component of the name refers, indeed, to a morphine-like chemical, though it is much milder than morphine itself. These gluteomorphins attach to opiate receptors in the brain and can result in diminished alertness, concentration and memory.[94] Not only is this important in patients with dementia, but it is also important in children with autism and other learning disorders.

How Autism and ADD Fit Into the Picture

Like dementia, autism is a complex brain disorder that has escaped a defined cause. Again, many theories exist, but, repeatedly, gluten seems to play at least a part in its presentation. In one study, a controlled trial placed one group of children with autism on a gluten-free diet while leaving the others with their regular, gluten-containing meals. After a year, the children were reassessed, and all the children on the gluten-free diet demonstrated benefits in behavior.[95] This is just one of many studies of autistic children that support a good response to gluten-free diets. Whether gluten is interacting in these children by immune mechanisms or whether it is through morphine-like metabolites is unknown. But, it is clear that gluten is having a negative effect regardless of the exact mechanism.

Other common neurological disorders affecting memory and attention have been reported as well. In a large study examining patients with gluten sensitivity, attention deficit disorder (ADD), learning disabilities and developmental delay conditions all were more common.[96] As we learn more about how the brain functions and how it responds to our diet, we will be better able to tailor our eating habits and lifestyles to promote good brain health.

It is well-supported, currently, that gluten can result in memory, attention and cognitive decline in sensitive individuals. Particularly for children suffering from ADD or autistic disorders, this is extremely important, as early intervention may allow significant strides in development and learning to occur, and perhaps an unnecessary label can be removed.

Seizures

Although fortunately less common, seizures can be a symptom of gluten sensitivity in a select few. And those who have seizures can be resistant to most common medications that make any positive results worth noting.

Gluten's Relationship to Seizures

An excellent study was evaluated with 171 patients who suffered seizures and likewise had gluten sensitivity/celiac disease and calcifications in the brain. The overwhelming majority had gliadin antibodies in the spinal fluid (which circulates around the brain and spinal cord), and, likewise, most had the gene for having gluten sensitivity.[97] Though many were unresponsive to treatment in general, it was notable that some did respond well to a gluten-free diet.

Why would gluten cause seizures? And are the calcium deposits in the brain related to gluten? Likely, the answer is "yes" to both questions. The presence of calcium deposits reflects chronic inflammation in some tissues. When inflammation has been present for years, calcium forms scars where the inflammation is located. Additionally, brain calcifications can form as a result of a folic acid (a B vitamin) deficiency, which may have been a contributing cause to the calcium deposits in these patients. Since gluten causes digestive malabsorption, then, folic acid may indeed have been low due to that.

The Mechanism Explained

Regardless, the root cause is most likely an immune system attack triggered by gluten sensitivity. Antibodies that are made to attack gluten get confused and attack normal tissue that looks similar to gluten's protein structure. In the brain, once the tissue is inflamed chronically, calcium can deposit and form a hardened scar.

Because of this scar, seizures develop and can be difficult to control with normal seizure medications. Seizures are basically short circuits of the brain. Suppose there were an electrical pole knocked down onto the ground. The electrical wires tore and were lying unprotected, sending out sparks from their broken ends. The electrical connection had been severed. Calcium deposits and scars in the brain essentially do the same thing. They send off electrical "sparks" that can develop into seizures if enough brain tissue becomes involved. Medication may help the sparks from spreading, but with gluten-related seizures, medicines work less well.

A Lovely Girl Who Leaves Her Seizures Behind

T.S. is a beautiful, vibrant, nine-year-old girl who had begun having seizures at the age of four. She had undergone standard medical testing without a cause of her seizures being found. We first saw her when she was four years old. Not only did we find that she was sensitive to gluten, but that she also had many intestinal infections, a Candida yeast infection, and an essential fatty acid imbalance. The infections were greater in number in her than in most adults we treat, and some were very resistant to treatment, requiring two rounds of antibiotics instead of the usual one. She was treated with fatty acids in addition to a gluten-free diet.

T.S. has had absolutely no seizures for two years. She told her mother recently that she knows that the gluten created her seizures, and she is more than happy to keep it out of her diet. It is noteworthy that her mother, also diagnosed by us as gluten-sensitive, never ate much gluten until her twenties because as a child, she had sensed that it bothered her. But, recalling when she was in college and consumed a lot of gluten, she remembered suffering from "brain fog" during that time.

Evidence of these inflammatory changes can be seen in some gluten-sensitive patients via MRI. This was supported in another study examining patients with gluten sensitivity and seizures, which demonstrated deep-tissue inflammation in at least twenty percent of the children studied who had seizures. In addition, none of these seizure patients had folic acid deficiency, which suggests that gluten was the primary cause of their problem.[98]

It's Worth Giving Gluten-Free a Try

While, thankfully, seizures are an uncommon manifestation of gluten sensitivity, it is extremely important to recognize it as a cause because the only effective treatment may be a gluten-free diet. If you never think of gluten as a cause, then you will never test for its presence. It would be miserable to have to suffer, or see someone else suffer, with seizures when a potential cure may exist with a simple dietary change.

Mood Disturbances—Depression, Anxiety, Etc.

It is well-established that mood symptoms occur in many patients with gluten sensitivity. These symptoms can include depression, anxiety and other, more serious behavioral disorders such as the ADD and autism described above. As with any illness, it is sometimes hard to distinguish whether the depression or anxiety is an emotional response to having chronic symptoms, but in gluten sensitivity, these mood problems are more common than would be expected. In addition, these mood disturbances respond well to gluten-free diets in most patients.[99] This suggests a separate problem that is specific to gluten itself rather than a psychological reaction to being ill.

How Does Gluten Cause Depression and Anxiety?

Theories as to why gluten causes depression and anxiety basically fall into two categories. Similar to other neurologic symptoms caused by gluten sensitivity, inflammatory damage to the deep portions of the brain's tissue, especially in the frontal areas, may very well be a significant factor. Many studies examining patients with mood disturbances demonstrate changes of circulation in the frontal areas of the brain. In one study examining blood flow to the brain, fifteen patients with untreated celiac disease were compared to fifteen patients treated with a gluten-free diet for a year. The findings were amazing.

Gluten Results in Reduced Blood Flow to the Brain

In the untreated group, seventy-three percent had abnormalities in brain circulation by testing, and only seven percent in the treated group had any disturbances. A number of these patients with abnormal brain circulation had depression and anxiety as well.[100].The blood flow reductions are most likely secondary to the inflammatory changes caused by gluten sensitivity.

June's Anxiety and Panic Attacks

June presented to our clinic with several complaints, but the most prominent were anxiety with intermittent panic attacks and intestinal symptoms. These symptoms were severe and often prevented her from carrying out her daily activities. She had undergone other medical tests without a diagnosis and likewise had tried behavioral and medication treatments for her anxiety and panic disorder. However, she had only received mild benefit.

Her exam was unremarkable, but her testing suggested intolerance to gluten. She was placed on an elimination diet including gluten restriction, and after being gluten-free for several weeks, her symptoms progressively improved. She has not had a panic attack since that time (it's been years), and her anxiety is much improved. It no longer interferes with her daily activities. Likewise, her digestive complaints have dissipated.

Gluten Is an Underappreciated Cause of Depression and Anxiety

Given the significant number of people with depression and anxiety, as well as the number who have no idea about its cause, gluten sensitivity is an underappreciated cause that deserves attention. In addition to circulation disturbances in the brain, other research suggests that gluten interferes with amino acid (protein) absorption. A reduced level of tryptophan (a protein in the brain responsible for a feeling of well-being, calm and relaxation) in the body causes mood disturbances to occur.[101] It is important to recognize diet and gluten as a cause.

In a society where it is customary to receive a prescription for mood complaints (despite the known, dangerous side effects associated with psychiatric drugs), we are neglecting to look at a basic, underlying cause. Be sure to look at your diet and lifestyle, and this implies gluten as well.

Fatigue and Weakness

While weakness and fatigue can certainly be symptoms of the nervous system, fatigue often results from effects on other systems as well. For this reason, fatigue will mostly be covered in the next section, under adrenal exhaustion.

However, within the scope of neurological complaints, weakness and hypotonia need to be mentioned. Hypotonia refers to a reduced level of muscle tone in the body—or, in other words, a "floppiness." Muscles have an inherent tension, or tone, that represents their readiness to contract. While hypotonia can occur in adults, it most commonly is seen in children.

Is Gluten Reducing the Tone and Strength of Your Muscles?

But what causes reduced muscle tone and weakness? In many cases, it is a reflection of dysfunction of the cerebellum. Remember, the cerebellum is that part of the brain that handles our coordination and balance. Well, it also maintains the tone in our muscles. It is likely that the same attack of gluten-related antibodies against the cells of the cerebellum not only causes imbalance but also hypotonia. In one report, hypotonia was one of the symptoms that indeed responded well to gluten-free diet intervention.[102] This situation can be a component of fatigue in some patients as well.

As you can see, in many individuals, the nervous system is affected by gluten intolerance. It is the second-most commonly affected part of the body, after the digestive system. However, because the nervous system is so complex, gluten is often overlooked as a potential cause.

Based on the above information, gluten affects the nervous system frequently due to the number of ways in which it influences the functions of the brain and nerves. Like other organ systems, the immune response to gluten causes injury to nervous tissue, resulting in many symptoms. Chemical effects through gluteomorphins can contribute to these symptoms, as can malabsorption of crucial vitamins, minerals and amino acids.

It Only Takes a Little Damage to Create a Variety of Symptoms

Because the nervous system is a major system that maintains functional balance within our bodies, it can take just subtle injuries to result in symptoms. These symptoms can be quite varied. Certain symptoms should always trigger an investigation for gluten sensitivity, such as ataxia, chronic headaches, seizures, attention and memory problems, numbness and loss of sensation. Not only does this group of symptoms have a track record of having unexplained causes in the majority of people, but it also statistically has a significant number that is related to gluten intolerance. Failing to assess for gluten sensitivity could commit you to chronic complaints for a lifetime, unnecessarily.

Be Relentless in Your Search for the Root Cause

It cannot be stressed enough that you should maintain vigilance in your search. Seek out causes to your symptoms through your diet and your lifestyle stressors, as well as through other health conditions you may be genetically predisposed to. Symptoms are our bodies' monitoring systems. Pay attention to all aspects of your health and what may worsen or appease your complaints.

It has been our experience that gluten sensitivity is an extremely common cause for many diverse symptoms. One reason for this is its interaction with the immune system, but another is the stress effects that it causes on the body in general. In the next chapter, we will address these mechanisms in detail, which will further explain gluten's broad scope of health effects.

This final case study encompasses many of the symptoms we've just discussed.

The Miserable Rocket Scientist

Several years ago L.A. came to see us. He's a famous scientist and travels the world lecturing to fellow scientists and researchers. L.A. had chronic, severe allergies since childhood and had suffered from a couple of heart attacks prior to his initial appointment. His family history wasn't "pretty," with his dad dying from a heart attack at the young age of forty-five and his grandfather dying at age forty-three with cardiovascular symptoms as well.

L.A. had his first heart attack at age forty-five and his second at age fifty-three, shortly before coming to HealthNOW. He had been told that the next heart attack would probably kill him. His initial complaints consisted of dizzy spells, nausea, chronic sleep problems, headaches and some numbness on his right side. He had suffered some depression and anxiety attacks, which a short bout of antidepressants had done nothing to improve. He had restricted animal protein from his diet for a few years but had seen no apparent benefit—especially considering that this had been prior to his second heart attack.

In his evaluation, we performed a test for gluten sensitivity that demonstrated, indeed, that he was gluten sensitive. In addition, tests revealed the presence of infectious organisms, which were subsequently treated successfully. After six weeks on the

HealthNOW method, L.A.'s blood work was the best it had ever been. In fact, he discontinued his cholesterol-lowering medication because his cholesterol was too low! His total cholesterol dropped from 213 to 134, his good cholesterol held steady at about 32, and his bad cholesterol dropped from a high of 177 to 81.

After staying on a gluten-free diet and watching his fat intake for several years, L.A.'s lipid numbers remain strong and healthy. In addition, his chronic sleep problem, headaches and severe allergy symptoms have resolved.

The standard medical approach would have been to "monitor" this patient's blood work and continue to treat him with increasing amounts of medications for his various symptoms. Instead, we chose to take a deeper look. We focus our interests on the root cause of the problem, not just the end result of the process, and L.A. says that he now feels better than he did ten years ago.

Six

Stress, Hormones and Gluten

The Attorney With a Long List of Complaints

K. is a lovely, intelligent, thirty-seven–year-old attorney who came to us two years ago with severe, chronic migraines that were resistant to even the strongest medication. The migraines could last for a week at times. They had first started when she was five months pregnant with her second child. She had never had any migraines prior to that time.

Asthma and allergies had also developed during her second pregnancy. She had mood swings associated with her migraines, and she stated that she had "never been the same" since her second pregnancy. She was completely exhausted, had little energy and got sick all the time. She complained of numbness, tingling and burning pain in her big toes. She had gained weight in her midsection, which she disliked, though she was very petite and not overweight. Additional symptoms included abdominal bloating, carpal tunnel symptoms of the hands, acid reflux and severe premenstrual syndrome

She came to see us in March and had been sick three times during the previous five months, and was suffering from a continuing illness for the previous six weeks. She had a stressful job as an attorney for a large corporation and admitted to poor dietary habits. She was on Lipitor, birth control pills and Zyrtec, but none had helped. She had a strong history of genetic heart disease in the family.

She was found to be gluten-intolerant through testing, which included positive anti-gliadin antibodies in both blood and saliva. She had parasitic infections, found by testing as well. She reacted to dairy products, rice and corn in addition to gluten.

When she was initially put on the hypoallergenic diet, which we call the modified elimination diet, she noticed a change in her migraines within a week. After being on the diet for one month, she accidentally ate gluten and dairy and suffered a migraine that lasted for eight days. Also, after a month on the modified elimination diet, she started to sleep better and have more energy.

Two months into the program, we received the results showing the parasitic infections and began treatment for this as well. Shortly after this, she was able to wean off all regular medications for her premenstrual syndrome and migraine conditions, and the intensity of her then-rare headaches were much milder.

Four months into program, she no longer needed even occasional medications for her headaches. The frequency of her headaches was down to twice a month, and her energy level was much improved. Her premenstrual symptoms had also improved. After six months, she had less bloating and after eight months, her headaches were essentially resolved totally. She was exercising three times a week, had good energy and had very rare acid reflux. Eleven months into the HealthNOW program, she checked in and was absolutely amazed at the restoration of health that she had received.

Consider This...

Here's a question: If you had a part of your body that was responsible for creating great energy levels, maintaining your ideal weight, encouraging restful sleep, balancing your mood, reducing pain and inflammation, preventing allergy symptoms, keeping your immune system strong and promoting anti-aging, would you want it to function properly? Of course, and we are in complete agreement with you. So, let's learn something about our adrenal glands.

Why Are Hormones So Important?

Of the various systems throughout your body, the hormonal system is probably one of the most important. What does it accomplish that makes it so important? Basically, it balances every other system in your body so you can maintain good health and function. Hormones are chemical messengers that carry signals, via the blood, from one area of your body to another in order to regulate function. This allows your body both to adapt to changes within the body and to your environment. Hormones enable you to remain flexible to all forms of stresses.

Are You Tired?

"I feel tired all the time" or "I have a really hard time getting up in the morning" are some of the most common complaints we hear in our office on a daily basis. These symptoms can be directly attributed to gluten sensitivity due to its effect on the body's adrenal glands. While hormone production occurs in many organs, the adrenal glands are one of the most important structures in regulating hormonal production and response.

Where Are My Adrenal Glands?

The adrenal glands are two small glands that sit just above your kidneys. They are immediately adjacent to some of your major blood vessels so that they can release hormones into the bloodstream and, likewise, respond to feedback information from other hormones and chemicals. In this way, they control how other systems operate. Hormones regulate your blood pressure, your ability to metabolize glucose, your weight distribution, your thyroid function, your moods and many, many other processes.

Adrenal Glands Have an Anti-Aging Effect

The adrenal glands are mainly involved in anabolic work—that is, repair and anti-aging effects. Their role is to keep the immune system properly functioning and, at the same time, balance other bodily systems to promote optimal health. When the adrenal glands become exhausted and overworked from chronic stress, they cannot keep up on all of their demands that are made of them. This results in catabolism, or a breakdown of systems. Think of catabolism as "cannibalism" because the body's health systems are unable themselves, and functions begin to deteriorate. This leads to fatigue, depression, loss of libido and frequent illnesses, to name a few.

Gluten Stresses Your Adrenal Glands

But what exactly does this have to do with gluten? In addition to the immune effects triggered by gluten in sensitive people, gluten also causes many symptoms through direct stress exerted on the adrenal gland. As you recall, gluten imparts an inflammatory reaction and an immune response at the intestinal level in individuals who are gluten-sensitive. The body's reaction to this is stress, a response from our hormonal system.

The balancing efforts of the hormonal pathways are constantly trying to "cool things off" when a stress occurs. Of all of the stresses that demand a response from the adrenals, it is inflammation (such as that created by gluten sensitivity) that demands a constant anti-inflammatory response.

Different Varieties of Stress

Stresses can come in many different varieties, other than from our diet. Some examples are sleep deprivation, emotional stress, infections, toxins and injuries. Gluten, specifically, stresses our immune system, our ability to absorb nutrients and other areas as a result of chemical and inflammatory changes. When this occurs chronically, our hormonal system begins to break down. The adrenals essentially become exhausted. This, in turn, causes a failure of the body's balancing mechanisms to function properly, and widespread symptoms develop.

While Adrenal Disease Is Rare, Adrenal Malfunction Is Extremely Common

In order to explain the symptoms related to gluten as it pertains to our hormonal systems, it is necessary to digress a bit and explain how the adrenal gland operates. For many of you (and for many clinicians), adrenal dysfunction is not readily appreciated. This is mainly due to the fact that it exerts effects on the body remotely, as the hormones the adrenals produce circulate to other areas of the body to do their job. Adrenal glands themselves rarely develop tumors or get diseased, but they malfunction often, which compromises their critical ability to regulate hormone balance. This helps explain why they can be a source of so many common symptoms and yet remain under-recognized by many health practitioners. Therefore, in order to have a better understanding of hormonal mechanisms, and, ultimately, how gluten affects these functions, we will give you a brief overview of how important this system is to our health.

For those of you who want to cut to the chase, you can jump ahead to the summary and symptoms section of this chapter. This area provides a less-detailed review of common complaints of adrenal dysfunction and the effects of gluten sensitivity. But for those of you interested in the science behind the symptoms—read on!

How Hormones Work in Your Body

Remember, hormones are molecules that travel from one place in your body, where they are produced, to another, where they exert their effect. This inherently allows for a feedback loop type of system. What is a feedback loop? An easy example of a feedback loop system is your thermostat in your home. The thermostat is set at seventy degrees. The temperature hits seventy-three degrees, and the air conditioner begins to cool the air of your home. Eventually, the temperature falls to seventy degrees. The thermostat recognizes this and shuts off the air conditioner. This is a feedback loop, and like the thermostat, many glands that produce hormones respond in this fashion. This includes the adrenal gland, the thyroid gland, the pituitary gland and others.

What Are the Major Hormones?

Major hormones in the body include cortisol, adrenaline and insulin. Cortisol is commonly referred to as our "stress hormone." It increases blood pressure and sugar levels, and it decreases the function of the immune system. Lesser hormones include estrogen, progesterone, testosterone, thyroid hormone and calcitriol. Calcitriol regulates the body's levels of calcium and phosphorus.

The important point is that through a complex system of interactions, our bodies respond to these chemicals called hormones by either increasing or decreasing certain functions. An easy example is the pancreas. You eat a meal, and the food is digested. Your blood sugar begins to rise, along with other nutrients. This stimulates the pancreas to produce and release the hormone insulin. Insulin allows the cells of your body to absorb the glucose so that your blood sugar reduces. Once it lowers, the pancreas responds (through a feedback loop) by shutting off insulin production. There are hundreds of these types of interactions, throughout your body, occurring all the time.

In discussing some of the hormones of the body, it is helpful to understand some key structures. For the purpose of this book, three areas will be discussed. These include the hypothalamic-pituitary axis (see below for definition.), the adrenal gland and the thyroid gland. These three are very important in the chronic stress effects they produce on the body in terms of symptoms. And, by defining these areas in more detail, it will be apparent how gluten causes symptoms and dysfunction to occur through hormonal effects.

The Hypothalamic-Pituitary Axis (HP Axis): A Critical Link Between Stress and Health

The name is daunting enough, so we'll call it the HP axis. That is much easier to digest. The name actually defines two small structures that are positioned just under the front part of your brain. The brain and nervous system regulate the function of the body in many ways. Likewise, the interplay between the brain and the hormonal system is crucial in keeping our health in balance. The HP axis, which represents a key interface between the brain and nervous systems, is divided into two parts: the hypothalamus and the pituitary gland.

The hypothalamus responds to many signals generated by the brain as well as by other hormone glands. In response to these signals, the hypothalamus releases hormones or molecules that stimulate or suppress the pituitary gland. The pituitary gland produces a hormone called ACTH, which is an abbreviation for a very long word (adrenocorticotrophic hormone) that isn't really necessary for you to know. But, since we're going to be referring to ACTH quite a bit in this chapter, you do need to know that it is produced by the pituitary gland and is an important player in how the brain and the adrenal glands interact.

Hormones Make More Hormones

ACTH (produced by the pituitary gland) is a powerful hormone that triggers many types of hormones to be produced by the adrenal gland. There's a different hormone produced by the pituitary gland, called TSH (thyroid stimulating hormone), that stimulates the thyroid gland to make thyroid hormone, which is important for your metabolism (how quickly and efficiently you burn your food to create energy). As thyroid hormones and the various adrenal hormones are subsequently produced, the hypothalamus and pituitary quit making their hormones and the cascade of events shuts down. Here's our feedback loop in action again. In normal health, this feedback loop keeps everything in balance for our metabolism, our immune system, our sexual functions, etc.

The HP axis, however, is not just responsive to the feedback of the hormones it triggers. It also is responsive to the effects of many stresses. These were mentioned previously, including infections, toxins, mental/emotional issues, etc.

Stress From Gluten Creates Adrenal Gland Weakness

When gluten creates stress on the body, it exerts effects on the hormonal system secondarily. When there are continual stresses present, the hypothalamus and pituitary gland respond by continuing to make ACTH, which, in turn, stimulates the adrenal gland to produce its hormones even when hormone levels are high. The feedback loop fails because the chronic stress overrides the system.

If the offending gluten is removed, then the chronic stress can be eliminated, and, eventually, the hormonal system and HP axis can recover. This is the reason why some symptoms do not immediately fade away when gluten is removed. It takes time and, usually, some nutritional assistance for these systems to get rebalanced.

A Many-Year Battle with Depression, Anxiety and Allergies

Conny is a forty-eight-year-old woman who came to see us suffering from severe allergies, depression and anxiety for eight years. She was on two different anti-depressant medications and still felt terrible. The anxiety that accompanied the depression caused her to overeat in order to combat how she was feeling. She was chronically fatigued and was tired of being sick all the time. She also had chronic muscle pain in her arms and hips, shooting pain in her feet and a chronic skin condition that caused her skin to be rough and irritated.

Her husband had attended a lecture at work and thought that perhaps we could help his wife. She was feeling discouraged when she first came into HealthNOW. Conny was originally from South America and liked the HealthNOW philosophy of getting to the underlying, root cause.

After the first week on the modified elimination diet, Conny noticed significant improvements. She had more energy, less depression, better sleep and improved allergy symptoms. Two weeks into the program, she had already lost seven pounds and was still improving on all fronts. While her lab tests showed borderline positive results for gluten sensitivity, she was convinced that gluten was a problem, based on her experience so far.

Her adrenal lab test was positive and she was in stage II adrenal exhaustion (there are three stages possible). She was put on a nutritional and lifestyle program to address this condition.

Three weeks later, she had lost ten pounds, her allergy symptoms were gone and she had stopped taking her allergy medication altogether. Her lab tests also showed that she had a parasitic infection, for which treatment was also begun. She continued to improve over the next month and desired to get off her antidepressants.

Despite explaining her recent course of events to her psychiatrist, he refused to accept gluten sensitivity as a diagnosis. Despite her frustration, she insisted on weaning off the antidepressants, and within two weeks, she had successfully stopped them with positive results.

Two months later, a follow-up visit found Conny still off all medications and pain-free. She literally couldn't believe how great she felt. She not only kept up with her two busy children, but she thoroughly enjoyed the many activities that previously she could not tolerate well. Since then, Conny has occasionally, inadvertently consumed gluten, and the response has been dramatic. She's felt bad for three or four days, with a return of her fatigue and shooting pains in her feet. She says she wouldn't have believed that the gluten would have caused such things if she hadn't experienced it for herself.

The Solution Wasn't Difficult

What was the root cause of Conny's eight-year battle? Gluten sensitivity resulting in adrenal exhaustion, hormonal imbalance and intestinal infection. Sounds simple, and it was, actually. But getting to the root cause is a more direct and simpler approach than chasing symptoms and masking them with drugs.

The Adrenal Glands: Perhaps the Most Misunderstood, Most Overlooked Parts of the Body

These two small glands are incredibly powerful, and they are responsible for how major hormones act within the body. Each has three outer layers and one inner layer. The inner layer produces our adrenaline hormone; the outermost layer makes aldosterone, which balances our electrolytes and fluid balance; the middle outer layer makes cortisol, which affects our immune system's function and our ability to deal with stress; and the innermost outer layer produces DHEA (short for dehydroepiandrosterone), which is a precursor of our sex hormones (estrogen, testosterone and progesterone).

Think for just a moment how these two walnut-sized glands are able to control so many functions. In essence, our immune system, our reproductive system, our metabolism and our survival responses are all housed within the adrenals.

Chronic Stress Can Beat Up Your Adrenal Glands

As you recall, the adrenal glands respond to the HP axis as it sends ACTH through the bloodstream. ACTH triggers the adrenal gland to make cortisol and DHEA, primarily. The stimulation of the adrenal gland by ACTH is so powerful that it will continue to attempt hormone production even when it nears the point of exhaustion.

When chronic stress is present, this is what occurs. The adrenal glands can no longer keep up with the demands of ACTH, and its ability to balance health functions throughout the body gradually declines. This can lead to all sorts of symptoms and medical disorders. We call this whole phenomenon "adrenal exhaustion" in our office.

The "Mother Hormone" Creates the Sex Hormones

When the adrenal glands are stimulated by ACTH, their main priority is to make cortisol. In normal conditions not influenced by stress, the adrenal glands take a molecule called pregnenolone and convert it into various hormones for release. Pregnenolone is the basic building block not only of cortisol, but also of DHEA, progesterone (a female sex hormone) and aldosterone. Pregnenolone is often called the "mother hormone" as it is a precursor to DHEA and progesterone. DHEA can then be converted into the sex hormones estrogen or testosterone. Through feedback loops, these hormones are released depending on the needs of our bodies in order to maintain ideal balance.

For example, under normal, healthy circumstances, cortisol is produced to create energy for survival under stress, to increase immunity to ward off infections, and to maintain balance in our bodies' metabolism. Cortisol also controls glucose metabolism (the breakdown of carbohydrates into fuel) by the many cells throughout the body.

Likewise, appropriate amounts of the sex hormones—estrogen, progesterone and testosterone—are made to balance our reproductive function, including menstrual cycling for women. And, necessary amounts of aldosterone are formed so that sodium, potassium and other electrolytes are normal for cellular operations. Aldosterone also helps you maintain healthy blood pressure. There is ample reserve within healthy adrenals to effortlessly handle these needs of our bodies.

What Happens When a Stressor Comes Along?

But suppose a short-term stress, like an infection, occurs. The infection will trigger an immune reaction. Then, inflammatory molecules and chemicals stimulate the HP axis to release ACTH in a stress response. Once ACTH reaches the adrenal glands, this stimulates increased production and release of cortisol. This hormone will create a short-term boost to the immune system and augment its ability to fight the infection.[103] Because there is a reserve within the healthy adrenal's ability to produce its hormones, there is no problem maintaining the body's balance as long as the stress is short-lived.

What if the Stress Is Chronic?

But suppose there is some form of chronic stress. In this case, let's assume you are gluten-sensitive, but you are eating a gluten-containing diet. The chronic stress on the immune system continues to trigger the release of ACTH from the HP axis as long as the gluten remains in the diet. The adrenals respond to ACTH over and over again the same way, but the chronicity of the stress and adrenal stimulation by ACTH begins to wear out the adrenal's ability to make all of its necessary hormones for the entire body.[104] In other words, something has to give.

Sex Hormone Production Goes by the Boards When Stress Is Chronic

A key point is that within the adrenal glands, when they are overworked by ACTH, the production of cortisol takes priority over all the other hormones that are made. Because all the adrenal hormones use pregnenolone as its basic precursor molecule, the production of cortisol selectively "steals" pregnenolone for its use. Subsequently, levels of

DHEA, aldosterone, testosterone, estrogen and progesterone fall.[105] The production of cortisol may be able to maintain adequate energy production to get the body through its basic daily obligations, but many other areas of the body begin to be affected because other hormone levels are insufficient for healthy balance.

Stress Exhausts the Adrenal Glands

"Pregnenolone steal" is the main mechanism of how chronic stress exhausts the adrenal glands and interferes with hormonal balance. Many of the symptoms that result, such as sleep disturbances, mood swings, weight gain and painful muscles and joints, affect many parts of the body. In this way, symptoms are alerting the body that something is wrong, but as they are remote from the source of the problem, it makes an accurate diagnosis difficult.

If gluten sensitivity is the chronic stress, then the resultant adrenal exhaustion can cause a plethora of complaints that may never be assumed to be a dietary issue. However, once you are familiar with the classic symptoms of adrenal exhaustion, the constellation of symptoms helps point to a chronic stress. Gluten should always be expected in this setting as a possibility.

Symptoms of Adrenal Exhaustion

- Interruptions in sleep
- Difficulty waking in morning
- Fatigue
- Joint and muscle aches
- Weight gain that is resistant to diet or exercise
- Frequent infections
- Lightheadedness/fainting
- Depression/mood swings
- Low blood sugar
- Poor concentration/memory

- Premenstrual syndromes
- Menstrual abnormalities
- Allergies (environmental)
- Asthma

Thyroid Malfunction and Gluten

In addition to the functions of the HP axis and the adrenal glands, the ability of your thyroid gland to function well is likewise important. Your thyroid gland regulates metabolism within the cells of your body. As a result, thyroid hormone influences heart rate, mood, body temperature, basal metabolism, memory, concentration, bowel movement and energy levels. Aberrations in thyroid function can cause these parameters to swing either too high or too low and cause significant complaints.

The Thyroid Gland Also Responds to Stress

As previously described, the HP axis also produces a hormone called TSH, which stands for thyroid stimulating hormone and which does just what its name implies. It stimulates the thyroid gland to make thyroid hormone. The thyroid actually makes two forms of thyroid hormone. One is called T4 and one is called T3. T3 is the active form of the body's thyroid hormone.[106] Similar to the adrenal glands, the thyroid has some reserve ability to handle stress and can increase or decrease thyroid hormone as the needs of the body require.

Unlike the adrenals, the thyroid is not directly affected by ACTH. However, when stress to our bodies occurs, a few changes result within the thyroid gland as well. Let's assume again that we have an infection, a stress that stimulates ACTH release and causes the adrenals to make cortisol. In a normal setting of balance, cortisol creates a brief boost to the immune system to fight the infection. Additionally, adrenaline, released from the adrenals, revs up the system, producing heightened concentration and a quick energy surge.

Thyroid Production Is Reduced While Adrenals Rev Up for Stress

In order for the thyroid hormone not to interfere with the adrenaline stimulation, two things happen. First, hormones released from the HP axis suppress production of TSH (thyroid stimulating hormone) from the pituitary. In turn, this decreases thyroid hormone production. Secondly, cortisol, made by the adrenals, directly suppresses the formation of T3 (active thyroid hormone) and its ability to have its full effect.[107]

If thyroid hormone release were increased instead of suppressed, the body's cells would be stimulated to increase their metabolism. This would compete with the body's energy stores, needed for adrenaline's response. Therefore, it is optimal for thyroid function to reduce, freeing up the body's energy for the stress response. In this way, adrenaline and the immune system optimally function to rid the body of the infection without thyroid function counteracting it.

Chronic Stress Causes Decline in Thyroid Function

But what happens as the stress becomes chronic? The chronic production of hormones by the HP axis and of cortisol by the adrenal glands chronically suppresses the thyroid gland. This results in a persistently low level of thyroid hormone throughout the body. While temporary suppression is fine for a short-term stress, long-term suppression is not. The body needs thyroid hormone to carry out its normal metabolism. If it is low for a long period of time, fatigue, low heart rate, dry skin, constipation and many other symptoms develop.

The adrenaline response to stress is usually short-lived, so it cannot maintain the body's health the same way that thyroid function can. This is where chronic stress results in a decline of healthy function. Adrenal exhaustion leads to decline in thyroid function. Considering that over forty-two million prescriptions for thyroid hormone replacement (levothyroxine) are prescribed every year in the United States, perhaps adrenal exhaustion could be considered a likely root cause of thyroid dysfunction.

Chronic Stress Comes at a Price to Your Health

While there are a variety of short-term stresses that affect us, the thyroid gland, along with other hormonal systems, is well-designed to handle them and allow our body to maintain a balance. But our bodies are not capable of sustaining long periods of stress without a resultant ill effect on our overall health. Priorities are given to immune function often over other areas, and this may affect many different organ systems. The result is a variety of complaints, and, depending on which systems may be most vulnerable, complaints will first develop in these areas. Gluten sensitivity may cause fatigue and sleep problems in one person, but cause headaches and weight gain in another.

The important point is to begin to appreciate the symptoms of adrenal exhaustion. Once these are identified by clinical history and lab testing, searches for chronic stresses (including gluten sensitivity) can be initiated.

Your Ability to Deal With Stress Is Compromised by Gluten

The purpose of the above explanation is not for you to pass your medical entrance exams, but for you to gain some concept of how a dietary reaction to gluten by your body can result in a host of symptoms far away from your digestive tract. A major mechanism in how this is accomplished is the immune system's reaction to gluten and the inflammation that follows. But, in addition, adrenal exhaustion is another significant pathway by which symptoms develop with chronic gluten sensitivity.

Putting It All Together

In summation, as gluten causes persistent immune reactions and inflammation, the body reacts by producing stress hormones. This begins in the brain, which then stimulates the adrenals to make stress hormones (cortisol). This cortisol production initially boosts the immune system for a brief period of time, but as more time passes, the adrenals become fatigued and exhausted. As this occurs, other adrenal hormones that regulate many other areas of the body drop in production.

Also, secondary effects on the thyroid gland cause it to produce lower levels of thyroid hormone. Eventually, symptoms develop related to the inability of our hormonal system to maintain healthy balance. Depending on which part of the body is most sensitive to these hormonal changes, complaints will first surface in that area. This defines adrenal exhaustion.

Gluten Can Be a Chronic Stressor of the Adrenal Glands

By eliminating gluten, the immune reaction can subside, as can the inflammation. Only then can the hormonal system begin to recover. This may well take a while, as the problems have developed over a significant period of time. However, until the stress is removed (in this case, gluten), there is no chance for improvement to occur.

Now that you are educated about the reactions of our hormonal systems to stress, the common symptoms that characterize this condition will be detailed.

Adrenal Exhaustion: The Root Cause of Many Common Symptoms

While the following list is not comprehensive, the majority of symptoms that can be present with adrenal exhaustion are summarized below. These include fatigue and lack of energy, weight changes (often weight gain around the midsection), joint pains, sleep disturbances, mood changes, menstrual symptoms and other sex hormone imbalances, stomach symptoms and memory/concentration problems.

The adrenal glands, when overly compromised, also affect the immune system by weakening it, which can lead to infections. These aspects will be addressed in the following chapter. Likewise, some symptoms have more than one mechanism of cause related to gluten (for instance, poor concentration and memory have adrenal exhaustion causes as well as neurological causes, as previously discussed in Chapter 5).

Fatigue and Loss of Energy

Fatigue can be difficult to define when you are trying to describe it. Generally, fatigue is described as a lack of energy sufficient to go through your normal, daily activities. We all have had this for short periods of time when we have cut our sleep, had too much to accomplish, etc. But chronic fatigue is a persistence of this lack of energy for long periods of time. For many, fatigue is related to sleep quality, but this is not always the case.

Fatigue Is Epidemic

Fatigue has become so prevalent in our society that currently, the CDC (Centers for Disease Control) reports that more than a million people suffer from chronic fatigue syndrome, and that a much higher number have symptoms of fatigue but fail to meet the full diagnostic criteria.[108] Why is this disorder, which has no definitive cause, so prevalent? From the standpoint of gluten and adrenal exhaustion, there are several factors that lead to feelings of fatigue and a lack of energy that may give an answer.

First, when gluten activates the immune system and triggers an inflammatory response, your body is expending energy. Of course, you are not aware of it any more than you would be aware of your body successfully fighting off bacteria in your digestive tract, but it is still ongoing. As the process becomes more chronic, the energy used begins to tap into the body's energy reserves, and fatigue becomes more likely. When you have a cold and a fever, generally, there is a greater desire to sleep. In part, this is due to your body's natural means of redirecting energy needs where they belong. In this case, your body directs energy to your immune system to help fight the infection.

Corinne's Chronic Fatigue

Corinne is a middle-aged woman who presented to our clinic with a prior diagnosis of chronic fatigue and fibromyalgia. Her blood tests showed a high ANA count (evidence of autoimmune disease), but the medication her doctor had put her on aggravated her depression. She also complained of joint pains and asthma.

Here at HealthNOW, we discovered that she had gluten sensitivity. When she removed gluten from her diet, she lost twenty pounds. She was subsequently found to have a parasitic infection and treatment to eradicate the infection also ended her joint pain and inflammation symptoms.

Corinne's cravings for sugar and simple carbohydrates were overwhelming her. When she removed gluten from her diet, the cravings disappeared. She didn't miss foods that contained gluten, and she actually placed them in the category of "rat poison." Her recent follow-up visit showed that her energy was markedly improved, and she had not had any recent bouts of asthma. Likewise, her joint aches had resolved totally. She only wished she had known of her gluten sensitivity sooner because it would have saved her years of discomfort!

This case demonstrates that more than one chronic stress can be present to result in adrenal exhaustion and symptoms. Failing to attend to all stresses will typically result in an incomplete response.

How Many Stressors Can the Adrenals Juggle?

As the stress of an inflammation becomes chronic, the adrenal glands begin to become fatigued. They have increased their production in one area to help the immune system, but other areas of maintenance in the body are being neglected. As an example, a drop in testosterone affects our libido and energy. And, specifically, the elevated cortisol production occurring interferes with our ability to sleep well. Sleep changes will be discussed later in detail, but poor sleep will definitely augment feelings of fatigue.

In chronic fatigue, it is suspected that the eventual drop in cortisol production from an exhausted adrenal gland causes many symptoms. In the final stage of adrenal gland dysfunction, it is unable to respond to ACTH and make adequate amounts of cortisol. This affects every facet of hormonal balance in the body, and the immune system, nervous system and reproductive systems are all affected.

In a research trial in 1999, low-dose steroids were given to a group of chronic fatigue syndrome (CFS) patients, and a significant response was seen in the short-term effect of administration.[109] This suggests that, indeed, the adrenal's inability to keep up with cortisol production has a role in the fatigue.

More Than Fourteen Percent of the Population Has Hypothyroid

Another major mechanism of fatigue lies within the function of the thyroid gland. Between fourteen and seventeen percent of the population has either overt hypothyroidism or borderline low thyroid function, and gluten is one of the known causes.[110] Autoimmune thyroid disease is the most common autoimmune disease in the U.S., affecting four times as many women as men. Information from a recent functional medicine conference supports that approximately twenty percent of menopausal women, twenty-four percent of allergic women and ten percent of postpartum women have thyroid disorders.

Gluten Puts You at Risk for Hypothyroid

In an Italian study examining celiac disease patients, the risk among celiac patients for having thyroid dysfunction was thirty percent, compared to only eleven percent for normal individuals. Additionally, of these patients with celiac disease and thyroid disorders, two-thirds normalized within a year of being on a gluten-free diet.[111] Low thyroid function, by reducing the metabolic rate, can certainly result in a drop of energy and cause fatigue.

As you will recall, adrenal exhaustion suppresses thyroid hormone production at more than one level, so as the demands for cortisol are raised, thyroid hormone levels fall. Gluten sensitivity can affect the thyroid's function not only by direct, autoimmune attack, but also through adrenal exhaustion by causing chronic stress to the body. As our metabolism slows in response to these falling thyroid hormone levels, fatigue becomes an overwhelming complaint.

Depression Can Be a Result of Adrenal Fatigue

Finally, fatigue is commonly associated with the symptom of depression. Depression and other mood symptoms will be discussed shortly, but depression can be a result of adrenal exhaustion. Adrenal exhaustion by failure to produce adequate cortisol can trigger depressive symptoms.[112]

As you can see, fatigue can present commonly with gluten-induced stress and adrenal exhaustion. This occurs at many levels, and even if gluten is removed from the diet, the lasting effects of adrenal exhaustion may take some time from which to recover. Thyroid function, mood disturbances, sleep aberrations and a lack of immune system integrity all contribute to the symptom of fatigue. Attention to all of these systems of our bodies is needed to help speed recovery.

Weight Gain and Obesity

Weight gain, generally, is a more common problem in people who are suffering from adrenal exhaustion. This occurs for a couple of reasons. Do you know of anyone who has been placed on steroids for medical treatment for a long period of time? If you do, you might have noticed that one of the side effects is weight gain. However, most of the time, the weight gain is not all over but instead in selective areas. Steroid-induced weight gain typically occurs in the abdominal area and in the hip and upper thigh areas. Therefore, an individual can be slender everywhere else but have these "problem areas." Does this sound familiar?

Stress, Adrenal Fatigue and Weight Gain

Cortisol is the body's natural steroid, and when it is overproduced in chronic stress, the same distribution of weight gain and obesity occurs. If you take a look at our society, this manner of weight gain is incredibly common. Does this mean that our society, as a whole, is suffering from chronic stress? If you consider all the stresses listed previously, almost all of them are more common today than they were several decades ago. By gluten's triggering of chronic stress, the adrenals continually produce cortisol, which results in weight gain.

When You're Under Stress, Fat Storage Rises

How does cortisol cause this? As cortisol levels rise in the body, certain interactions occur. The largest effect is that the cells, which normally respond to insulin, become less receptive to insulin's influence. This is called insulin resistance. Once cells are resistant to insulin, glucose in the bloodstream is not used by our bodies' cells.

Where does this glucose go? Unfortunately, it is stored by the body as fat, thus the weight gain. Also, because the transformation of glucose into fat takes a little time, the glucose levels in the blood may, over time, elevate, which can lead to diabetes.[113] Again, going back to your friend who takes steroids, elevated sugar levels in the blood is another common side effect of these medicines.

Chronic Stress Sabotages Weight Loss Programs

So far, your body's cells cannot use the glucose you eat when cortisol is high because they cannot respond well to insulin, and the blood sugar levels rise as a result, eventually leading to fat accumulation. This is why, no matter how well you may diet, if you are suffering from chronic stress, you may continue to keep that extra weight. Also, because the cells cannot use the glucose in the bloodstream, they begin to take your body's protein and convert it to glucose (because it is easier for them to make glucose from protein than from the fat that just formed). This means that you may lose your muscle mass as your cells try to meet their needs.[114] The loss of muscle mass only complicates the weight problem, as you need muscle mass to burn calories.

No, I'm Not Pregnant!

J. W. is a classic example of weight complaints typical of adrenal exhaustion. She had developed a big belly that she could not get rid of. She felt bloated all the time, and no matter how often she exercised or how closely she watched her caloric intake, her weight remained the same. She felt constantly four months pregnant.

We diagnosed her with gluten sensitivity, and after being off gluten for several months, she went from a size fourteen to a size six, with a thirty-pound weight loss. She not only lost the weight, but it came off her "problem areas" first—her stomach and her face. She now had a flat belly, which she had never enjoyed before. J.W. also noted that her bloating was gone, and that she felt "clean" inside.

We diagnosed several infections, which were treated successfully as well, which also removed other chronic stressors from her system. In J.W.'s case, the distribution of weight around the mid-region of the body was typical of excessive cortisol production with adrenal exhaustion. Once gluten was removed, the stress on her body subsided, and a normal weight distribution returned.

Adrenal Fatigue = Slower Metabolism

Another means by which adrenal exhaustion manifests as weight gain is through the effects on the thyroid gland. As previously discussed, elevated ACTH and cortisol levels result in suppression of both the production and function of thyroid hormone. As this occurs, our metabolic rate declines, and we burn fewer calories. This is simply the rule of "ins" and "outs." If your diet has the same intake of calories, and your metabolism slows, the extra calories will be stored as fat in your body when they are not used. The end result, again, is weight gain and fat deposition.

While obesity and weight gain are most common, some individuals experience weight loss. This may be a manifestation of poor nutrient absorption secondary to gluten's effect on the digestive tract. Rarely, weight loss can also occur with stress-induced appetite suppression.

Joint Pains—Why Do I Hurt?

The average person weights approximately 155 pounds, and as we maneuver through our day, the musculoskeletal system has to handle a great deal of mechanical stress. This includes the muscles and tendons, but even more so, the actual joints and ligaments of our bodies.

Natural Anti-Inflammatories Lessen With Adrenal Stress

In a normal, healthy body, the wear and tear on the joints is offset by natural cortisol as the adrenal glands naturally respond to minor inflammations of the joints that occur with the production of natural anti-inflammatories. But what happens when the adrenals are overwhelmed?

As you might imagine, the minor inflammation that is produced persists and eventually causes significant swelling and/or pain in the joint areas. The ligaments that keep our joints in good alignment and ready to react to movement become more lax. Imagine that ligaments are like rubber bands, and they lose their elasticity with damage from inflammation. As time advances, joint pains, muscle spasms and limitations of movement can occur. In this fashion, adrenal exhaustion fails to keep up with balancing the health of the musculoskeletal system.

Nine Years of Pain

N.F. presented with nine years of complaints before coming to the clinic for evaluation. Her main complaint had been diffuse body aches with inflammatory pain around her joints, especially in her fingers. Concomitantly, she had progressive fatigue with difficulty waking in the morning, and had weight gain that she attributed to her lack of energy and joint aches.

She had been diagnosed with an autoimmune disorder of some type by another doctor, but there was no specific diagnosis. She was taken off gluten, and despite her almost decade-long chronic complaints, she dramatically improved over the ensuing months. The aches and pains throughout her body resolved, and her dexterity and energy improved, allowing her to resume work full-time. She now gets out of bed without an alarm and has lost twenty-five pounds in the process. While it is difficult to rule out solely a gluten-related immune reaction when accounting for her joint pains, the constellation of weight gain, fatigue and sleep changes support adrenal dysfunction as well.

Is Fibromyalgia Related to Adrenal Fatigue?

As of 2005, there were more than five million people suffering from fibromyalgia,[115] and this disorder is still without a clearly defined etiology or cause in traditional medical arenas. The disorder is named according to its symptom, which is pain in the muscles and ligaments. In relationship to adrenal dysfunction, patients with fibromyalgia have been found to have consistently elevated levels of cortisol and low levels of thyroid hormone.[116] Both of these findings support adrenal exhaustion as a factor in these individuals, and that is definitely in alignment with what we've found clinically over the past two decades among our patients.

Gluten sensitivity can cause arthritis syndromes to occur through the immune system, such as rheumatoid arthritis and others. This mechanism has been well-established and will be described later. But gluten, by causing adrenal exhaustion, can be the root cause of fibromyalgia and other aches and pains of the joints. Identifying gluten as the trigger, and eliminating it from the diet, will begin a process whereby a healthy balance in joint function can resume.

Sleep Disturbances

Stacey's Sleep Trouble and Exhaustion

Stacey T. came into the clinic because she was so tired. Her afternoon fatigue made work difficult, and her early evening fatigue made it tough to be an attentive mom to her young children. Stacey was also frustrated by what she called the "hit or miss" reactions she had with food. Sometimes she ate beef and seemed fine. Other times she wouldn't make it out of a restaurant before she had to run to the bathroom with diarrhea. She also had similar reactions to dairy products. She couldn't drink milk, but some cheeses were tolerated some of the time.

For more than ten years (basically, for as long as she could remember), she would get a "second wind" at night, about 10:00 p.m. When she finally went to bed after midnight, it would take her a minimum of forty-five minutes to fall asleep. Because she had always slept this way, as had her family, she had never considered this a treatable condition. This was just her normal sleep pattern.

If only every patient's body responded as well as Stacey's did, compliance would never be a problem. Literally three days after stopping gluten, her sleep problem disappeared. She fell asleep immediately upon going to bed and her energy secondarily improved. Her lab test showed a positive gluten sensitivity, and her adrenal testing supported adrenal stress. Stacey is now doing very well, and her "hit or miss" reactions to beef have resolved. She doesn't tolerate milk yet, and time will tell if this is a true allergy or a secondary reaction to her gluten sensitivity.

Good Sleep Is Needed for Health on Many Levels

Sleep is a multi-faceted process in which many parts of your body must balance just right in order to operate smoothly. Sleep is also very important in order to allow other systems to regulate themselves and restore function daily. The brain, the heart, the intestinal tract, the immune system and the musculoskeletal system are just a few examples of these.

When sleep is cut short chronically, it causes stress to many parts of your body, including your adrenal system.[117] As the adrenals become more dysfunctional and exhausted, they no longer control the sleep cycle as well. This results in a dwindling spiral of decreasing adrenal function and declining health.

Gluten Sensitivity Affects Sleep

Gluten can affect sleep in other ways besides weakening the adrenal system. Gluten-related antibodies can cause deeper portions of the brain to be inflamed, resulting in sleep disturbances. The brain regulates both our wake and sleep cycles. However, when gluten triggers adrenal exhaustion, the chronic elevation of cortisol at night can keep the body too alert and result in awakenings affecting sleep duration. This typically occurs around 2:00 to 4:00 a.m. and cuts the night short in terms of sleep.

Awake at Night and Tired During the Day

If you are lucky enough to go back to sleep, it is then incredibly hard to awaken on time. This is not only because of sleep deprivation but due to variations in the cortisol levels. They are high at night, causing an interruption of sleep, and low in the morning, causing you to not want to get up—the exact reverse of what they should be.

What happens, then, can be a vicious cycle. Cortisol-induced insomnia causes sleep deprivation that then continues chronic stress, thus elevating cortisol production further. The normal, counter-balancing effect of the sleep hormone melatonin on cortisol does not occur, and sleep becomes more and more difficult.

The More Chronic the Stress, the More Assistance the Adrenals Need

If gluten is the underlying cause of the stress and adrenal dysfunction, removing it will eventually allow cortisol levels to decline and sleep to resume uninterrupted. Typically, if the stress has been long-term, the body is not able to reset itself without the assistance of nutritional, dietary and lifestyle changes. This type of program usually takes about ninety days and is one of the mainstays of the HealthNOW Method.

While gluten is often a major culprit in adrenal fatigue, it is not the only one. We will discuss typical treatment protocols later, but suffice it to say that restoring the delicate balance among these hormones is vital to restoring health.

Interrupted Sleep and Exhaustion

S.W. had chronic complaints of fatigue as well as sleep difficulties. Sleep was constantly interrupted, especially in the latter half of the night. However, despite accumulating ten hours of interrupted sleep on many nights, she still found it very difficult to get out of bed in the morning. No matter how many hours she slept, her fatigue was unchanged.

She was identified as being gluten-sensitive, and gluten was eliminated from her diet. Amazingly, her fatigue completely resolved and her sleeping patterns normalized to an uninterrupted eight to nine hours. Best of all, getting out of bed in the morning became effortless, as she was so well-rested.

When she now accidentally eats gluten, her fatigue returns. In her case, gluten may have been causing fatigue through some direct sedating effects of gluteomorphins (partially digested proteins from the incomplete digestion of gluten, which have opiate-like effects in the body). However, the sleep interruptions she described point to high cortisol production during the night, resulting from adrenal stress. Once gluten was removed, her symptoms dissipated, indicating a direct cause and effect.

Mood Disturbances: Depression, Irritability and Anxiety

Gluten intolerance indeed can result in depression and anxiety as well as other mood disturbances. Some studies indicate that inflammation from gluten-induced immune reactions may be a cause.[118] But, in addition, the effects gluten imposes through the hormonal system can result in symptoms of depression and anxiety. By far, depression symptoms tend to be more common with adrenal exhaustion. This likely has to do with direct effects that create an imbalance of hormones.

With short-term stresses, as you will recall, adrenaline rises. Adrenaline is part of our bodies' stress response systems. It raises our heart rates, elevates our blood pressure and prepares our bodies for whatever is about to happen or is happening. The balance between adrenaline and another chemical, serotonin, often balance our moods.

Chronic Stress Affects Mood

If chronic stress occurs, this balance between adrenaline and serotonin can be affected, resulting in depression and other mood disorders. As the adrenals become fatigued, cortisol is made at the expense of other hormones, including adrenaline.[119] Adrenaline's depletion causes an imbalance with serotonin, which can lead to changes such as depression, anxiety and rapid mood swings.

Many other features associated with gluten sensitivity can trigger depression as well. Chronic discomfort due to digestive upset, malnutrition, poor sleep and altered lifestyle are just a few related features. However, it is apparent that adrenal effects play a strong role in depressive complaints.

There is tremendous interplay between the hormonal system, the brain and the immune system that is significantly challenged under chronic stress. Depression can result from malfunctions in any of these systems, and, when present, can often cause a further decline in function.[120] While depression is a common symptom of many disorders, gluten and adrenal exhaustion warrant consideration as root causes.

Fertility Problems and Menstrual Cycle Symptoms

Gluten sensitivity appears to exert most of its menstrual effects through the hormonal system, though its effects on folic acid absorption may likewise be pertinent. Folic acid is an important nutrient for the development of a fetus, and its deficiency can cause miscarriages and birth defects. Its malabsorption does not alone explain the dramatic increase in infertility among women with gluten sensitivity, or the other menstrual symptoms that can be quite common, but it is likely a component.

Gluten Sensitivity Affects Fertility

A recent study of women with celiac disease demonstrated that those on gluten-containing diets had shorter fertile periods, greater spontaneous abortions and greater overall infertility compared to those on gluten-free diets.[121] Some gluten-related immune mechanisms were likely at play, in addition to folic acid deficiency, in accounting for this spectrum of reproductive problems.

PMS and Menopause

More commonly, premenstrual syndrome and menopausal symptoms are issues that bother many women with gluten disorders. To simplify this as best as possible, let's reconsider the adrenal gland and its production of reproductive hormones. As you will recall, pregnenolone is the basic molecule that serves as the building block of all the hormones made by the adrenals. Under normal conditions, ample pregnenolone exists for conversion to cortisol and DHEA, but when stressed, pregnenolone is diverted preferentially to cortisol.

Something's Gotta Give

When your body is under stress, it's as if it has to make a decision: It can get you through the day, putting one foot in front of the other, or it can make adequate amounts of sex hormones. It can't do both. It's too stressed. When in this situation, your body decides that the most pro-survival thing to do is to get you through the day, to the detriment of making sex hormones.

Even though DHEA is reduced under adrenal exhaustion circumstances, it still produces estrogen to a degree. However, progesterone (which balances estrogen in its effects in the body) falls significantly. This results in estrogen dominance because there is no longer a balance between estrogen and progesterone.[122] It is estrogen dominance that causes symptoms of cramping, heavy bleeding, menstrual irregularity, endometriosis, polycystic ovaries, fibrocystic breasts, migraines and PMS. Because the adrenals are fatigued, they cannot maintain the balance needed between estrogen and progesterone in the cycle each month.

Tired Adrenals Can Make Menopause a Nightmare

Additionally, the adrenals are supposed to take over as the gradual decline in ovarian function occurs during peri-menopause and menopause. Adrenal fatigue can result in severe menopausal symptoms due to the inability of the fatigued adrenals to take over hormonal production for the ovaries. Symptoms of hot flashes, night sweats, irritability, decreased libido and weight gain are not experienced when a peri-menopausal woman has normally functioning adrenal glands.

While gluten intolerance causes menstrual complaints and infertility through hormonal mechanisms as described, other dietary factors also may be important in supplying excess exogenous (coming from our diet or environment) estrogens that further create or exacerbate estrogen dominance. Beef and milk, unless organic, may contain estrogen compounds that were fed to cattle to fatten them. Additionally, synthetic hormones in birth control pills, hormone replacement therapy, pesticides, herbicides and fungicides are all sources of dangerous synthetic estrogens. This stresses the importance of diet and lifestyle, once again, in achieving optimal health.

My Stomach Hurts

What? Gluten causing stomach complaints? Yes, we realize that we covered this in detail previously, but it is noteworthy to realize that hormonal imbalances cause gastric problems as well. While most of the hormonal conversation has been about the HP axis and the adrenal glands, many other areas of our bodies produce hormonal substances. The pancreas produces the hormone insulin, but the intestinal tract produces many hormonal molecules that influence digestion as well as the immune system.

Hormones of the GI Tract

Hormones that exist in the intestines include gastrin, secretin and cholecystokinin. Don't worry about their names, but it is important realize that hormones do help the intestines function. Each of these affects digestion as various food types enter the stomach.

But, in addition, another hormone produced in the digestive tract, called ghrelin, is directly influenced by cortisol levels. Ghrelin stimulates appetite and appears to be related to growth hormone release.[123] If cortisol levels increase, ghrelin levels decrease, which suppresses appetite and possibly growth hormone. With chronic stress and cortisol release, this can affect one's ability to grow normally. This is, of course, particularly important in children.

On occasion, the removal of gluten from the diet may not result in quick results, even when it comes to intestinal symptoms. Most individuals respond within several weeks to removal of gluten from the diet, but if adrenal exhaustion and chronic stress have resulted in additional insults to the system, it may take longer for the body to recover and for symptoms to abate.

Poor Memory and Loss of Concentration

Impairment of memory and concentration has many mechanisms of development in gluten-sensitive individuals. When gluten results in chronic physical stress to the body and subsequent adrenal exhaustion, memory and concentration difficulties can result. In a study on memory, nerve cells were shown to be damaged as a result of chronic stress and the elevation of cortisol.[124]

Adrenal Fatigue Affects Memory

Fluctuations in estrogen can also cause memory loss, which is affected negatively in adrenal stress. Many peri-menopausal and menopausal women will attest to this fact. And, of course, lower thyroid hormone levels from adrenal dysfunction cause focus and concentration to decline. In a simplified summary, the stress to our adrenals and hormonal system results in fluctuations and imbalances that cause failure of our bodies' regulatory processes, and abilities to concentrate and remember can show decline.

Adrenal Fatigue and Gluten Sensitivity: Not a Pretty Combination

Would you ever have imagined that so many symptoms could result from a decline in your body's hormonal regulation? And would you have thought that a simple protein found in wheat, rye and barley would have the potential to create such distress? It really is no different than the ability a tiny virus or bacteria has to reek havoc on the body, but we often don't think of our diets as being that powerful. Certainly, we understand that high-fat foods and a lack of vitamins have effects on our health, but we don't anticipate chronic fatigue syndrome, fibromyalgia, a weakened immune system or hormonal imbalance to come from indirect effects of gluten.

While the immune system and nutritional issues factor in, to a large degree, in gluten's effects throughout the entire body, the chronic stress imposed by gluten sensitivity hinders our bodies' abilities to regulate hormonal balance. The nervous system, the immune system and the hormonal systems are the most important control systems for our optimal health. And when one is impaired for long periods of time, dysfunctions in all three systems eventually result. Because of the interplay among all three, the delicate balance of good health becomes compromised.

Adrenal Fatigue Is Very Treatable

Fortunately, as with gluten, adrenal exhaustion can be identified and treated by attending to the underlying root cause and supplying the body with nutrition and individualized measures that allow healing. The first step is to be aware of common symptoms related to gluten intolerance and symptoms that also may be caused by adrenal dysfunction. In this manner, appropriate examinations and interventions can verify the suspicions. The symptoms lead you in the right direction if you simply listen rather than try to suppress them or mask them temporarily with drugs.

Evaluation of adrenal gland function is an integral part of the HealthNOW Method because the adrenals are a gauge of the body's ability to cope with stress. If the adrenals are exhausted, we know that there has to be an underlying cause. Searching for that cause is what led us to the discovery that gluten was a very common contributor to adrenal exhaustion.

Seven

Autoimmune Diseases and a Weak Immune System

You probably don't go to your doctor and say, "Hey, doc, my immune system is killing me today!" You might know what your immune system does, but identifying the complaints you are having as related to an immune dysfunction is difficult.

Your Immune System Does More Than Protect You From Infection

Our immune systems are there to protect us from disease and illness. This includes protection from infections due to various bacteria and other organisms, but also includes protection from cancers and malignancies. Because of this, when your immune system is not functioning well, many different parts of your body can be affected.

To review a bit, understand that there are certain people who have a genetic risk for having gluten sensitivity. They have certain HLA genes that, when exposed to gluten, cause production of antibodies from the immune system, which then attacks gluten as well as their body's own tissues. The component wherein the body's own tissue is attacked is referred to as autoimmune disease.

Autoimmune Disease—Your Body Attacking Itself

There are many different types of autoimmune disease, and gluten can trigger many of them.[125] In this chapter, we will cover the symptoms of many of these disorders. Gluten sensitivity is a complex inflammatory disorder that, in essence, has many components. While there is an immune susceptibility in some people for having gluten sensitivity,[126] in others, it occurs for other reasons. For instance, irritation of the bowel's lining from viruses, bacteria, toxins and stress can cause a leaky lining. Because the lining is too permeable, gluten and other proteins cross through without proper digestion. In many people, this is a mechanism by which gluten also triggers an immune and inflammatory response.

In earlier chapters, we described how the immune system develops during embryonic and childhood development. In a normal, healthy immune system, tissues of the body and "good" bacteria, as well as dietary foods, are all labeled as "safe" by the body and do not trigger immune reactions. However, when these mechanisms go awry, autoimmune disorders and food reactions can develop. In the case of gluten intolerance, one of two major possibilities can happen.

The Happy Story of a Lupus Patient

T.T. is a lovely young woman from the Philippines who worked with us for over a year. She had a constellation of symptoms that included complaints of bloating, constipation, fatigue, wheezing, anemia, weakness and light-headedness. She had been suffering from this myriad of complaints most of her life.

Examination and lab tests revealed a gluten sensitivity and a number of infections. T.T. was very sensitive to gluten, as well as diary products and other grains, but when she stuck to her diet, she felt well. She was feeling very well physically, and as life went onwards, she came off her gluten-free diet. She ate minimal gluten, but she did eat it. She also started eating more dairy products, sugary desserts and caffeine.

Unfortunately, the next time we saw her was two years later, and she was in bad shape. She had been diagnosed with lupus and had been on several immunosuppressive drugs including prednisone and Plaquenil. Both drugs had severe side effects, and she was very depressed at the prospect of having to be on them forever.

It was upsetting to see how much her health had deteriorated in such a short period of time. The sad part of the story is the question that can never be answered: Would she have developed lupus if she had stuck with the initial program? We will never know.

But now to the good news. Despite being diagnosed with a supposedly incurable autoimmune disease, seven years after her diagnosis, T.T. is completely off all medications. Her lab tests show her to be stable, and her rheumatologist is pleased (and surprised) by how well she is doing. He's happy to have her continue her current program and just monitor her periodically. Needless to say, she NEVER consumes gluten. She just turned forty and is planning, for the next four decades, to be much healthier.

Gluten Creates a "Leaky Gut"

When gluten sensitivity is present, immune reactions occur at the level of the intestinal lining. Antibodies are made against gliadin (which, as you'll remember, is the major protein in gluten), which result in inflammation and damage to the lining cells. The lining becomes leaky and additional gluten crosses the lining, as do other possible viruses, bacteria, partially digested foods and other proteins.

In addition, substances like alcohol, heavy exercise, and viruses can also directly cause inflammation of the intestinal wall and result in a leaky bowel lining even before an immune reaction occurs. But once the bowel is leaky, the poorly digested proteins, foods, etc. then trigger immune reactions. Either way, eventually, an immune reaction is triggered against gliadin (gluten), the enzymes that metabolize gluten (the transaminases), or other molecules sneaking across.

Proteins of Your Body Are Similar to Gluten... Unfortunately

These antibodies not only attack the intestinal lining and gluten, but they also travel to other tissues of the body, where they cause inflammation as well. This is very significant. The immune system creates large amounts of antibodies to attack the gluten protein. However, because there are other proteins in the body that are similar in molecular structure to gluten, these same antibodies end up attacking healthy tissues. The term that is used to describe this phenomenon is "cross-reactivity" or "cross-reaction."

This cross-reaction in other organs outside of the digestive tract can cause a vast array of autoimmune disorders that result in complaints such as clumsiness, headaches, joint pains, skin rashes and many others.[127] This is a major mechanism of how gluten causes autoimmune disorders.

Healthy Adrenals Prevent Self-Cannibalism

Secondly, as discussed in the last chapter on adrenal exhaustion, autoimmune disorders can occur when chronic stress results in poor immune system control. Cortisol, our stress hormone, is initially produced by our adrenals to keep our normal immune reactions from overreacting. However, when the adrenals fail from the chronic stimulation of stress, this regulation declines. In some cases, this results in autoimmune disorders as the immune system goes unchecked. In other words, cortisol (produced by the adrenals) prevents our immune systems from self-cannibalizing our own bodies' tissues. That is the function of the adrenal glands' role in controlling the degree of the immune system's reaction.

Fatigued Adrenals Lead to Autoimmune Diseases

If the adrenal glands are exhausted, then cortisol is insufficient and autoimmune disorders develop. In other words, self-cannibalizing of the body's systems occurs unchecked. In gluten sensitivity, there are a number of different autoimmune disorders that occur. Additionally, the longer you have gluten sensitivity untreated, the higher your risk for developing these disorders.[128]

Families With Gluten Sensitivity See a Five-Time Greater Risk of Autoimmune Disease

Regardless of whether autoimmune disorders develop through direct immune triggers by gluten or indirectly through stress on the adrenal glands, it is evident that these disorders require both the genetic risk and the gluten trigger. Even in close family members of gluten-sensitive patients who have no intestinal symptoms, the rate of having autoimmune disorders is more than five times greater than in normal subjects.[129] It is likely that these relatives have silent gluten sensitivity (no symptoms, but are still likely to be gluten-intolerant). It is therefore difficult to know how large a role gluten plays in these individuals in terms of triggering autoimmune disorders.

Gluten Sensitivity and Adrenal Fatigue: A Risky Combination for Autoimmune Disease

The HLA genes typical of gluten sensitivity risk predispose individuals to autoimmune dysfunction, but at the same time, we also know that gluten triggers autoimmune conditions directly. Either way, gluten should be avoided so that the risk of developing autoimmune disease can be minimized.

To make this point with a case study, one research report describes a twelve-year-old girl who was diagnosed with celiac disease and who had developed leukemia. As a result of her leukemia diagnosis, she underwent a bone marrow transplant. (If you recall, the bone marrow is one of the major sites where the immune cells are made.) After her transplant, her celiac disease seemed to completely resolve.[130] Assumedly, by removing the immune cells with the HLA genes typical of gluten sensitivity, her gluten intolerance was eliminated.

Don't think that this report implies that you should go out and have your bone marrow transplanted. This is not a fun procedure, and it has very high risks. But the example does support the immune system's role in gluten-related disorders.

Here's the Good News!

There is good news even if you have the "gluten" genes, however. In studies examining autoimmune disease in gluten-sensitive disorders, a gluten-free diet is effective in decreasing the risk.[131] Also, the duration of gluten sensitivity, even if silent in terms of symptoms, matters. If the diagnosis is made and treatment is begun earlier in life, there is a lower occurrence of autoimmune disease.[132] This stresses the importance of seeking a diagnosis of gluten sensitivity for yourself or your children even before symptoms develop, if you have family members with the disorder.

Symptoms Suggesting Immune Disorders

Because autoimmune disorders can affect so many different organ systems, symptoms are quite varied, as you might imagine. The common autoimmune disorders associated with gluten sensitivity include diabetes, asthma, thyroid disease, skin disorders and conditions affecting joints and muscles.[133] There are a few others, but they are less frequent.

Symptoms Deserve Your Attention

Common symptoms that can occur with these conditions will be summarized, but detailed descriptions of the actual diseases will be covered later in this book. Because symptom-based assessment is extremely important in detecting early bodily dysfunction, this remains our primary focus. Symptoms deserve our attention even when diagnostic testing fails to show a problem because they impact our quality of living,[134] and help us treat disease earlier, before complications or irreversibility develop. In doing so, health can be preserved and serious illness can be averted.

In addition to the various inflammatory conditions caused by the immune system in gluten disorders, immune dysfunction can also result in some malignancies. Of the various cancers, lymphoma is the most common,[135] and it will be discussed later as well. Fortunately, compared to other autoimmune problems, lymphoma and other malignancies are fairly rare.

Eighty Percent of Patients With Lymphoma Are Gluten-Sensitive

It is noteworthy to mention that research reports that more than eighty percent of patients with lymphoma have positive gluten antibody testing but no evidence of injury to the intestinal lining.[136] Lymphoma, therefore, seems to fall into the category of silent gluten intolerance. No digestive disturbances are present, but the damage to the immune system is occurring to the point that, eventually, cancer occurs. Therefore, pay attention to your symptoms and keep the possibilities open in terms of cause. Gluten may be the cause even when no digestive problems are evident.

Two-Thirds of the Time, Gluten-Sensitive Patients Have No Digestive Complaints

Remember, digestive complaints associated with gluten intolerance occur only one-third of the time. Two-thirds of all patients with gluten intolerance have no digestive symptoms. Gluten is causing damage elsewhere in their bodies, and it can be many years before the nature of that damage is appreciated, as evidenced in the case of lymphoma.

Susan's Nine-Year Nightmare

Susan S. had been seeing dermatologists for nine years for a persistent skin condition. She had been diagnosed with papullar eczema and was taking an oral allergy tablet daily, along with frequent applications of a topical cream for her rash and itch. Essentially, her entire body was covered with angry red, bumps, except for her face. Despite being very attractive woman, she was forced to remain covered continuously to hide her rash.

The cycle of symptoms usually began with irritation of and itching on an area of skin, followed by a red bump that formed and then erupted. Because of the uncontrollable itching, she would succumb to scratching, which then caused the bump to open, bleed and ooze. It would then scab over and heal, leaving an area between four and six millimeters in diameter with a raised, red lump. Then, the cycle would start again in another area.

The constant, unrelenting itchiness disturbed her sleep and caused her to suffer from anxiety. Susan could only sleep for a couple of hours before the itch awakened her. She would read for a while and then sleep for a couple more hours. Her sleep pattern had been this way for four years.

Despite the fact that Susan had seen many dermatologists, we felt strongly about our diagnosis of dermatitis herpetiformis, a skin condition frequently associated with gluten sensitivity. Her diet contained an abundance of gluten-containing foods in every meal and snack, and her lab tests showed borderline-positive gluten-related antibodies. Susan had tried changing her diet previously and had eliminated chocolate, caffeine, nuts, dairy and soy. It had made no difference. Susan also had absolutely no digestive complaints. This made our suggestion of gluten sensitivity none too popular when we initially suggested it. But after a couple of heartfelt consultations, she decided to give it a try.

Once she began a gluten-free diet, she started to feel better overall. Her skin didn't change initially, but she definitely detected a positive overall change in her health, which included improved sleep and less anxiety. Within five weeks, her breakouts became much less frequent, and over the course of the next few months, her red bumps began to fade. Her inflammation reduced and she was much less itchy.

She slept through the night with no interruptions. Her anxiety also improved markedly since changing her diet and embarking on a nutritional program to improve her adrenal and hormonal balance. As support to the theory that healing a leaky gut will improve food allergies, she recently ate some nuts, to which she had previously been highly allergic, with no symptoms or consequence.

Susan has to be very careful with her diet and has recently discovered that she does best on a grain-free diet. She wanted us to include, for all you vegetable haters, that she can't believe how much she enjoys a big bowl of dark green, leafy vegetables. She relates that while she was told to eat them initially, now she loves eating them and feels great for having done so. It still amazes her because she was initially rather vegetable-phobic!

Interestingly, she has a sister who is very ill with several medical problems. Susan is trying to have her sister evaluated for gluten sensitivity based on her own rapid improvement on a gluten-free diet.

Rashes and Itchy Skin

One of the more common autoimmune disorders associated with gluten sensitivity is dermatitis herpetiformis (DH). This disorder is selectively associated with gluten sensitivity and can be the major presenting symptom. It consists of small blisters that often develop over the buttocks, lower back, knees, elbows and back of the head. Usually, itching and burning of the skin is significant.[137]

The Proper Diagnosis Is Often Missed

What typically occurs is that a specific type of antibody made by the immune system reacts against gluten and is deposited in the skin's layers.[138] This can be seen on biopsy, and this confirms the diagnosis. Most of the time, when the rash is classic, the diagnosis is easily made. But, all too often, it's still missed. If the patient is not aware of gluten sensitivity, this diagnosis should always prompt immediate steps to test for gluten intolerance and to place them on a gluten-free diet.

But what if you don't have classic symptoms? Some patients have intense itching or rashes, and skin biopsies fail to confirm a cause. Sometimes, in a patchy presentation of DH, a skin biopsy may miss the tell-tale signs. This is where the persistent symptoms still indicate a problem even though the tests are negative.

Interestingly, in a study comparing DH to celiac disease ten years ago, it was noted that both conditions shared similar patterns of attracting other autoimmune disorders. In this study, patients had either DH or celiac disease.[139] While many people have gluten sensitivity and do not have DH, those with DH almost always have gluten intolerance.

His Skin Felt Like It Had Kerosene Burning Beneath It

R.H. was a pleasant gentleman who had been suffering for more than seven years from an incredible itchiness and burning of his skin. He described what he suffered as similar to having kerosene burning beneath his skin. His sleep was interrupted, and he had become mildly depressed as a result.

In addition, he had extreme intolerance to allergens in the environment. He could not stand to be around freshly cut grass, and even dust at a neighbor's home irritated his allergies terribly. His spouse had to keep his home immaculately clean and his ability to go anywhere outside his home was severely restricted due to the intense reactions he would suffer from.

He had seen two allergists who could not define a condition, and skin scratch testing was negative even for the grass that he knew bothered him. The last allergy specialist he saw suggested antidepressants because he felt that that R.H. didn't really have anything wrong with him, and that it was "all in his head."

After coming into our office, he was found to have both positive saliva and blood testing for gluten sensitivity. We also found that he had an intestinal infection. After several weeks of being gluten-free and eradicating his infection, his itching had resolved, he was sleeping better, and his quality of life was dramatically better. Additionally, he no longer had to guard against dust and grass exposure, making his wife extremely happy as she no longer has to keep their home like a "clean room." If he accidentally ate some gluten, his skin would start to burn. Otherwise, the symptom had completely resolved. As he described it, his freedom to live had been restored.

Psoriasis, Eczema and Vitiligo Related to Gluten Sensitivity

Other rashes and itchy conditions can be caused by gluten-related disorders. Rashes vary according to the condition, but psoriasis, vitilgo, eczema and other skin diseases are reported as being due to autoimmunity and being associated with gluten intolerance.[140] The main point is that skin rashes are not uncommonly affiliated with gluten sensitivity. If you suffer from a chronic rash or itching, it would be worthwhile to investigate gluten or other dietary factors as a root cause.

While creams and inflammation-suppressing treatments may help your symptoms, they are not focusing on the underlying trigger. Finding that trigger can be very rewarding, not to mention help you in avoiding future health problems down the road.

Joint Pains and Swelling

As mentioned in earlier sections, gluten can indeed trigger joint pains and muscle aches through a few different mechanisms. However, there are several autoimmune conditions that primarily involve the musculoskeletal system and cause joint pains and joint swelling. Some of the more common ones include Sjogren's syndrome, lupus and rheumatoid arthritis.[141] Each of these has varied degrees of joint pain and swelling associated with their disease features in addition to other characteristic symptoms.

Autoimmune Diseases Affecting Joints Are Common With Gluten Sensitivity

Large studies have, amazingly, demonstrated that more than ten percent of celiac disease patients have autoimmune disorders affecting their musculoskeletal systems.[142] This is an incredibly high figure that warrants that all patients with immune arthritic conditions be tested for gluten sensitivity. Another study of 335 celiac patients reported a similar figure of 10.5 percent having immune-related arthritis conditions like rheumatoid arthritis, lupus and others.[143] While arthritis can develop as a result of adrenal fatigue and a poorly controlled immune system, direct autoimmune attack from gluten-related antibodies can also be a common cause of these conditions. This makes symptoms of joint pain and swelling highly significant in considering gluten as a root cause.

Which joints are affected is also important. Symmetric involvement of the hands, wrists and knees may suggest rheumatoid arthritis. If all your joints are affected, and there is a waxing and waning, it might suggest lupus. Likewise, other non-joint symptoms that are present help you and your clinician categorize this further.

Medications That Only Treat Symptoms Are Not Enough

Often, however, blood tests are inconclusive, and you are left waiting for a diagnosis while treatments or medications are given to appease your complaints. Because the frequency of gluten-related joint conditions are so high, gluten sensitivity should be considered as part of the investigation routinely.

An Eight-Year Battle With Arthritis Is Won

N.F. presented with an eight-year history of joint aches all over, but with prominence in her fingers. In addition, she had a feeling of diffuse swelling, and she had difficulty moving and completing her usual workday activities. Her doctor had found a positive autoimmune marker in the blood, but it was insufficient to make a diagnosis of a particular condition. Other symptoms included poor sleep and fatigue.

With the elimination of gluten from her diet, she had a significant improvement. Her aches were markedly improved, and she had no problem getting through her workday without discomfort or fatigue. She also sprang out of bed without an alarm every morning and felt great. Gluten intolerance appeared to have been the primary etiology of her arthritic symptoms. The abnormal immune blood test was most likely a reflection of how gluten was causing joint-related complaints through inflammation.

It's Difficult to Maintain Health When You Can't Move Easily

Stiffness can also accompany these conditions, as can limitations of movement. These can certainly result in a decline in the overall quality of life and limit your ability to complete the tasks of your day, not to mention make you feel like you're getting old. Often, the reduced activity level can lead to weight gain, which places further strain on your joints, ligaments and muscles. This can perpetuate a vicious cycle that is never-ending until a root cause is found.

Osteoporosis Has Immune and Gluten Components

Pain can also occur with other bone conditions like osteoporosis. When silent bone fractures occur as a result of weakened bones, pain can be significant. Causes of osteoporosis have been discussed briefly in relationship to malabsorption of vitamin D and calcium, but recent findings support autoimmune causes as well.[144] If you recall, one of the antibodies formed in gluten sensitivity is directed against a gliadin-related enzyme called tissue transaminases (tTG), which helps metabolize gliadin as it crosses the intestinal lining. Together, gliadin and tTG form a protein complex. The immune system actually targets the tTG molecule in its autoimmune attack, and, therefore, the antibodies can be directed at not only gliadin but also the transaminase.

More Than Fifty Percent of Gluten-Sensitive Patients Had Antibodies Against Their Own Bone

It so happens that there are also transaminases in the bone matrix that are responsible for making your bones strong and mature through proper bone formation. In more than fifty percent of the gluten-sensitive patients tested, antibodies directed at bone transaminases were found. The higher the antibody levels against bone transaminases in these patients, the worse their osteoporosis.

A Gluten-Free Diet Showed a Positive Response

Also of note was that a gluten-free diet showed a positive response for these individuals. The study postulated that gluten antibodies formed in the intestine, directed against tTG transaminases, cross-reacted with the transaminases in the bone, causing weakening.[145] These findings are quite significant in linking the cause of osteoporosis to gluten intolerance in a large number of people. Likewise, these results are certainly consistent with what we see in our practice.

Look for Gluten Sensitivity if Osteoporosis Is in Your Family

Because of this high percentage, and because osteoporosis is common in gluten sensitivity, bone density scans are recommended for all people who are intolerant to gluten. Likewise, the reverse is true. If you have osteoporosis or osteopenia, gluten sensitivity should be screened. If you have developed symptoms of bone pain, stooped posturing or unexplained fractures, these should alert you to gluten as a possible cause. Osteoporosis is an incredibly debilitating disease prevalent worldwide, and it leads to tremendous problems including pain, physical limitations, spinal problems of mobility, and a general decline in the quality of life.

Osteoporosis Medications Can Make Bone Less Healthy

To complicate matters further, the major medications prescribed for osteoporosis, such as Fosamax (Merck & Co.) and Boniva (Roche), can actually cause gastrointestinal side effects and make bones more brittle over time. These medications make bones more dense by preventing breakdown of old bone matrix, but, at the same time, inhibit new bone growth. For healthy bones, we need a balance between new bone formation and old bone remodeling, and, therefore, these drugs actually lead to bone difficulties.[146] This can then cause bone discomfort, joint pains and stiffness. These symptoms may then prompt treatment with anti-inflammatories, which can hinder the health of the intestinal lining further.

Let's Follow the Trail

You can see the chain of events from this. The root of the problem is gluten sensitivity. This causes irritation of the intestinal lining and results in changes in the immune system and nutrition that affect bone formation and healthy bones. Osteoporosis develops, and you get treated with one of these medications. Bones become more brittle, resulting in bone pain and stiffness, so you are prescribed an anti-inflammatory. This further causes intestinal irritation, making the gluten effects even worse. And the cycle continues.

Poor Absorption of Nutrients Plus Autoimmune Damage: A Nasty Combination

Certainly, poor absorption of calcium and vitamin D in gluten sensitivity is a cause for osteoporosis as well, but data indicates that this only compounds what is caused by autoimmune damage to the bone. This results in a "double whammy," so to speak. Increasing calcium supplements and vitamin D in your diet may help to a degree, but does not get to the root cause. As a result, its effect will only be partial and certainly not curative. If gluten sensitivity is found to be the underlying problem, a gluten-free diet can make dramatic improvements in your complaints and also slow or stop further bone loss and deterioration.

An Elderly Woman Improves Her Bone Density

Dorothy M. was an elderly woman diagnosed with osteoporosis many years ago. Her bone loss was significant but shortly after being diagnosed with osteoporosis, we also found her to be gluten-sensitive, through lab testing. Dorothy stopped gluten immediately and noticed many positive changes in her health. The most dramatic change was an improvement in her bone density upon her next bone scan! Her doctor was so surprised that he rechecked the dates of the exams. An increase in bone density was not something he was used to seeing in such an elderly patient.

Allergies and Wheezing

You may not appreciate the impact your diet can have on your health, but as you read about the potential impact of gluten on your health, you hopefully are beginning to appreciate how far-reaching the effects can be. Respiratory symptoms are another example of the remote effects of gluten sensitivity outside the digestive tract. While these symptoms are less common than other gluten-related symptoms, they are, indeed, quite common among our population. Wheezing and sinus allergies affect a huge number of people, and can be from mild to severe. All you have to do is peruse the aisles of your local pharmacy and examine all the over-the-counter allergy medications available to purchase to appreciate this.

Can Gluten Affect Allergies and Wheezing?

By nature, allergies and wheezing are both inflammatory disorders. Something in the environment triggers your nose to run or become congested. This can be an infectious particle, a non-infectious allergen or even something in your diet. Likewise, wheezing can result from the same triggers. Something stimulates your immune system to inflame your airways, making it difficult to breathe. But these typical triggers are usually only molds, viruses and dust mites, right? What does this have to do with gluten?

Life-Long Allergies, Asthma and Eczema Go by the Boards

N.D. had been suffering with respiratory allergies as well as mild asthma since she was an infant. She had been on medications for both conditions for many years. Her symptoms were suppressed partially by the medication, but she had to take it regularly. Additional symptoms included an eczema rash, which flared intermittently and was worse on her elbows.

In the process of eliminating potential foods from her diet, it was found that she was gluten-sensitive. Although it took some time for her to commit to the diet, eventually, she was able to be medication-free without any recurrence of allergies or asthma. As an added benefit, her eczema was much improved.

Studies in Children Show a Dietary Link to Allergies

There are several large population studies that looked at the appearance of allergies and wheezing in relationship to diet. One involved 2,290 fifth graders, and it found that sweetened beverages and eggs increased their allergy symptoms, while soy and fruit reduced their occurrence.[147] Another demonstrated, in 690 children, that fruits, vegetables and nuts provided a beneficial effect on both asthma and allergies.[148] Lastly, a third examined over 5,000 children and found similar effects for vegetables and fruits, but also found that bread and margarine increased the occurrence of wheezing.[149]

This last study, most revealingly, supported gluten as a trigger for asthma and sinus allergy symptoms. Gluten comprises the majority of the protein content in wheat, barley and rye, and, therefore, it is likely the main trigger in bread that would stimulate respiratory symptoms.

Food Affects Your Respiratory System

The other significant finding in these three studies is the impact diet can have on our respiratory symptoms. Interestingly, fruits and vegetables have many natural antioxidants and nutrients (called phytonutrients) that our bodies need. These may have protective effects compared to other foods.

But, in addition, fruits and vegetables also provide our bodies with natural exposure to many molds, bacteria and other organisms. Some theories suggest that our immune systems need exposure to different foods and organisms to help them develop oral tolerance and effective defense mechanisms that aren't overactive.[150] Changes in our dietary habits, which have reduced the variety of foods we consume, as well as our frequent use of sanitizers can hinder oral tolerance mechanisms and make autoimmune disorders more common.

Adrenal Fatigue Ties In to Allergies

In addition, adrenal exhaustion plays a role in many gluten-sensitive patients. As you may recall from the preceding chapter, the adrenal glands produce cortisol, which is our stress hormone. Cortisol keeps the immune system in check, and a major way it accomplishes this is by cooling down the inflammation caused by the immune system.

The histamine and other inflammatory chemicals released by our immune systems during minor allergy exposure are usually balanced by cortisol. But when the adrenals are no longer able to produce enough cortisol, this balance shifts in favor of inflammation. As a result, minor allergens in our diets and environments become major hassles.

The key point is that, indeed, diet affects our respiratory systems. There may be autoimmune effects from gluten yet to be defined that cause wheezing and sinus allergies, but we do know that our immune systems' reactions to our environments is influenced by what we eat. Gluten, indeed, can be a cause of these symptoms.

Weight Changes

Excessive weight is a growing problem in our society. Most people, and most doctors, do not think that a gluten-sensitive patient will be overweight, however. Descriptions of celiac patients usually describe malnourished, thin people with abundant diarrhea and abdominal pain. Much to the contrary, this is definitely not the case, although it speaks to one of the many reasons why celiac disease and gluten sensitivity are so underdiagnosed.

Gluten-Sensitive Patients Are Usually NOT Underweight

Doctors have a fixed idea that if a patient isn't very thin with unrelenting diarrhea, he or she couldn't possibly have a problem with gluten. In a study of 371 recently diagnosed celiac patients, thirty-nine percent were legitimately overweight, and a third of these were obese. In addition, less than ten percent had below-normal weight.[151] Gluten-related disorders cause weight gain more commonly than weight loss, by far.

When Your Cells Are "Starving," Your Body's Metabolic Rate Goes Down

Weight changes can be a reflection of gluten sensitivity due to a few mechanisms. One of the ways in which weight can be affected by gluten is through the gastrointestinal system and its inflammatory damage. As a result of being malnourished, with reduced nutrients reaching our bodies' cells, the cells adapt and go into starvation mode. As a result, the metabolic rate slows down and fewer calories are burned. A slowed metabolic rate results in weight gain.

Also, in many cellular mechanisms, important vitamins and minerals are needed for metabolism to proceed well. If these are deficient because the intestinal wall is inflamed from gluten intolerance, then metabolic pathways are affected. This also slows down our metabolic rates and leads to weight gain. The immune reaction at the intestinal level results in these eventual weight increases over time.

Tired Adrenal Glands Result in Weight Gain

Also, as mentioned in the last chapter, adrenal changes can cause weight distribution to change. Excess cortisol production from the chronic stress of gluten intolerance leads to fatty tissue being deposited around the midsection. Cortisol also results in cells resisting insulin, and, therefore, the cells cannot use the glucose. It ends up being converted to fat, and, thus, weight increases. In this fashion, ongoing autoimmune disorders related to gluten further add to the stress and demands on the adrenal glands. As a result, the vicious cycle of stress, adrenal exhaustion and symptoms continue.

There are some specific, immune-related conditions that also affect your weight if you are gluten-intolerant. While not all forms of diabetes have autoimmune bases, diabetics who require insulin early in life usually have the autoimmune form. Unfortunately, one of the autoimmune disorders associated with gluten sensitivity is, indeed, diabetes. In two separate studies, both of which examined over 300 people with celiac disease, the occurrence of diabetes was over five percent.[152] This is significantly higher than in the normal population, which is approximately one percent, according to the Centers for Disease Control.

Diabetes and Weight Gain Resolve Successfully

J.D. was a middle-aged woman who was an insulin-dependent diabetic. Her diabetes was relatively stable but she required insulin, and weight gain was a problem, as were some digestive complaints and allergies. Her tests for gluten sensitivity were positive, and she had a dramatically positive response to gluten's elimination from her diet. She lost thirty-five pounds, her digestive complaints resolved, and she noticed clearer thinking as well as an improvement in her allergies and congestion. Her diabetes became more stable, and after five months on the HealthNOW Method, she had to stop taking insulin completely because her blood sugar was going too low.

Your Risk of Diabetes Increases If You're Gluten Sensitive

Diabetes results in higher levels of glucose in the blood as the ability to produce insulin, or the body's response to insulin, becomes less effective.

This, subsequently, can lead to weight gain unless sugar levels are tightly controlled. Higher levels of glucose in the blood eventually are converted to fat, which causes weight gain (similar to adrenal-induced insulin resistance).

Whether autoimmune forms of diabetes result directly from gluten-related antibodies or they're due to another mechanism of autoimmunity such as genetics, leaky bowel wall or others, diabetes is increased in gluten sensitivity and can result in weight-related changes.

Thyroid Problems Cause Weight Gain

Autoimmune attack on the thyroid gland also can affect your weight. Sometimes autoimmune thyroid disorders can make thyroid levels higher, but, most commonly, thyroid hormone levels fall. Lower thyroid hormone slows the metabolism, so fewer calories are burned; thus, weight may increase. Similar to diabetes, the occurrence of autoimmune thyroid dysfunction in celiac disease is reported to be around five percent.[153]

Diabetes, Thyroid Disease and Gluten Sensitivity Show a Genetic Link

In addition, in large groups of thyroid disorder patients without known gluten intolerance, more than five percent had gluten-related antibodies. This same study also demonstrated that patients with both diabetes and autoimmune thyroids had typical HLA gene patterns for gluten sensitivity risk.[154] This would suggest that there is a basic genetic risk for both conditions, which are closely related.

If You Have Thyroid Problems, Get Screened For Gluten Sensitivity

In a study done in 2000, fourteen percent of men and women had hypothyroid disorders,[155] suggesting that the prevalence of all types of thyroid disorders is well over fifteen percent. This is significant in terms of the number of people affected daily by thyroid dysfunction. If your weight is chronically elevated, or chronically low, thyroid testing should be evaluated. If thyroid dysfunction is found, these study findings strongly encourage an assessment for gluten sensitivity.

Non-Hodgkin's Lymphoma and Gluten Are Related

If weight loss is a bigger concern despite receiving adequate nutrition, certainly gluten can cause this through malabsorption syndromes. But, keeping the immune system in mind, some malignancies need to be considered as well. Of malignancies, non-Hodgkin's lymphoma (NHL) is the most common in gluten disorders, with colon cancer being the second most common. The notable thing about NHL in gluten-related disorders is that often, it is present without any digestive symptoms.

In a study of eighty patients with NHL, eight patients (ten percent) had gluten-related antibodies.[156] Of these eight, seven had no digestive symptoms at all. Fortunately, cancer is uncommon. However, weight loss symptoms, if present, should, of course, prompt attention to discovering the cause. Likewise, because of the frequency of colon cancer in our population, any family history of colon cancer should urge you to be tested for gluten sensitivity.

I'm So Tired...

When your body does not tolerate gluten, fatigue hits you from all angles. This can be due to nutritional issues, diffuse inflammation in the digestive tract, adrenal exhaustion, poor sleep, etc.

In regard to the immune system, fatigue can be a prominent symptom of some autoimmune disorders. Low thyroid function from autoimmune thyroid disease can certainly diminish your energy level and cause a feeling of tiredness, as can malignancies. These have been covered above and, therefore, knowing that these disorders can cause fatigue is important.

Discover Where Your Fatigue Is Coming From

Keep in mind that fatigue does indicate an abnormality in your health. It may be simply an immediate reaction to diet and lifestyle, or it could be more serious.

One other autoimmune condition is worth noting under the category of fatigue and autoimmune disease. Our bodies require glucose as well as oxygen to function well. Our cells depend on this for normal function, and it enables us to feel energetic. In order for cells to get oxygen, it has to come in through the lungs and attach to red blood cells. These cells then circulate to the tissues, providing oxygen for energy demands. This is why respiratory problems, anemia and poor circulation all can cause fatigue.

Gluten Can Attack the Heart As Well

In addition, the pump for the circulation must operate well. This is, of course, the heart. Research has demonstrated that in patients with myocarditis (an autoimmune attack causing inflammation of the heart), those who have gluten sensitivity as well account for almost six percent. In addition, in comparing gluten antibodies to antibodies directed against the inner lining of the heart, there is a high degree of similarity.

These findings have led to the theory that in some patients with myocarditis, gluten antibodies cross-react with the heart and cause damage.[157] As a result, if the heart is inflamed, its muscle cannot pump as well. This, then, leads to fatigue.

Fatigue and Lack of Energy May Be Common, But They're NOT Normal

Many people complain of lack of energy and fatigue much of the time. They are among the most frequent symptoms we doctors hear from patients. Excuses such as too little sleep, too much stress, poor diet and not enough exercise are postulated as the cause, and, indeed, all of this may be true. But pay attention to the symptom. Don't write it off or ignore it just because you know that it is a common complaint. "Common" doesn't mean "normal." If it persists despite the needed lifestyle changes, then other problems are present.

Gluten Can Trigger Problems via Several Mechanisms

Gluten has the ability to cause a multitude of symptoms, based on various mechanisms, by which it can affect our health. While the digestive system is a primary area of influence (and, likewise, changes in the body's hormonal system), the immune system remains a means by which gluten causes multiple symptoms. Some immune disorders are due to cross-reactivity with gluten-related antibodies, some related to immune system dysfunction from chronic stress and some from genetic patterns that cause a lower threshold to immune disorders. While several mechanisms may be at work, in the end, gluten remains a trigger and a root cause.

Your Symptoms Are Not Normal— Stop Putting Up With Them

From this information, it is most important that you take the symptoms you have and consider them to be manifestations of altered health. Investigate their causes, and, if nothing surfaces, don't give up. Symptoms are real and indicate a problem. Consider dietary causes, lifestyle changes and environmental influences even if standard examinations fail. If you have a family history of gluten intolerance, a family history of autoimmune disorders, or classic gluten-related symptoms, please take the challenge to evaluate gluten as an underlying cause.

Statistically, gluten is associated with a tremendous number of symptoms, yet gluten sensitivity remains tremendously underdiagnosed. Autoimmune disorders are just another example of gluten's wide-reaching health effects.

SECTION THREE

The Mainstream Gluten Disorders

Hopefully, we are making the case that gluten has far-reaching effects on the health of one's body. For some disorders, like Celiac disease, gluten has been the known cause for a long time. But, for a myriad of other conditions, it is less well-appreciated.

The symptoms of these gluten-related disorders have been covered extensively in the preceding chapters because it is our belief that one should be very aware of their symptoms. Symptoms are the body's alarm system, telling you something is wrong. Whether medical tests and exams confirm this or not, this simple fact still holds true.

Many Common Health Disorders Share a Known Gluten Relationship

However, in order to provide a complete understanding of all gluten-related conditions, we will cover specific disorders by name in this section and the next. For the sake of clarity, we will describe the mainstream disorders first in this section, and in Section IV, outline the ones that are less commonly known as gluten-related conditions.

It is also important that you understand that substantial evidence supports the association between these conditions and gluten. In all the conditions listed, we have had first-hand, clinical experience supporting gluten as the cause in many cases—not to mention that there are ample scientific papers that also clearly support the association.

With each gluten-related condition, three components will be addressed. First, an overview of the disorder will be given. Second, what your doctor is likely to tell you based on current traditional medical practices will be described. And, finally, what you may not know as the condition relates to gluten.

Scientific Evidence Supports the Relationship to Gluten

As with the preceding chapters, scientific and clinical evidence will be provided to support the relationships between gluten and your health. In this fashion, you can understand that we really have just scratched the surface in identifying the ways in which gluten can be a root cause of several disorders.

To start with, we will discuss the most well-accepted gluten-related disorder, which is celiac disease. But even with celiac disease, the best-known disorder associated with gluten intolerance, there are likely some things that may come as a surprise to you. From the previous sections, you have a good understanding of how gluten can affect our bodies through the digestive, immunologic and hormonal systems. These will be reviewed when necessary, as a reminder, to conceptualize how exactly gluten is causing the problem. Sometimes, it may be predominantly one mechanism, and at other times, several mechanisms may be at work. In order to further increase your awareness and understanding, we will point out these specific mechanisms in each particular disorder as it relates to gluten.

Feel Free To Look Ahead and Find the Disorder That Concerns You

If you identified certain disorders that may interest you in the section on symptoms, you can also use these sections to target a specific disorder or condition for better understanding. For instance, if fatigue and obesity are your main concerns, and from preceding chapters, you suspect thyroid or adrenal dysfunction, you may wish to jump ahead to read about those conditions first. Others may wish to cover all the known gluten disorders to see if certain conditions apply more specifically to their loved ones' overall complaints. Either way, the descriptions of the specific gluten disorders are to serve as educational tools to increase your understanding of gluten's ability to be the main cause of your health problems.

Eight

Celiac Disease

Overview

Celiac disease is the most commonly accepted condition of gluten intolerance. You may have previously thought that celiac disease was the only disorder that gluten caused, but this is far from the truth. Celiac disease is simply a major manifestation of gluten intolerance as it relates to the digestive system.

In essence, gluten results in damage to the intestinal lining by causing inflammation, and then, secondarily results in poor absorption of nutrients. This leads to a variety of other conditions related to malnutrition and the spread of inflammation to other tissues. This can include osteoporosis, arthritis, thyroid dysfunction and others.

Celiac Disease Is Highly Underdiagnosed

Women are diagnosed more commonly than men, and the disorder tends to be diagnosed most commonly in adulthood. Despite current estimates that celiac disease affects one in every 133 people, many clinicians feel that this is a large underestimation. Current ability to diagnose celiac disease, as this book will support, is just the tip of the iceberg when it comes to the actual number of celiac patients present.[158]

Celiac disease was first described in the second century A.D. by Arteus of Cappadocia,[159] and later by Gee in the late nineteenth century.[160] Artaeus' books were initially published in Latin and the word "coeliac" was used to translate the Greek word for "abdominal." The "o" in "coeliac" was dropped in certain cultures, forming the "celiac" we now use. But, in Great Britain and other countries, you will still see it spelled with an "o" today.[161]

Gluten Is Known to Cause Intestinal Damage

It was after this that the symptoms of celiac disease were linked to gluten, and more specifically gliadin, which is the major protein within wheat, rye and barley products. As a result, elimination of gluten from the diet resolves the intestinal injury and allows the body to heal over several weeks or months, depending on the severity of the damage. The widely accepted mechanism by which gluten causes celiac disease is an immune reaction against gliadin. This immune reaction not only attacks gliadin but also causes damage to the small structures on the surface of the intestinal lining. This results in intestinal dysfunction.[162]

Criteria for Diagnosis Varies Widely

Celiac disease varies tremendously within the terms of its definition. Some doctors require small bowel biopsies to show classic gluten-related damage to make a formal diagnosis; others require only classic symptoms with positive blood tests; and others accept common and uncommon symptoms that simply respond to gluten elimination from the diet. For this reason, labeling celiac disease as "celiac disease" or as "gluten sensitivity" can vary depending on each person's opinion. It is also the reason why common gluten-related symptoms can go undiagnosed.

The following will depict what many patients are routinely told by their physicians, as well as what they may not be told.

What Your Doctor Likely Told You About Celiac Disease

Conditions Considered "Rare" Are Not Often Diagnosed

Celiac disease patients who come to our office undiagnosed have often undergone extensive testing and evaluations with several other doctors. Indeed, the average time from symptom onset to diagnosis for celiac patients is eleven years.[163] Generally, doctors are looking for classic symptoms such as fatigue, weight loss, diarrhea, abdominal pain and anemia. If these are not present (and sometimes even when they are), many physicians fail to think about celiac disease as a possibility. It has been shown that the greatest likelihood of making an accurate diagnosis of celiac disease is the level of suspicion a clinician has about the condition.[164]

Positive and Negative Lab Tests— Mixed Results and Inconsistent Diagnoses

If classic symptoms are present, most physicians will then check blood tests for various antibodies to gluten or related enzymes, like tTG, that attach to gluten during metabolism. While the sensitivity of these tests is reported to be more than ninety-percent accurate,[165] this only truly pertains to celiac disease. If someone has gluten sensitivity without intestinal biopsy changes, the blood tests can still be positive, yet with a negative intestinal biopsy.

If the blood tests are positive and symptoms are classic, then many physicians will diagnose celiac disease and implement a gluten-free diet. However, there are several physicians who will not make a diagnosis of celiac disease without a positive small-bowel biopsy.[166] These clinicians believe that without a biopsy to support the diagnosis, the inconvenience of a gluten-free diet is not justified. What about the inconvenience of all those chronic, gluten-related complaints? And, truly, a gluten-free diet is minor compared to gambling with your health.

Negative Tests Don't Always Rule Out the Problem

The other problem that might occur is that the blood tests may come back negative or normal. In this situation, many doctors will state that celiac disease is not present and move on to other investigations. If symptoms are classic, a minority of physicians will still consider a small-bowel biopsy. Even fewer will consider a trial of a gluten-free diet to see how a person responds.

Delaying Diagnosis Wastes Precious Time

When clinicians prefer a small intestinal biopsy and wait for classic symptoms before ordering it, precious time elapses. Delayed diagnosis not only allows further intestinal damage to occur, but it also increases the risk of developing irreversible autoimmune disorders. According to the *New England Journal of Medicine* in 2007, a gluten-free diet is a valid means for diagnosis of gluten intolerance.[167] Waiting for classic symptoms before considering celiac disease or gluten sensitivity is like waiting for a heart attack before making the diagnosis of heart disease.

If your symptoms are not classic and severe, then your chances of being accurately diagnosed with celiac disease are poor. Many of our patients present in just this fashion, frustrated by years of symptoms without a definitive answer.

She Was Told She Just Had to Live With It

A.G. was a young woman who reached our clinic as a last resort. She complained that her belly felt bloated constantly and was enlarged, and she had suffered stomachaches since she was just a small child. She had seen pediatricians, internists and stomach specialists, but no diagnosis had ever occurred. She had been told just to live with it.

Fortunately, she persevered. When she also began getting colds every other week and missing work, she presented to our clinic. Her blood tests for gluten sensitivity were in a "suspicious" range of being positive, and she went on a gluten-free diet. Almost immediately, her energy improved and her belly flattened. She described being able to concentrate better at work, and over the next several months, she only suffered one additional cold. A.G. also lost twenty-five pounds and was back to her ideal weight. Currently, as long as she remains off gluten, she feels perfectly healthy.

Traditional Understanding of Celiac Disease Needs Updating

The disease process of celiac disease, from a traditional perspective, occurs as the body's immune system attacks gluten/gliadin and the related enzymes that metabolize it, such as tTG (tissue transglutaminase).[168] This is, indeed, a major pathway by which gluten causes symptoms in the digestive tract.

As we will discuss below, however, it is not the only mechanism. The immune pathway is well-accepted, and it is now accepted that celiac patients have higher risks for other immune conditions. These include diabetes, thyroid disease, lymphoma, lupus, rheumatoid arthritis and others. It is also accepted that there is a genetic risk for acquiring celiac disease. Patients who have first-degree relatives with insulin-dependent diabetes and celiac disease are recommended for celiac screening.[169] However, this has been a recent trend, appearing only in the last five years.

If Symptoms Are Not Classic the Diagnosis Is Often Missed

Overall, the standard approach for many clinicians in making a diagnosis of celiac disease hangs on hard evidence and factual findings in the setting of common symptoms. If any of these are absent, then the chance of diagnosis drops significantly. This is the difference between a symptom-based approach to health and a result-based approach.

What You Need to Know About Celiac Disease

If you have classic symptoms of celiac disease and positive test results from your doctor's office, then you are unlikely to be reading this book. However, if you fall into the majority of people who suffer "silent" celiac disease, then this book, and particularly this chapter, is definitely for you.

Using Digestive Symptoms Alone Is a Poor Marker and Misdiagnosis Is the Result

It has been shown that the number of patients with celiac disease and digestive symptoms is significantly less than those who have celiac disease but no digestive symptoms.[170] This was not simply supported based on suspicion, but actually confirmed by biopsy. Therefore, if the majority of people suffering from celiac disease have no digestive complaints, they are not exhibiting classic symptoms; therefore, their likelihood of receiving a correct diagnosis is dramatically reduced.

Many Celiac Patients Have "Silent" Celiac With No Symptoms

Did you know that the number of celiac disease patients who have no symptoms at all is eight times greater than those with symptoms? These patients are called "silent" celiacs. This statistic was supported through widespread lab testing for typical celiac disease antibodies in patients with gluten-related complaints.[171] You can put together the figures, but if a majority of celiac disease patients are without any symptoms, and, of the ones who do have symptoms, more than half do not have digestive complaints, then why are digestive symptoms supposed to be so typical of the disease?

Good question. Failing to have digestive symptoms is not a reason to ignore the damage that can be ongoing. This can lead to health problems later in life that could have been prevented. If you have family members with autoimmune disorders or gluten intolerance, you need to be tested for gluten intolerance whether symptoms are present or not.

Study Shows Weight Loss Is Not a "Classic Symptom"

Other symptoms that are supposed to be "classic" also include weight loss. In a study of newly diagnosed celiac patients, fifty-nine percent had normal weight and thirty-seven percent were overweight[172]—hardly a typical symptom either.

By reviewing the symptoms that can be associated with gluten sensitivity previously, it is our hope to change the definition of what really is a typical constellation of gluten-related complaints. These can include weight gain, joint aches, sleep disruption, depression, numbness, neurological symptoms, autoimmune disease and many others. It is apparent that many celiac disease patients have a variety of symptoms. Unless we can expand the definition to accommodate the less well-known complaints with the "typical" ones, we will continue to underestimate this disorder significantly.

Her Symptoms Were Ruining Her Life

C.T. had been seeing doctor after doctor with her complaints. Her main complaint was back pain as well as a feeling of tightness in her muscles diffusely. For twenty years, she had undergone spinal manipulations, physical therapy, medications, etc. None had ever provided any long-lasting relief, and she had become incredibly frustrated.

Her other symptoms included a tremendous lack of energy. She previously had been very active, but gradually, she had become quite sedentary as her health problems had worsened. She also had gained thirty-five pounds over several years.

Though her tests in our clinic were not definitive, she responded well when she went on a modified elimination diet. Gluten was the culprit. Over the next several weeks, C.T. had complete resolution of her back pain, and her energy returned. She stated, "I have my life back again." Additionally, she lost the weight she had gained.

We Must Expand Our Definition of Celiac Symptoms

While it is not clear whether she had basic gluten sensitivity or overt celiac disease, the point needs to be made that we shouldn't wait for typical symptoms that never come. It is important that we expand our list of complaints to better reflect what celiac disease truly is.

Eating Gluten Can Be Hazardous to Your Health

Having to tolerate symptoms with celiac disease years before the actual diagnosis is bad enough, but, in addition, there are significant risks to your health the longer you remain on gluten. In a pediatric study, a delay in the diagnosis substantially increased the presence of other autoimmune disorders over a period of years.[173] Typical autoimmune disorders in this study included thyroid disease, immune arthritis conditions and diabetes.

In another large study of more than 10,000 patients, the presence of heart disease was sixty percent greater in celiac patients than in people without the disorder.[174] The longer it takes to reach a diagnosis of celiac disease, the greater the risk to your health.

Gluten Is a Stress That Takes Its Toll on Your Health

The chronic stress of gluten sensitivity on your body takes its toll. That is why we feel it is so important for you to think about gluten-related disorders earlier rather than later. If you have risks for having celiac disease, or possible symptoms related to gluten, then early testing and diagnosis are important.

One of the reasons why many physicians fail to diagnose celiac disease is that the intestinal biopsy does not show the "typical" damage to the intestinal lining. The villi, which are small, finger-like structures on the lining, help absorb nutrients into the body. In a biopsy of a celiac disease patient, these villi are typically flattened and damaged.[175]

Gluten Damages the Intestine in More Than One Way

But gluten causes damage to the lining in other ways as well in celiac disease. In many people, gluten damages the digestive lining by causing direct irritation. This inflammation loosens the junctions between the lining cells, resulting in a leaky intestinal wall and thus allowing gluten and other food particles to enter the body prematurely before full digestion occurs.[176] In this type of scenario, the immune reaction occurs inside the lining of the intestine, so damage to the villi on the surface is not seen.

A Negative Biopsy May Mean Nothing

This and the fact that damage can be patchy at times is why biopsies can be negative in many celiac disease patients. Gluten is hard to digest in the best of circumstances, and even though an immune reaction is a most common mechanism of injury, gluten also can directly injure the intestinal lining before the immune reaction starts. This can account for why people who don't have a genetic risk of having celiac disease can still suffer from the disorder.

Waiting for a Positive Biopsy Is a Dangerous Gamble With Your Health

If you and your physician are waiting for a positive biopsy, in the face of gluten-related symptoms, before starting treatment, this is an undue delay and a truly dangerous delay. If you are waiting for positive lab tests before thinking about a gluten-free diet, these may never occur. If you are high-risk for having celiac disease and are waiting for complaints before being tested, your health may be at risk.

A Gluten-Free Diet That Improves Your Symptoms May Be Your Best Test

What we know currently is that there is a broader group of symptoms than previously realized with celiac disease, and that medical tests miss a great number of people with celiac disease. The easiest diagnostic test is to eliminate gluten from your diet and see if symptoms abate. If they do, regardless of other test results, celiac disease or gluten sensitivity is the cause of your condition.

Summary

Celiac disease is the best-known gluten-related health condition. For many years in the past, it was the only known gluten-related disorder. But, over the last several decades, evidence has supported many other health conditions that are due to this hard-to-digest protein. There is no question that lab testing has advanced significantly in identifying celiac disease, but even so, many people are never tested for the disorder. The lack of typical symptoms and a general lack of awareness of the vast number of complaints gluten can cause are the reasons.

Awareness of This Disorder Needs to Increase

From our perspective, gluten is the root cause of many complaints well outside the digestive system. But, even among individuals with gastrointestinal symptoms, celiac disease is infrequently suspected. Increasing the awareness of the number of "silent" celiacs can help increase detection rates. Likewise, if tests such as labs and biopsies fail to make a definitive diagnosis, a trial of being off gluten for a few weeks is well worth it. Abatement of your symptoms makes for a legitimate diagnosis even when other tests fail.

While statistics report one in every 250 people with celiac disease currently, the reality is that the occurrence is much, much higher. We help people every week in our clinic with previously undiagnosed celiac disease, and it is evident that, indeed, we are just exposing the tip of the iceberg. If you have symptoms, consider gluten as the cause. And if your have a family history of celiac disease or other disorders that make gluten intolerance more likely, make plans to be tested. The earlier celiac disease is diagnosed and treated, the healthier you will be.

Nine

Autism, ADD, ADHD

Overview

Autism, "attention deficit disorder" ("ADD") and "attention deficit hyperactivity disorder" ("ADHD") represent neurological and behavioral disorders that first present in childhood. Why do we put "ADD" and "ADHD" in quotes? Because we don't consider them to be actual medical conditions as purported by the psychiatric community, even though symptoms associated with these conditions are extremely legitimate, and we have experienced first-hand in our clinic the irritable child who couldn't sit still or control his body's movements.

Medications Commonly Used Are Ineffective and Dangerous

But we've also experienced remarkable benefits from adjusting dietary and lifestyle factors in treating these symptoms, and, unfortunately, witnessed the many dangerous side effects of medications prescribed by others for "ADD" and "ADHD" symptoms.

In this chapter, we will discuss all three conditions since they have

177

gluten-related influences in their causes and in their treatments. In comparing these conditions, you will see that there is a great deal of unknown in the medical and psychiatric communities about these disorders. As a result, medications have been thrown at the symptoms with disregard to side effects and without good understanding of the underlying cause. In regards to "ADD" and "ADHD," there is actually no real support that these labels represent actual medical disorders.[177]

Autism Incidence Has Increased More Than 500 Percent

Autism is an unfortunate condition that has rapidly advanced in the last two decades, increasing by more than 500 percent. Autism is a disorder of childhood brain development that affects social interactions, abilities to communicate and various behaviors. Autism is typically noted in children before the age of three years, and autistic disorders affect boys more than girls at a ratio of four to one.

Recent data from the Centers for Disease Control indicates that one in every 150 children is affected, as of 2002. While genetic risks for developing autism may be present, there appears to be a significant environmental factors as well, which have yet to be securely defined.[178]

"ADD"and "ADHD": Illegitimate Labels?

"ADD" and "ADHD" also present in childhood, but the symptoms associated with these conditions often develop later, during preschool to early school years. While both are described as being overt medical disorders in the psychiatric community, there is no evidence that biologic, chemical, neurologic or genetic markers are present to substantiate these as legitimate diseases.

Psychiatric accounts describes three to five percent of all children as suffering from "ADD" or "ADHD," which totals about two million children in the Unites States.[179] Basic symptoms include an inability to pay attention and control their movements and behaviors for long periods of time, and boys are affected more than girls.[180] While these figures are quite concerning, more concerning is the number of children medicated for "ADD" and "ADHD." Approximately 8.5 million children are prescribed stimulants, antidepressants or psychiatric drugs for these symptoms, and the side effects associated with these drugs are tremendous.[181]

What Your Doctor Likely Told You About Autism

Because of its rising occurrence and unknown definitive cause, autism has received a great deal of attention. From a genetic standpoint, identical twins support an inherited risk. If one twin has autism, the chance that the other twin also has autism is sixty to eighty percent. Because this figure is not 100 percent between identical twins, however, there must be environmental factors as well. This has also been supported by the dramatic increase in autistic disorders in the last twenty years.[182] Genetic disorders do not advance this rapidly.

Medications for Autism Have Dangerous Side Effects

Most treatments are geared toward early diagnosis with intervention as soon as possible through speech therapists and occupational therapists. These measures have been shown to improve developmental abilities, but they are far from a cure. Outside of these interventions, options are quite limited to date in the traditional medical arena. Medications may, unfortunately, be used for behavioral control, but no benefit has been reported with medication in autistic disorders, and the risk of side effects is significant.

Gluten and Dairy May Be Problems in Autistic Children

While many autism organizations support elimination of gluten and casein in the diet, this has not been a standard among medical clinicians so far. Casein is the major protein in milk, and there is evidence that both gluten and casein are metabolized to proteins that worsen function in autistic children. This information will be described later in the chapter.

Mercury in Vaccinations May Be a Risk Factor

Regarding possible environmental factors that may cause autism, some have included the MMR vaccine (for measles, mumps and rubella) as well as thimerosal, which can be a preservative in many vaccines. Because of thimerosal's association with autism, the United States encouraged vaccine manufacturers to remove thimerosal from all vaccines. However, some vaccines still contain trace amounts of thimerosal, and flu vaccines as of 2005 still used this preservative, even in children's flu vaccines.[183] Thimerosal contains mercury, which can be toxic to the nervous system.

Nutritional Deficiencies May Be a Cause

Other than gluten and casein, other dietary factors in potential causes for autism include nutritional deficiencies. Vitamin deficiencies in B-complex vitamins and other minerals have been suggested, but, again, are not routinely accepted by the medical community in general. Other researchers have suggested chronic yeast infections as a cause.[184]

Despite these theories, traditional medicine has yet to truly embrace any particular cause of autistic disorders. It remains a mystery that urgently needs to be solved.

A Brilliant Young Boy Gets Some Relief

J.P. was initially diagnosed with Asperger's syndrome in school. This is a common form of autism. Up until age three and a half, he was a brilliant child with no behavioral problems. The first things his parents noticed, in addition to his social and behavioral changes, were weight loss and repeated infections. Most bothersome were the development of severe canker sores in his mouth that further limited his ability to eat.

Over the ensuing year, J.P. also developed feelings of anxiety and difficulty passing bowel movements (later, this was attributed to bowel inflammation). Prior to coming to our clinic, his mother did eliminate gluten from his diet. Within three weeks, the canker sores all healed and his appetite was much better. She later gave him a popover as a trial, and the next day, he had five canker sores that were raw and bleeding. Once gluten was completely avoided again, his eating habits, weight and bowel function returned to normal.

Many months later, he was sending letters to his grandparents. He licked the envelopes and stamps (the glue had gluten) and once again broke out in canker sores for a week, and was unable to consume anything but very cold liquids. It was a tiny dose, but it didn't stop his body from reacting.

When he came to HealthNOW, he was already off gluten, but due to some continuing symptoms, we put him on a hypoallergenic diet to see if he was reacting to anything else. He turned out to be severely allergic to soy, and removal of soy even resulted in resolution of his "cradle cap," which he had always had. His chronic, hacking cough was gone as well. Lab tests revealed a bacterial infection in his stomach, which was successfully treated.

His pediatric gastroenterologist wanted to test him for celiac disease after the mother told him of their experience. His recommendation was that J. consume gluten for three weeks and then have a small bowel biopsy. J.'s mother told the specialist about the severe reactions he had to minute amounts of gluten, but he insisted that his recommendation was the only definitive option for diagnosis. She chose not to proceed, needless to say.

Regarding his autism, he continues to have features of the disorder, but he has improved in his behavior and his learning abilities since being off gluten. Interestingly, he has a brother with autism as well, and his mother has been found to be gluten-intolerant.

What You Need to Know About Autism

Study Shows Dietary Changes Have a Positive Effect

While there is no question that genetics play a part in the risk of having autism, clearly, environmental factors play a large role. And, there is ample evidence that gluten is a common factor that augments autism in many children. Originally, this was found through dietary changes, but antibody testing now supports this as well. In a 2002 study out of Norway, ten of twenty autistic children began gluten-free and casein-free diets while the other ten stayed on regular diets. After a year, the group on gluten-free and casein-free diets had significant improvements in development over the other children.[185] These findings have been repeated in other studies, and many advocacy groups for autism have recommend gluten-free diets for autistic children as early as possible.[186]

Fifty Percent of Autistic Children Showed a Reaction to Gluten

From the immune system side of investigation, others have found gluten-related antibodies in autistic children. In 2006, one study evaluated thirty autistic children and compared them to thirty non-autistic children. In the autistic group, fifty percent had gluten-related antibodies while less than seven percent had these antibodies in the non-autistic children's group.[187]

Autistic Children Show a Higher Incidence of Gluten-Related Immune Reactions

In another study, children with autism had a significant number of anti-gliadin and anti-Purkinje cell antibodies compared to normal children. These are the antibodies, as previously discussed, that are directed at gliadin (a protein within gluten) and Purkinje cells (nerve cells in the brain that regulate balance). These findings support that gluten sensitivity can indeed cause autistic symptoms through auto-antibody reactions.[188]

Despite many physicians being resistant to accepting gluten as a cause in autism, the above studies show that eliminating gluten can improve development in autistic children and that the mechanism of how gluten affects autism is through the immune system. There may also be additional causes through nutritional deficiencies if gluten affects the intestinal lining as well.

Children Should Be Tested for Gluten Sensitivity

Vitamins such B6, B2 and B12 can have beneficial effects in treating autism, as can calcium and the minerals chromium and molybdenum. While gluten is not likely the only environmental factor in autism, it definitely is a component. Because autism develops early in a child's life, early testing, if others in the family have gluten sensitivity, is strongly encouraged.

What Your Doctor Likely Told You About "ADD" and "ADHD"

"ADD" and "ADHD" classically consist of symptoms of hyperactivity, impulsivity and poor attention, with the key distinction between the two being symptoms of uncontrolled activity. The psychiatric community supports these both as diagnoses, as outlined in the *Diagnostic Statistical Manual IV*. ADD and ADHD were added as formal diagnoses in 1987, and since that time, there has been a 900-percent increase in the number of children who carry these labels.[189]

Diagnosis Is Made Without True Medically Objective Criteria

Psychiatric criteria for these diagnoses require some features of historical information about the child, some behavioral features on exam, and standardized testing. In essence, the labels of

"ADD" and "ADHD" are given without objective criteria involving actual biologic, chemical or neurologic findings. While this may simply be the state of some conditions, the concern is that these labels are used to prescribe seriously toxic medications.[190]

Similar to autism, "ADD" and "ADHD" have strong genetic influences, as identical twins have higher rates of occurrence than non-twins. Likewise, family members of persons with these symptom complexes have a twenty-five-percent risk of having "ADD" or "ADHD" symptoms, while the occurrence in the general population is only five percent.[191]

While again, this supports a genetic risk, environmental factors are also at play. Potential environmental influences have included the use of alcohol and tobacco during pregnancy, lead intoxication, sugar and food additives and brain injury from trauma. Despite these suspicions, there has not been enough evidence for traditional medicine to list any of these factors as contributing causes to the symptoms described by these psychiatric labels.[192]

Treatment for "ADD" and "ADHD": Help or Harm?

Treatments for "ADD" and "ADHD" have been multiple and include many medications that have an abundance of dangerous side effects. These, of course, include methylphenidate (Ritalin), but also many others that fall into a category of stimulants, antidepressants and psychotics. Worldwide, six million children are taking stimulants for control of "ADD" and "ADHD" symptoms. Likewise, in children under five years of age, there was a 580-percent increase in the use of antidepressants between 1995 and 1999. This is the largest growing segment of the population using antidepressant drugs.[193]

In short, psychiatric focus is geared toward treating the symptoms of "ADD" and "ADHD" without necessarily focusing on the root causes. The criteria for diagnosis of these conditions do not hold to rigid findings, as with other medical diseases, and even more worrisome is the accepted basis for which drugs are prescribed for these diagnoses. Considering the vast number of children and adults affected by "ADD" and "ADHD," it certainly warrants a continued search for other causes. Routinely, no definitive root cause has been assigned to "ADD" or "ADHD," other than having a genetic susceptibility.

What You Need to Know About "ADD" and "ADHD"

Gluten's role in "ADD" and "ADHD" has been even less well-accepted despite evidence to the contrary. In more than one study, patients with gluten sensitivity have a higher chance of having "ADD" and "ADHD" than those individuals without gluten intolerance. In a large study by Zelnick, the number of gluten-sensitive persons with either "ADD," "ADHD" or a learning disability was much higher than subjects who were not gluten-sensitive.[194]

Higher Incidence of "ADHD" Found in Gluten-Sensitive Population

In another study in 2006, 132 patients who had gluten sensitivity were examined for the presence of "ADHD." In the results, "ADHD" was over-represented among these patients, compared to the general population. Additionally, after these identified patients were placed on a gluten-free diet, a significant improvement in behavior was noted within six months.[195]

Drugs Given to Children Have High Addictive Potential

One of the greatest concerns with the current treatment of "ADD" and "ADHD" is the widespread use of toxic medication to treat these symptom patterns. While there is no evidence to support biologic or chemical causes of "ADD" and "ADHD" as supported by psychiatric theory, medications are prescribed in huge volumes to children. The most common type of medication used is stimulant medication. This includes Ritalin, Dexedrine, Concerta and some other, less-common ones. These are controlled substances in the same category as opiates, and have addictive potential. In fact, ten percent of all teenagers are known to abuse stimulants.[196]

Concerns Raised Over Ethical Practices of Well-Known Psychiatrist

Recent evidence further raises concern over the ethical practices of medication prescriptions for behavioral disorders in children. Many physicians are involved in pharmaceutical studies of pediatric patients that are funded by drug companies that manufacture stimulant medications and anti-psychotic drugs. *The New York Times* recently described a story about a well-known Harvard psychiatrist, Dr. Joseph Biederman, who received $1.6 million in various fees, for consulting and pharmaceutical research, from companies designing these psychiatric medicines. While the focus in this article was his lack of reporting this sizable income, additional concerns were raised over the ethics behind such reimbursement.

Questionable Findings in Small Studies Using Psychiatric Medications

Over several years, Biederman had conducted several small group studies supporting the benefit of using psychiatric medication for disorders in children labeled with "ADD," "ADHD" and bipolar disorder. Despite what appears to be questionable findings, his studies account for a significant increase in the use of these potent medications in children. These studies, combined with lobbyist power from major pharmaceutical companies, can facilitate Food and Drug Administration approval of medications. This is where we, as patients and clinicians, must be very wary of published results and drug approvals.

Our Children Suffer...

This is a frightening glimpse into the psychiatric profession, which still controls autism treatment for many, and the power of the pharmaceutical industry. Millions of American kids are on powerful drugs, recommended by their neurologists, psychiatrists and pediatricians every day, for autism, ADHD, bipolar and other diagnoses because pharmaceutical companies and physicians with conflicts of interest influence widespread opinions.

Stimulants may make behavioral symptoms easier to control, but reports that these medications help academic performance have not been substantiated.[197] In addition, stimulants can cause a variety of dangerous side effects. Deaths from heart attacks have been most notable with these drugs, affecting otherwise healthy children.[198] Other stimulant side effects can include violent behavior, psychosis and hallucination, nervousness, insomnia, weight loss, poor appetite, increased blood pressure and poor growth.[199]

Psychiatric Drugs Have Side Effect of Suicide

The use of antidepressants in children with "ADD" and "ADHD" is likewise a tremendous concern. Some antidepressants, such as Prozac and Straterra, have been associated with suicidal thoughts and actual suicides.[200] Straterra has also been associated with serious liver damage.[201] These medications are ubiquitous in our society in general, but now they are prevalent in our children as well. These medications have many other side effects including poor concentration, poor sleep patterns, changes in mood patterns, weight gain and heart effects.

Holland Court Rules That "ADD" Is Not an Actual Disease

In Holland, a court ruled that there was insufficient evidence to support that "ADD" was an actual disease. After reviewing abundant information between the prosecution and defense, there was a lack of biological, chemical or physical evidence to support psychiatric theory and treatment.[202] Despite this, in the United States, not only do we embrace these diagnoses without adequate support, but we support a billion-dollar drug industry to treat our children with dangerous medications and drugs.

It is time to look at the real cause of these symptoms rather than placing an arbitrary label on them. The labels of "ADD" and "ADHD" simply provide a means by which to treat symptoms without getting to the underlying causes of the situation. It is similar to treating a broken bone with pain medications but not worrying about the fracture.

MRI Studies Show Reduced Size of Brain

While it is not known whether children with "ADD" or "ADHD" have immune reactions to gluten similar to those seen in autism, it is a likely situation. In MRI studies looking at children with "ADHD," parts of the cerebella (where Purkinje cells are predominant) were smaller compared to MRI scans of individuals who did not have "ADHD."[203] If gliadin and gluten antibodies cross-react with Purkinje cells in ADHD as they do in autism, this supports an immune mechanism of action based on the MRI findings. In other words, gluten would trigger an immune reaction that makes Purkinje cell antibodies, which then attack the cerebellum, making it smaller. This, in turn, causes the "ADD" or "ADHD" symptoms.

Other mechanisms could also include metabolites of gluten causing difficulties in brain function. Gluten, as was previously mentioned, can be metabolized into the gluteomorphins.[204] These molecules can then stimulate opiate receptors in the brain and cause sedation, poor attention, poor memory and learning difficulties. In this way, gluten can also affect autism symptoms as well. As with many conditions, gluten can have more than one way of causing symptoms and complaints.

Summary

Autism, "ADD" and "ADHD" affect large numbers of children each year. Unfortunately, these effects can last a lifetime, and the opportunity to intervene in the causation appears to come very early in life. Genetics play a role in both disorders, but environmental effects seem to be a larger portion of the problem. This gives us the chance to make a difference, if the environmental causes can be found.

Gluten-Free Diet Is Shown to Help

In these disorders, evidence that gluten plays a part in the root cause is overwhelming. Gluten's elimination from the diet helps all of the conditions, and there is progressive evidence that gluten-related antibodies and gluten metabolites affect the brain's function negatively. By adhering to a gluten-free diet, autism, "ADD" and "ADHD" can improve in severity, allowing for a much better quality of life. But how do you know when to consider a gluten-free diet or a gluten-related cause?

Test Children Early, Please...

If you or your family have anyone with a gluten-related condition or overt gluten sensitivity, it is better to be safe than sorry. Have your children tested earlier rather than later. The longer you wait, the higher the risk of an autoimmune disorder, and the more likely it is that conditions like autism and "ADD" or "ADHD" can develop and be more severe.

A Gluten-Free Trial Is a Good Idea

If your child already suffers from these conditions, you should eliminate gluten from his or her diet immediately. The evidence supports that the presence of gluten in the diet can prevent possible improvements from occurring, and for children with "ADD" or "ADHD," removal of gluten can prevent the high-risk side effects associated with prescribed medications.

Ten

Arthritis Syndromes: Osteoarthritis, Rheumatoid Arthritis and Sjogren's Syndrome

Norma's Chronic Joint Pain

Norma had felt ill for almost nine years, complaining of aches all over her body and a generalized feeling of being swollen. Specifically, her fingers felt swollen. She had gone to see several doctors, including some specialists, over the years, but a definitive diagnosis had not been made.

Her doctor felt as though she may have some type of immune disease affecting her joints, but her tests and exam findings did not fit her into any disease category. Likewise, she had a blood test (an ANA) that was positive, suggestive of immune system overactivity, but this alone could not confirm a disorder.

After arriving in our clinic, she tried an elimination diet, and while off gluten, her symptoms improved. Within weeks she lost weight, had more energy, was much more productive and, most importantly, had relief from her constant aches and pains. Even the swelling and inflammation resolved. Norma felt better than she had in almost a decade after going off gluten.

Overview

Arthritis is a condition that is quite varied in its description. From a very basic standpoint, it simply means inflammation of the joints of the body. But, as a general term, "arthritis" can refer to a great many subtypes of conditions. Most individuals, when they state that they have arthritis, refer to a chronic condition rather than a recently injured joint. But this comes in several varieties, with the common categories including osteoarthritis, rheumatoid arthritis, systemic lupus erythematosis and a few others.

For the purposes of this chapter, we will focus mainly on three of these categories as they relate to gluten. This will include osteoarthritis, rheumatoid arthritis and Sjogren's syndrome.

Arthritis Affects Twenty-One Percent of the Population

As an umbrella term, "arthritis" affects about twenty-one percent of the population by conservative estimation, which means that more than forty-six million people are affected in the Unites States alone. These numbers increase even further with advancing age, with more than fifty percent of people over age sixty-five being affected.

Arthritis Is Costly

Women tend to be affected slightly more than men. The best guess as to the actual costs to our society is $128 billion from medical care, lost productivity and secondary complications.[205] These numbers alone should attract our attention.

Osteoarthritis is also known as degenerative joint disease, and this disorder accounts for more than half of all cases of arthritis. It is unique in that weight-bearing joints are typically affected (hips, knees and spine) as well as the hands. Rheumatoid arthritis (RA) is much less common, but is more debilitating. RA is an autoimmune disorder that has both genetic and environmental risk factors. It is three times more common in women than men, and its juvenile form is the most common arthritis in childhood.[206]

Sjogren's syndrome is not solely an arthritic disorder, but it does involve the joints when present, and it can occur secondarily with other forms of arthritis like rheumatoid arthritis or lupus. Sjogren's syndrome is an autoimmune disease as well, and it attacks the tear ducts and salivary glands, resulting in dry eyes and a dry mouth. It is nine times more common in women than men.[207]

These Diseases Are Well-Linked to Gluten

Of the various connective tissue and arthritis disorders, these three have been well-linked to gluten sensitivity. Other arthritic syndromes have been less commonly associated, and these will be covered in the following section. Regardless, even many patients who present to our clinic rarely know about the association between gluten and arthritis. Considering the available evidence, this is quite a surprise.

What Your Doctor Likely Told You About Arthritis Syndromes

Osteoarthritis

With osteoarthritis, there is a general acceptance that it occurs as a result of two factors. One is aging and the other is wear and tear. Indeed, the occurrence of osteoarthritis increases as we get older, and it affects the joints that bear the most weight or stress. This includes the knees, hips, spine and hands. In other words, the cause is felt to be simply a matter of physics and mechanics. The more weight you bear on a joint and the older it gets, the more likely it is that you will have osteoarthritis.[208] But, overall, this doesn't go far enough to explain the cause.

Why do some people in their thirties develop osteoarthritis and others in their eighties fail to have any features of it at all? In short, the exact reason is not known. What is known is that the joint shows deterioration of the cartilage over the bony surfaces of the joints and a reduced joint space. Also, inflammatory cells (immune cells) and fluid occupy the joint space.[209] With time, this erodes the joint itself, causing pain, limitation of movement and limited function.

Treatment for osteoarthritis is aimed at reducing the weight-bearing stress on the affected joints and reducing the inflammation in the joint space. To this extent, it is targeting some of the causes and not just symptoms. Weight loss, strengthening of supporting muscles and ligaments, and medicines such as anti-inflammatories are invoked for this purpose. If these therapies fail over time, some joints can be surgically replaced.[210]

Current treatments are very limited overall in reducing the actual occurrence of this condition, but they have increased the functional ability of many who suffer from osteoarthritis.

Rheumatoid Arthritis

While joints in rheumatoid arthritis also become inflamed, the process of disease is completely different. Usually, smaller joints (not weight-bearing joints) are affected first such as the feet, ankles, wrists and hands. Severity varies greatly and can be progressive and constant, or the disorder can come in waves, with periods of minimal symptoms in between.

Pain, limited movements, redness and swelling of the joints are the key symptoms, and, most commonly, it develops in middle age. However, in children, a juvenile variant of rheumatoid arthritis can be quite severe.[211]

Rheumatoid Arthritis Has a Known Immune Component

While osteoarthritis is related to wear and tear, rheumatoid arthritis is not. The cause is felt to be autoimmune, with antibodies and immune cells attacking selective joints. In addition, a genetic risk predisposes individuals to the disorder, but something in their lifestyle or environment triggers the disorder to develop. Environmental triggers that are suspected can include tobacco use or viral infections, but none of this has been definitive to date.[212]

Treatment, in general, is mainly medication, with two main categories of drugs. One category includes medications that reduce the inflammatory response at the joint so that damage is reduced and symptoms improved. The other category is medications that suppress the immune system. By suppressing the immune system, the inflammatory response is called off, and the joint can begin to heal.[213] While these treatments do help, most have significant side effects and expense.

Is It a Good Idea to Suppress Your Immune System With Drugs?

Some examples of these medications that suppress the immune system include prednisone and some oral chemotherapy drugs. While these medications accomplish the suppression of an overactive immune system in autoimmune disease, the suppression is not selective. This means that all of the immune system is suppressed, not just the part causing rheumatoid arthritis. As a result, you can suffer infections, develop a drop in your blood counts and even be at a higher risk for cancer by chronically suppressing your immune system's function.

Therefore, while these medications are helpful, they are not identifying the root cause and can lead to other problems. Clearly identifying the primary triggers in rheumatoid arthritis would be a great advantage in providing a better treatment.

Sjogren's Syndrome

Named after an ophthalmologist in the early 1900s, Sjogren's syndrome is an autoimmune disorder that primarily attacks the tear glands of the eyes and the salivary glands of the mouth. It is included in this chapter for a few reasons. First, arthritis can be an extra-glandular symptom of the disorder. Extra-glandular symptoms refer to those symptoms outside of the tear glands and the saliva glands of the eyes and mouth.

Sjogren's Is Related to Other Autoimmune Disorders

Secondly, Sjogren's is often associated with other autoimmune joint conditions such as rheumatoid arthritis, systemic lupus erythematosis and others. The cause of the autoimmune attack is unknown, but genetics play a role, partially. While it can run in families, more commonly, Sjogren's syndrome is likely to be present if other autoimmune disorders are in a family in general.[214]

By far, women are affected much more commonly than men, and symptoms, predominantly, are dry eyes and dry mouth that can lead to eye abrasions and gum disease. Other symptoms can include arthritis of many joints throughout the body as well as inflammation of the body's blood vessels, called vasculitis.

Treatment Is Aimed at Reducing Symptoms

In terms of risk factors, none are known. No triggers or environmental influences have been defined. Treatment is aimed at symptomatically relieving the dry eyes and dry mouth while alleviating the arthritis pains with anti-inflammatories. If the condition fails to respond to these measures, medications that suppress the immune system's activity are used.[215] Overall, Sjogren's syndrome is fairly uncommon, but for those who have it, symptoms can be miserable.

What You Need to Know About Arthritis Syndromes

OSTEOARTHRITIS

If you recall, osteoarthritis is due to wear and tear of the weight-bearing joints and simple aging, but questions why some people develop it early and some not at all fail to be answered by this theory. By looking a little deeper, it seems likely that other influences are the reason.

Gluten Sensitivity Is Well-Represented in Arthritic Patients

Gluten itself has been implicated as a root cause in several research studies. For example, in one study, 200 consecutive patients with gluten sensitivity were examined for arthritis. Of the group, twenty-six percent had arthritis while only 7.5 percent of a group of normal individuals suffered from the condition.[216] In another case report study, two patients were described as having progressive arthritis (one with involvement of the knee and the other with the hip), both of whom responded completely to a gluten-free diet.[217]

What Is Gluten's Role in Arthritis?

But how does gluten result in arthritis? A few theories exist. For one, gluten is thought to trigger the immune system to form auto-antibodies that then attack the joint's lining. This leads to inflammation and swelling. Some suspect that gluten's irritation of the intestinal lining allows molecules and food particles to gain access to our bodies without full digestion. These particles then appear foreign to our immune systems, which launches an attack against them.

Why Antibodies Against Your Own Tissues Form

As the immune system creates antibodies against these food particles, some are already attached to your body's enzymes and tissues. Therefore, the immune attack can create not only anti-bodies against foreign food materials but also auto-antibodies against your body's own tissues or enzymes as well. This is how auto-antibodies in autoimmune disease develop.[218]

The larger weight-bearing joints may be more susceptible to an immune system attack because of wear and tear. Because these joints are more stressed, microscopic tears in the joint lining may allow greater access of auto-antibodies into the joint. In this fashion, gluten can be a root cause.

To support this further, another investigator describes an eleven-year-old boy who had a single joint inflamed for years. It would come and go, but no cause could be found. Eventually, he was tested for anti-gliadin antibodies, which were found to be present. After being placed on a gluten-free diet, the arthritis resolved completely. He was confirmed to have gluten sensitivity and celiac disease by intestinal biopsy.[219]

Therefore, if obvious causes are not present, and you suffer from osteoarthritis, gluten can be a trigger for its development. Diet and lifestyle do significantly influence our bodies' abilities to stay healthy.

RHEUMATOID ARTHRITIS

Gluten Is a Risk Factor

Considering that rheumatoid arthritis is an immune disorder, its relationship to gluten is even stronger. Gluten sensitivity increases the risk of having rheumatoid arthritis significantly. In a 1995 study, a group of patients with rheumatoid arthritis was compared to a healthy group of individuals. Of the healthy group, twelve percent had anti-gliadin antibodies, compared to thirty-seven percent in the rheumatoid arthritis group.[220] The risk of having one condition therefore increases the chances of having the other.

Gluten-Free Diet Results in Decline of Symptoms

Is this just a case of an overactive immune system causing more than one autoimmune disorder? Possibly, but other studies suggest more of a direct correlation between gluten and rheumatoid arthritis. One investigation reports sixty-six rheumatoid arthritis patients who were divided into different diet groups. Thirty-eight ate a gluten-free, vegan diet and twenty-eight ate a normal diet. In the gluten-free diet group, not only did anti-gliadin antibodies decline over time, but so did rheumatoid-arthritis-related antibodies. This did not happen in the normal-diet group.

The authors concluded that gluten (and possibly other foods) can trigger the immune system into making auto-antibodies.221 We know this to definitively be the case with gluten in particular.

Sjogren's Syndrome

Sjogren's syndrome has been associated with gluten sensitivity for a long time. A study in 1984 demonstrated that in twenty-five patients with Sjogren's syndrome, in comparison to nineteen lupus patients, a significant increase in anti-gliadin antibodies and gluten antibodies was noted.222

Sjogren's Patients Have a Higher Risk of Gluten Sensitivity

More recently, a much larger study, with 110 patients with Sjogren's syndrome, found that five percent had anti-gliadin antibodies, and all but one of these anti-gliadin antibody individuals had positive intestinal biopsies for celiac disease.223 This information does not confirm that gluten is a trigger for Sjogren's syndrome, but it does support a higher risk of gluten sensitivity if Sjogren's is present. The chance of having gluten-related antibodies is elevated, as is intestinal damage, if you have Sjogren's syndrome and include gluten in your diet.

To make this point further, another study challenged patients with a gluten diet and then measured intestinal changes for intolerance. Twenty Sjogren's syndrome patients were sampled along with eighteen healthy individuals. In the Sjogren's group, twenty-five percent had bad reactions to gluten in the diet. These patients were not previously known to be gluten sensitive.[224]

While gluten may be a dietary trigger for developing Sjogren's syndrome, it clearly is contraindicated if you have Sjogren's syndrome already. The addition of gluten to your diet will only create new problems through potential malnutrition, increased immune system activity and, eventually, adrenal exhaustion. While traditional medical advice neglects this important message, science clearly indicates that gluten should be avoided if you suffer from Sjogren's syndrome.

Summary

The interplay between gluten and our joint system is certainly strong. From current information available, gluten appears to cause or worsen arthritis syndromes through reactions in our immune systems. Gluten causes disruption of our intestinal lining, which can then lead to gluten and other undigested material gaining access to our bodies prematurely. This then triggers an immune reaction that affects the lining surfaces of our joints. Swelling and redness from the inflammation develops and, eventually, damage to the cartilage and bone occurs, resulting in arthritis symptoms. These symptoms typically include pain, limitation of movements and swelling.

If You Have a Risk Factor for Arthritis, Consider Gluten Sensitivity

If you are at genetic risk for having disorders like rheumatoid arthritis or Sjogren's syndrome, gluten is even more risky. Gluten can cause these conditions to develop as a dietary, environmental trigger. While gluten is not stressed at all by traditional medicine as a cause of these conditions, the medical evidence suggests that it should be a strong consideration in causation.

If you have osteoarthritis, rheumatoid arthritis or Sjogren's syndrome, gluten sensitivity needs to be evaluated. This can be done through formal testing for gluten-related antibodies, or you can eliminate gluten from your diet to assess a response over several weeks. You are likely to be surprised by what you find.

Eleven

Gluten and Diabetes

Diabetes Eliminated in Seventy-Four-Year-Old

S.L. was a lovely, Chinese lady, seventy-four years old. While she had diabetes (her mom and dad had it as well), she came to us for digestive problems. She was quite thin and had suffered for many years from digestive discomfort consisting of fullness, indigestion and acid reflux. The less she ate, the better she felt digestively. She had suffered from chronic constipation her whole life, complained of chronic fatigue, and had been diagnosed with high cholesterol. She had been diagnosed with diabetes four years before coming to see us.

She was found to be gluten-intolerant and also had an H. pylori infection of her intestines. Additionally, her adrenals were in stage III exhaustion. After being put on the modified elimination diet and having the H. pylori infection treated, she had to reduce her diabetic medications by fifty percent. After six weeks, she had to stop them altogether because her glucose numbers were too low!

> Her chronic constipation was gone and her energy was better. Her stomach pain disappeared and she was sleeping better. She considered the change in her blood sugar "amazing." Her doctor had some disbelief about her blood sugar, but couldn't argue with the fact that she was completely stable while off medication.
>
> A recent conversation with her daughter-in-law confirmed that after several years she is still diabetes-free!

Overview

As you likely realize, diabetes is a common disorder that affects many Americans, compromising their health significantly. But you may not know about the association between diabetes and gluten. Repeatedly, gluten has been shown to be a factor in the development as well as the severity of diabetes. Diet is, of course, a big part of diabetic risk and control, but the importance of gluten in the diet is rarely stressed.

Type I Diabetes Associated With Gluten

Diabetes affects seven percent of the population, which amounts to approximately twenty-one million people in the United States alone. This results in a total cost of $132 billion, with $92 billion going to direct medical care and $40 billion to indirect productivity losses. There are two major types of diabetes, which include type I and type II. Type I diabetes is an autoimmune disease wherein the body's immune system attacks cells in the pancreas that produce insulin. Type II diabetes is much more common and is the result of the body's cells' resistance to responding to insulin. In terms of gluten sensitivity, type I diabetes is the condition directly associated with its intolerance.[225]

Type I diabetes is less common than type II diabetes, accounting for ten percent of all diabetics. It affects males and females equally, but tends to present earlier in life, often being diagnosed in childhood. Diabetes is basically a disorder of the body's metabolism. Glucose is our body's main source of energy. Our food is digested and broken down into glucose, and then glucose is absorbed into the bloodstream for our cells to use. In order for the glucose to go from the bloodstream to inside our cells, the hormone insulin is required. Insulin is produced by special cells, called beta cells, in the pancreas in response to a rise of glucose in the bloodstream. The insulin response is perfectly balanced, making sure that the glucose level in the blood doesn't get too low or too high.[226]

When type I diabetes develops, the immune system makes auto-antibodies against the beta cells of the pancreas. Once they are destroyed and reduced to a critically low number, the amount of insulin produced is insufficient to keep up with the glucose in the system. As a result, glucose increases in the bloodstream and causes many health problems. In patients with type I diabetes, insulin administration is required to survive.[227]

What Your Doctor Likely Told You About Diabetes

If you or somebody you know has type I diabetes, you are aware of the daily struggle of trying to keep glucose meticulously controlled. Having diabetes can lead to many other health problems including loss of vision, kidney failure, heart disease, strokes and nerve damage. Studies support that rigid control with insulin, diet and exercise reduce the chances of developing these serious health conditions.[228] Diabetes is one of the top causes of death, and sixty-five percent of diabetics die of heart disease.[229]

Environmental Factors Play a Part

Even though type I diabetes is known to be an autoimmune disorder, your doctor has likely not been able to tell you a reason for its develop-ment. Indeed, genetics play a part, but so do environmental factors such as diet and potential viral infections. The goals are to make the diag-nosis early and keep glucose controlled to normal levels as much as possible. This is monitored through daily glucose checks, wherein patients will sample their blood to see the glucose content. This helps them adjust their insulin dose so that hopefully, glucose can stay close to normal and reduce the risk of health complications.[230]

Dietary instructions are routinely aimed at preventing glucose overloads. Simple sugars, such as those found in many sweets, and simple starches can easily result in a rapid rise in glucose in the bloodstream, so these are monitored more closely. Complex carbohydrates, such as vegetables, some fruits and beans, are preferred in the diet because they allow a slower build up of glucose.

In looking toward future therapies, beta cell transplants are being investigated to allow a means for the body to start reproducing insulin again in adequate quantities.[231] Because type I diabetes affects many children and commits them to long lives of medical demands, it is important to find better treatments.

What You Need to Know About Type I Diabetes

While your doctor may have told you many things about your diabetes, gluten intolerance is not likely to have been one of them. However, there is a substantial amount of information linking the two conditions together. This makes intuitive sense since both gluten sensitivity and type I diabetes have autoimmune dysfunction at the root of their disease mechanisms. But gluten is more than just an associated autoimmune disorder. Gluten affects the onset and severity of type I diabetes, which suggests that it is more than just a casual association.

Type I Diabetics Are at Higher Risk of Gluten Sensitivity

Many research studies done on patients with celiac disease demonstrate a much higher risk of celiac disease in patients with type I diabetes compared to the normal population. As you may recall, celiac disease, a small subdivision of gluten sensitivity, is found in one percent of the general population. One researcher studied 261 people with type I diabetes and found that at least eight percent had celiac disease.[232] Another evaluated 269 children with type I diabetes, finding that 12.3 percent had celiac disease.[233] Two other studies using intestinal biopsies as their gold standard for diagnosing celiac disease found that 9.4 percent[234] and 8.8 percent[235] had celiac disease in large groups of type I diabetics.

While the occurrence of type II diabetes is over six percent of the population, type I diabetes occurs in less than one percent.[236] These findings clearly demonstrate the association of gluten sensitivity and type I diabetes as being well above the normal occurrence.

Timing and Length of Exposure to Gluten Increases Risk of Developing Type I Diabetes

To take it a step further, there is also good evidence that the timing and length of exposure to gluten affects the risk of developing type I diabetes. In a study of over 1,600 newborns of parents who had type I diabetes, the children given gluten foods prior to three months of age had much higher development of beta cell antibodies.[237] These are the cells that produce insulin, and so their destruction results, eventually, in type I diabetes. This suggests that early dosing with gluten in children at risk for diabetes can increase their risk of developing diabetes.

Non-Compliance to a Gluten-Free Diet Is a Bad Idea

But what about length of exposure? In one study, 158 patients with gluten sensitivity who were noncompliant with a gluten-free diet were compared to a group of gluten-sensitive patients who remained faithful to their gluten avoidance. The noncompliant group was found to have a significantly higher number of beta cell auto-antibodies.[238]

In a 2008 research report, another investigator found that gluten exposure increased the risk of type I diabetes in people at risk for diabetes.[239] He also found that these diabetic patients had early intestinal inflammation at the time of diagnosis. This intestinal inflammation was presumably caused by gluten and may explain how gluten increases the risk of type I diabetes. By disrupting the intestinal lining, gluten and other undigested food substances get across the lining, triggering immune reactions.

Study Recommends All Type I Diabetic Children Be Evaluated for Gluten Sensitivity

While the exact mechanism remains undefined, it is clear that gluten exposure in patients at risk for type I diabetes is a bad idea. A researcher in France, after studying 950 children with type I diabetes, recommended that all children with type I diabetes be tested for gluten sensitivity.[240] Other researchers, based on their own independent testing, likewise agree with this recommendation.[241]

Certainly, intestinal biopsies are not necessary, and these may fail to identify gluten-sensitive patients who don't have intestinal involvement. Lab testing of saliva and/or blood is the preferred method, and some support that testing for anti-tTG antibodies (those directed against the enzyme transglutaminase, which metabolizes gluten) is the most sensitive for diabetic patients.[242] The important point is to check, and to check early. Time is of the essence.

Diabetes Was Just One of Her Complaints

Annette W. was a pleasant, young lady who came to see us plagued by many complaints. Her symptoms ranged from tendonitis to diarrhea to high blood pressure, but she also was found to have an elevated blood glucose level, adding a diagnosis of diabetes to her list of health problems.

While her testing for gluten sensitivity was borderline and therefore not conclusive, she became convinced of her gluten sensitivity after eliminating gluten from her diet. Once off gluten, her blood glucose levels returned to normal, her joint pains resolved and she cut her blood pressure medications in half.

She started eating gluten again about two years later and once again experienced bad joint pain, in addition to weight gain. As a result, she stopped gluten, ate five small meals per day (she had been eating just lunch and dinner) and lost forty pounds over the course of nine months. She has now been effectively off gluten for five years and has had no further problems with diabetic symptoms.

In Annette's case, it is not clear if her diabetes was type I or type II. Since she was not taking insulin, it is less likely that it was type I, though early type I diabetics may simply have elevated blood sugar levels. Whether elimination of gluten allowed beta cells of the pancreas to recover, or whether associated weight loss prevented type II diabetes, gluten's role in her diabetic condition is clear.

Can Gluten-Free Diets Protect Against Diabetes?

While we have stressed the need to be tested early and avoid gluten if a diabetic risk exists, we have not yet spoken about the effects of a gluten-free diet on treating diabetes. Again, this appears to be mostly an issue of timing. If a patient has yet to develop diabetes, but is at risk, gluten-free diets appear protective. One study placed people at risk for type I diabetes on a gluten-free diet and compared them to people with similar risks on a gluten-containing diet. The outcome did show a beneficial, protective effect in the gluten-free group.[243]

Gluten-Free Diets Can Keep Diabetes Under Better Control

Other studies show different results if diabetes has already developed. In patients who already had beta cell antibodies, a gluten-free diet had no benefit in reducing the antibody level.[244] However, gluten-free diets in children who already have type I diabetes do allow for normal growth patterns and better ability to control the diabetes with insulin.[245]

Gluten's Causal Association With Type II Diabetes

While gluten may not have the same direct association with type II diabetes, gluten is often associated with being overweight. This can occur with adrenal gland exhaustion and with fat deposition in the abdominal area as the body deals with the chronic stress of gluten intolerance. Weight gain is the biggest risk factor, other than age, for developing type II diabetes.[246] So, in this fashion, gluten can also trigger type II diabetes. As mentioned earlier, multiple research studies demonstrate a much higher risk of gluten sensitivity in patients with type I diabetes compared to the normal population.

Gluten Can Cause Your Immune System to Attack Your Pancreas

In type I diabetes, the gluten's mechanism of causation likely involves the immune system, either directly or indirectly. Because gluten sensitivity is an autoimmune disorder, antibodies that are formed against gluten may cross-react against beta cells of the pancreas. This would result in attack and damage to these cells, eventually causing diabetes because insulin could not be adequately produced.

There Are Several Possible Mechanisms

For instance, it has been shown that antibodies formed against gluten by your body cross-react with brain tissues to cause some neurological disorders. This mechanism is also present in the bone, causing osteoporosis in gluten sensitivity. More research is needed to conclusively prove this mechanism between gluten and type I diabetes.

One researcher believes that gluten intolerance causes type I diabetes through the failure of the oral tolerance mechanism to develop early in life.[247] As we discussed earlier, when our immune systems are developing, they learn to ignore foods and "good" bacteria in our digestive tracts that are beneficial to us. This is defined as oral tolerance.

When this doesn't develop normally, immune reactions against foods such as gluten can develop. This failure of oral tolerance then leads to an overactive immune system not only attacking some food particles and beneficial bacteria but also tissues of the body, causing autoimmune disease. This would be another mechanism of how gluten could trigger diabetes.

Another likely mechanism is through direct inflammation of the intestinal lining. This lets gluten, as well as other food materials that are not properly digested, cross the lining into our bodies. Because they are not adequately digested, they can trigger immune responses, resulting in autoimmune disorders like type I diabetes.

Genetic Risk Shared Between Type I Diabetes and Gluten Sensitivity

And, lastly, because both type I diabetes and gluten sensitivity have genetic causes in part, the two conditions may share some genetic risks. Recent scientific research, published in *Nature Genetics* in March 2008, demonstrates that some gene segments associated with celiac disease share some of the gene segments responsible for type I diabetes. Like-wise, many of these same segments are felt to be critical for developing good immune system function. Therefore, having certain types of gene patterns would increase your risk of having both disorders.

It is surprising that, with this amount of solid information between gluten sensitivity and type I diabetes, more of this knowledge isn't main-stream. It has been our experience that gluten certainly is a factor in the development of diabetes, and the better this fact is realized, the better we can reduce the occurrence of diabetic disorders.

Summary

You realize how prevalent diabetes is within our society, and, by now, we hope you are beginning to appreciate how common gluten sensitivity is as well. There is a strong correlation between gluten sensitivity and type I diabetes, and every patient who is at risk for diabetes or already has diabetes should be tested for gluten intolerance. Simply having no digestive symptoms is not a reason to delay investigation.

In fact, the lack of any symptom is not a reason either, if you have family members with diabetes or gluten disorders. From the information above, you can clearly see that delaying the diagnosis while including gluten in your diet can lead to increased risk of diabetes as well as autoimmune disorders in general.

Gluten: "The Great Imitator of Our Time"

Gluten is a difficult protein to digest, and for many, this leads to intestinal lining inflammation and immune dysfunction. The number of people affected by gluten sensitivity is significantly underestimated. It has been called "the great imitator of our time" by some researchers.[248] Because gluten causes a variety of symptoms and affects so many bodily systems, it can mimic many other medical conditions.

For instance, gluten can cause joint symptoms, mimicking many types of arthritis; it can result in skin conditions, mimicking many varieties of rashes. It can cause sleep disturbances, mimicking primary sleep disorders. And, it can cause diabetes. If you are not aware of the association between gluten and diabetes, you will fail to seek gluten as the underlying problem. Don't wait for further research to demonstrate what is already apparent. Diabetes is just one of many health conditions that is influenced by gluten in the diet.

Twelve

Irritable Bowel Syndrome

Overview

Irritable bowel syndrome is another common health condition affecting a progressive number of people but without a clearly defined cause. As the name implies, irritable bowel syndrome, or IBS, is an uncomfortable syndrome resulting in abdominal complaints such as cramping, bloating, constipation and diarrhea. The basic premise is that altered bowel motility results in bowel function that is either too fast or too slow. Theories exist as to the cause, but to date, definitive reasons why this disorder is so prevalent are not known.

IBS Affects Up to Twenty Percent of Our Population

IBS develops before the age of thirty-five in more than half the cases, so, therefore, it is a disorder of young individuals. Women are affected much more than men, and the overall prevalence in our population is about ten to twenty percent. What is even more astounding is that approximately seventy percent of people with IBS have not sought any help or medical attention. In other words, they simply live with their symptoms.[249]

Up to Twenty-Five Percent of Gluten-Sensitive Patients Suffer From IBS

Studies looking at the occurrence of irritable bowel syndrome have shown that the risk of IBS in gluten sensitivity is quite high. Between twenty and fifty-five percent of all gluten-sensitive patients suffer IBS complaints. This is in contrast to a range of five to ten percent of the normal controls studied that met IBS criteria.[250]

Overlap of symptoms can occur between IBS and gluten sensitivity because abdominal pain, bowel irregularity and food intolerance can be common to both. In these studies, accepted criteria that define irritable bowel syndrome were utilized to help make a distinction as best as possible. The results of these studies indicate that a much higher number of gluten-sensitive people have IBS symptoms than the population in general; therefore, assessing anyone with IBS complaints for gluten intolerance is recommended.

IBS Significantly Impacts Quality of Life

Irritable bowel syndrome can be intermittent and mild or it can be relentlessly progressive and severe. The first goal is simply to seek medical attention. Without proper assessment, evaluation for root causes such as gluten sensitivity cannot be evaluated. IBS has a significant impact on quality of life and certainly should not be ignored.[251] While the disorder itself has not been linked to more malignant disorders such as intestinal cancers or other immune conditions, if it is secondary to gluten sensitivity, it certainly can be. Understanding that gluten is a potentially treatable condition for those who suffer IBS should encourage you to have an evaluation as soon as possible.

What Your Doctor Likely Told You About Irritable Bowel Syndrome

Irritable bowel syndrome can be a very frustrating condition. Like many conditions in medicine, the distinct cause is not well-defined for many individuals. Additionally, the symptoms of cramping, abdominal pain and bloating are nonspecific and can be related to many other disorders of the digestive tract.

The hallmark of IBS is a bowel pattern of diarrhea alternating with constipation intermittently, although variations exist with either constipation or diarrhea being predominant. Because of this, a set of criteria called the Rome criteria has been developed to help validate who has IBS and who does not.

The Rome criteria of IBS are as follows:

- Abdominal discomfort present at least twelve weeks out of the last twelve months
- Abdominal pain has at least two of these three features: pain relieved with bowel movement, a bowel movement at pain onset, or a change in bowel function with pain
- Change in bowel movement frequency present
- Change in bowel movement appearance present
- Uncontrolled urgency to have a bowel movement
- Difficulty passing bowel movement
- Mucus in your stool
- Bloating

These features should be present over the preceding year to meet IBS criteria. In addition, exacerbating factors such as large meals, medications, dietary factors, caffeine, stress and menstruation are typically described by most patients.[252]

The True Root Cause of IBS Is Often Missed

Many physicians focus on stress and conflict as being the main precipitants of irritable bowel syndrome. Different tests are ordered to determine if other conditions are causing the symptoms, but, oftentimes, these fail to show a cause. Medications are tried for relief of symptoms, but these may or may not be effective, depending on severity of the complaints. Both patients and doctors become frustrated with the lack of response, and a greater amount of attention is focused on psychological stress than often should be. This leaves you feeling as if your IBS problems are "all in your head."

As far as dietary factors, traditional medicine has recognized that gluten, casein (a milk protein), lactose and alcohol exacerbate IBS symptoms in many patients; however, very few doctors recommend an assessment of gluten sensitivity by lab testing or by elimination diet. In fact, we cannot recall a single patient in our clinic carrying a label of irritable bowel syndrome who had been previously told that gluten sensitivity might be their problem.

Many Theories but Few Cures

Obvious instructions to avoid dietary foods that trigger symptoms are the main approach, but formal gluten-free diet trials are rare. Most of the theories about irritable bowel syndrome stem from causes of impaired bowel wall motility and movement. Common theories include an impaired receptor for serotonin along the bowel wall. Ninety-five percent of the body's serotonin is in the digestive tract, and it is important for proper bowel function. If these serotonin receptors on the bowel wall are defective, serotonin is not transported back into the body. This results in increased amounts of serotonin in the bowel, which cause movement dysfunction of the bowel wall and increased sensitivity to pain.[253]

Other theories include immune attacks on the bowel wall as well as secondary injuries to the bowel after viral infections. These theories are less commonly held because IBS studies have failed to show damage to the bowel wall lining by endoscopy. Treatments mainly employed include medications that reduce the bowel wall muscle activity and movement. These include anti-spasmodics and anti-diarrheals.

Changing diet to include more or less fiber depending on the main complaints is also recommended. Smaller meals are usually recommended, as is avoiding triggering foods and situations. Many patients can end up being referred to psychologists to deal with stress issues as a last resort, when other treatments fail.[254]

She Had IBS for Thirty Years... and She Was Only Thirty-Two!

J.C. was a pleasant young lady, but by the time she arrived at our clinic, she was feeling much less than pleasant. She had suffered with stomachaches and a diagnosis of irritable bowel syndrome for thirty years. J. was only thirty-two years old.

Her lifelong symptoms included abdominal pain, recurring constipation and acid reflux. In addition, she complained of many other problems including fatigue, insomnia, joint aches and headaches. We diagnosed her with gluten sensitivity and after being off gluten for several weeks, she was able to discontinue the Zantac, for her acid reflux, as well as the ibuprofen, which she took for her joint pains and headaches. Her bowel complaints resolved entirely, her energy increased and her insomnia was gone. She could not believe that after three decades of suffering IBS, her symptoms were all secondary to gluten sensitivity!

What You Need To Know About IBS

As mentioned, the medical community is well aware that a significant percentage of patients with irritable bowel syndrome have gluten sensitivity as the root cause. But this continues to receive little attention. From reading the other sections of this book, you know that identifying gluten as a cause can be a challenge since the ill effects from the time you eat gluten-containing food can occur days, weeks and even months afterwards. Therefore, the traditional approach of avoiding foods that trigger your IBS is unlikely to include gluten in patients with irritable bowel syndrome since a relationship between gluten and IBS symptoms is often not apparent.

Study Recommends All IBS Patients Be Evaluated for Gluten Sensitivity

How many patients with IBS actually have gluten sensitivity? In a study examining 105 IBS patients, twelve were found to have biopsy-proven celiac disease. Roughly, this suggests that at least twelve percent have gluten sensitivity, though many gluten-sensitive patients have negative biopsies, as we know. Therefore, this statistic is likely higher. In this same study, all of these positive biopsy patients responded to a gluten-free diet. The authors recommended that all patients with irritable bowel syndrome be evaluated for gluten sensitivity on a regular basis.[255]

Gluten-Free Diet Benefits IBS Sufferers

Other researchers have also found similar results in terms of IBS patients and beneficial responses to gluten-free diets. One study sampled several irritable bowel syndrome patients and evaluated them for HLA DQ2 antigens and intestinal IgA antibodies. If you recall, gluten-sensitive patients commonly have the HLA gene and intestinal IgA antibodies against gluten. In the subsets of the IBS patients who had this HLA gene and positive intestinal antibodies, a beneficial response was noted in their IBS symptoms on a gluten-free diet.[256] Again, this supports that a percentage of IBS patients have gluten sensitivity as their root cause.

Routine Screening for Gluten Sensitivity Is Beneficial and Cost-Effective

Other IBS researchers have also suggested that routine testing for gluten sensitivity in irritable bowel syndrome is appropriate.[257] Cost analyses by some have shown that if more than one percent of the IBS patient population has gluten sensitivity, the screening for gluten intolerance is cost-effective. The amount of money saved on medical costs and lost productivity clearly substantiates this position.

Even from the standpoint of treating IBS in general without cost considerations, it was concluded that generalized screening for gluten sensitivity was warranted if more than eight percent of IBS patients had the disorder.[258] As referenced above, studies support that approximately twelve percent of IBS sufferers have gluten sensitivity, if not more.

A Blood Test Is a Good Screening Tool

One of the best screening tests for gluten sensitivity remains blood antibody testing. While this test do have expense, the benefit obtained clinically by defining the root cause and the amount of savings on future medical care are tremendous. If the prevalence of gluten sensitivity in irritable bowel syndrome is three percent or greater (which we know it is), then even antibody testing with anti-tTG antibodies on patients' blood is cost-effective as a generalized screening tool.[259]

It is well-established that of the many symptoms that can occur in gluten sensitivity, those symptoms of irritable bowel syndrome can significantly affect people's quality of life.[260] Identifying gluten sensitivity then becomes the only obstacle to implementing necessary treatment to provide significant benefit to these many patients.

Donna's IBS Linked Conclusively to Gluten

Donna S. came into our office with a five-year history of severe abdominal pain that typically occurred after eating. However, because the timing was extremely variable between eating and her symptoms, she had been unable to associate her complaints with any particular food. She had been diagnosed by her regular physician as having irritable bowel syndrome. Whenever she was in pain from her IBS, she ate innocuous foods like bagels and crackers.

Once she started a gluten elimination diet, and had a concurrent intestinal infection treated, she had no abdominal complaints at all. She also had suffered from severe environmental allergies, which had created constantly watery eyes. This, too, cleared up when she eliminated gluten.

About one year later, she had a relapse, with her symptoms returning. Her gluten lab test was repeated and her antibodies were found to be markedly elevated again. As it turned out, she was drinking a nutritional health drink that contained gluten and she occasionally was "cheating" with dessert. Once she stopped this, her symptoms once again abated.

A Negative Biopsy Does Not Rule Out Gluten Sensitivity

As previously noted, many gluten-sensitive patients will not have positive intestinal biopsies, but they will have positive blood lab testing more commonly. It is important to remember that a negative biopsy does not rule out gluten sensitivity and is not required for a diagnosis. In a sample of twenty-two patients with irritable bowel syndrome who had negative biopsies of the small intestine, yet positive results for blood antibody testing for gluten sensitivity, all demonstrated a beneficial response to a gluten-free diet. And all had resolution of their IBS symptoms.[261] This supports the need for better blood testing of IBS patients for gluten sensitivity as well as providing these patients with a clear benefit from appropriate treatment.

Summary

Although abdominal and bowel symptoms are common to many medical disorders, unique features do exist that enable the diagnosis of irritable bowel syndrome on a consistent basis. From research information, it appears that IBS is extremely common, with a range of ten to twenty percent in the general population. Additionally, it significantly affects quality of life and affects people in their younger, productive years. From this standpoint, it is important that causes of IBS are found and treated effectively.

While gluten may not represent the only cause of IBS symptoms, it clearly accounts for at least twelve percent of all irritable bowel syndrome cases. For this reason, checking for gluten sensitivity as a root cause is critical. Consistently, as with other gluten disorders, avoidance of gluten restores the normal bowel function in this subset of IBS individuals. The sooner the diagnosis is made, the sooner relief and quality of life can be restored.

Gluten Sensitivity Creates Many Problems Beyond IBS

While IBS has not been directly linked to other immune conditions or cancers of the digestive system, gluten intolerance has. Therefore, if gluten sensitivity is the cause of a person's IBS complaints, it is important for his or her long-term health to identify gluten as the culprit.

If you have been frustrated with the symptoms of irritable bowel syndrome, the lack of a defined cause, and the limited benefit of treatments, be sure your clinician considers gluten sensitivity as a potential cause of your complaints. Whether this is evaluated by blood testing or if a trial off gluten for several weeks is needed, finding gluten sensitivity as the problem can result in dramatic improvements in a very short time. While stress may play a role, irritable bowel syndrome is definitely not just "in your head." You may be pleasantly surprised when the elimination of gluten causes your symptoms to evaporate and restores your well being.

Thirteen

Thyroid Disorders

Overview

Thyroid dysfunction is an underestimated disease affecting millions of Americans. By recent assessments, hypothyroidism affects 8.9 percent of the population and hyperthyroidism is found in 1.1 percent. Therefore, ten percent of all Americans have some type of thyroid dysfunction, which amounts to about thirteen million people.[262]

Many people are unaware that they have a thyroid condition since many times, symptoms may be mild or lacking. Low thyroid function, or hypothyroidism, commonly can present with fatigue only. Many people will attribute this to poor sleep, stress, etc. but never consider a thyroid condition. The most common cause of thyroid disorders is immune system dysfunction. Autoimmune disorders, as you will soon see, can cause the thyroid gland to make too little or too much thyroid hormone.

Gluten Sensitivity Correlates to Thyroid Disorders

This is where gluten comes into play. Despite ample literature demonstrating the correlation between gluten sensitivity and thyroid disease, you aren't likely aware of this correlation. Patients who present to our clinic on thyroid medication or having been diagnosed with thyroid disorders consistently have not been told by their clinicians that gluten may be the root cause. Even in routine clinical practice, many doctors are not aware of these important research findings.

Gluten Plays an Important Role in Prevention

Thyroid disease is a very treatable condition with medication, but if undiagnosed, it can lead to serious complications. This can develop if the thyroid hormone levels are excessively high or low. While gluten may not prevent the need for thyroid dysfunction treatments, it does play a role in prevention. And this is where isolating gluten sensitivity can have a significant impact on you and your children.

Both Hypo- and Hyperthyroid Conditions Relate to Gluten Sensitivity

In the subsequent sections, you will learn about the two main types of thyroid disorders associated with gluten sensitivity, which are also the two most common thyroid disorders. One is Hashimoto's disease, which results in low thyroid function. The other is Grave's disease, which results in high thyroid function, or hyperthyroidism. Both of these are autoimmune disorders, and both are associated with gluten intolerance in many individuals. By understanding the basics of each and how they relate to gluten and your diet, you will appreciate the importance of gluten-intolerance testing.

For us, we see gluten-related thyroid dysfunction frequently in our clinic, and there is ample scientific evidence that supports the association as well. We will first inform you of what is common knowledge regarding these thyroid conditions, and then we will describe their specific relationships to gluten. By this chapter's conclusion, you will clearly see that gluten sensitivity screening should be performed on anyone at risk for thyroid disease.

What Your Doctor Likely Told You About Grave's Disease

Grave's disease is an autoimmune disorder that attacks the thyroid gland, resulting in hyperthyroidism. Classically, it affects more women than men and presents after the age of twenty years. Normally, you would suspect that a direct attack on the thyroid gland would cause less thyroid hormone to be made, but this is not the case in Grave's disease. The autoimmune antibodies produced in this instance target a thyroid gland receptor. Once the antibody attaches to the receptor, it stimulates the thyroid gland to make more thyroid hormone, resulting in a hyperthyroid condition.[263]

The Many Symptoms of Hyperthyroidism

Because your thyroid hormone controls your body's rate of metabolism, higher thyroid levels cause your metabolic rate to rise. This results in many symptoms that include anxiety, fast heart rate, irritability, insomnia, weight loss, diarrhea and brittle hair. Every process in your body is accelerated including your heart beat, your digestion, your brain activity, daily calorie usage, etc. This is why the various symptoms listed above develop.[264]

Other complications with Grave's disease also develop. A condition known as exophthalmos is common, wherein the tissues and muscles behind the eyes swell and enlarge when thyroid hormone is chronically elevated. This causes the eyes to protrude excessively from the eye sockets. This can lead to excessive eye tearing, light sensitivity and eye irritation. Other complications include brittle bones and osteoporosis as bone destruction accelerates with increased metabolism. When severe, even heart rhythm disturbances and heart failure can develop.[265]

There Is No Established Cause

Causes of this autoimmune disorder are unknown. Thyroid disorders do run in families and genetic risks are present, but these do not explain the entire reason for developing Grave's disease. Viral infections, stress and other factors have been suggested but poorly validated to date; therefore, an accepted cause is not uniformly described.[266]

Diagnosis Is Straightforward

Diagnosis of Grave's disease is fairly straightforward. Lab tests define an elevation of thyroid hormone (called thyroxin) and a low TSH level (thyroid stimulating hormone). If you recall from earlier chapters, TSH stimulates the thyroid gland to make thyroid hormone, but when thyroid hormone level is high, the production of TSH is shut off through a feedback loop. So, if TSH is low and thyroxin is high, a diagnosis of hyperthyroidism is made.

Another way to diagnose thyroid disease is through radioactive iodine uptake. Iodine is required for the production of thyroxin. If production of thyroxin is increased, more iodine will be needed and used by the thyroid gland. Using radioactive iodine allows radiology tests to measure this uptake and can likewise support a diagnosis of hyperthyroidism.[267]

Treatments Are Symptomatic

Generally, treatment comes in three forms. First there are medications that suppress the production of thyroid hormone. Secondly, higher doses of radioactive iodine can be given, which eventually destroys enough of the thyroid gland to reduce thyroxin levels. Lastly, surgical removal of the thyroid gland in total or in part can be effective.[268] Any of these therapies are quite effective, but nothing targets the reason for the underlying autoimmune reaction. In this regard, the treatments are mainly symptomatic.

Hashimoto's Disease

The most common autoimmune disorder causing low thyroid function, or hypothyroidism, is Hashimoto's disease. While the autoimmune attack in Grave's disease causes activation of a receptor and increased thyroid hormone production, the autoimmune attack in Hashimoto's results in destruction of the thyroid gland and eventually drops thyroxin production. This disorder occurs most commonly in middle-aged women, though anyone may develop it, and it often runs in families, suggesting a genetic component in its causation.[269]

The Symptoms of Hypothyroidism

Because the immune attack gradually damages the thyroid gland, symptoms are often very slow in developing. Likewise, many people may have low thyroid by blood testing but have no symptoms at all early in the disorder. Generally, fatigue and sluggishness are most common at the beginning, but because these are nonspecific, many people simply attribute these complaints to poor sleep, being overweight or aging. As thyroid hormone slowly declines, so does the body's metabolic rate. This reduction eventually results in symptoms.[270]

Other symptoms that then develop can include intolerance to cold temperatures, constipation, hoarseness of the voice, dry skin, weight gain, muscle aches and joint pains. When significant, even depression and memory loss can develop as brain activity also begins to slow. One of the least-known symptoms associated with Hashimoto's disease is high cholesterol.[271] A slower metabolism results in an accumulation of cholesterol in the blood as the liver does not process these fatty substances as well.

Chronically, Hashimoto's disease can lead to more serious complications. Goiter, which is an enlargement of the thyroid gland, develops as the low levels of thyroid hormone trigger TSH to be continually produced. TSH is trying to stimulate the thyroid gland to make more thyroxin, even though it cannot. As a result, the thyroid tissue gradually grows in size under the constant stimulation of TSH, which causes goiter.

There's a Risk of Developing Heart Disease and Depression

Also, having elevated cholesterol can lead to heart disease and heart attacks if untreated. Depression has been mentioned, but when low thyroid function is severe, even confusion and delirium can develop.[272] Fortunately, thyroid hormone replacement is very effective in alleviating the symptoms and complications of Hashimoto's disease. Again, it is not getting to the root of the problem but instead replacing thyroid hormone, in the form of a tablet, that the thyroid gland can no longer make.

Hashimoto's disease is diagnosed by blood testing. The actual antibody that causes Hashimoto's can be measured to verify the disease, and the levels of thyroxin and TSH help complete the picture, identifying how low thyroid function has become. This also helps determine the dose of thyroid hormone replacement needed.[273] Thyroid replacement has become quite common, as has the occurrence of thyroid disorders. But it is time to focus on the underlying cause rather than on medication replacement only.

What You Need to Know About Thyroid Disease

If it is so well-known that gluten sensitivity is associated with autoimmune thyroid diseases, then why isn't testing for gluten-related problems part of a thyroid medical workup? Good question, but there is no good answer. Numerous studies link the two disorders together, and, likewise, studies support that family members of individuals with autoimmune thyroid disorders should be tested for gluten sensitivity as well. This lack of awareness was one of the reasons why we chose to write this book.

Gluten Sensitivity Markedly Raises Your Risk for Thyroid Disease

Let's go back to the association between gluten sensitivity and autoimmune thyroid diseases. First, how many patients with gluten sensitivity have autoimmune thyroid disease? In other words, if gluten sensitivity is a known condition in a person, what are the chances they also have thyroid disease compared to the normal population?

From the data listed in this chapter's overview, we know that about ten percent of the normal population has thyroid disorders. In a study examining fifty-two patients with gluten sensitivity, 19.2 percent were found to have clinical hypothyroidism, and another 21.2 percent were found to have subclinical hypothyroid disease. "Subclinical" means that their blood tests supported low thyroid function even though they had no complaints. This study, therefore, found that forty percent of gluten patients have thyroid dysfunction.[274]

Patients With Autoimmune Disease Show a Prevalence of Gluten Sensitivity

In contrast, how many patients with autoimmune thyroid disorders have gluten sensitivity? Here, many studies have provided good, and consistent, statistics. In a study of 276 patients with autoimmune thyroid disease, 5.4 percent had celiac disease based on gluten antibody testing or intestinal biopsy.[275] Another study reported that thirty-one patients out of 113 thyroid patients (twenty-seven percent) had gluten sensitivity by gluten antibody testing.[276] And yet another study of 400 patients with either Grave's disease or Hashimoto's disease demonstrated that 5.5 percent had anti-gliadin antibodies.[277] There are additional studies, but most report around a five-percent prevalence of celiac disease if autoimmune thyroid disease is present.

The question, of course, is whether five percent is a high percentage or not. Another study compared 456 patients with autoimmune thyroid disease with blood samples from a normal control population. The patients' blood samples, as well as the normal blood samples, were evaluated for anti-endomysial antibodies (EM-Ab), which is one of the sensitive, gluten-related antibody tests. In the normal samples, the test was positive in only 0.5 percent, but in the thyroid disease group, the test was positive in 2.2 percent.[278] This means that gluten sensitivity is between four and five times more common in patients with autoimmune thyroid disorders.

Thyroid Disease, Diabetes and Gluten Sensitivity—All Linked

In researching this association between thyroid disorders and gluten sensitivity, you may wonder why these two disorders would be linked together. It appears that this is due to common risks for developing autoimmune disease. In a condition known as autoimmune polyglandular syndrome, gluten sensitivity, diabetes and thyroid disease are often linked together. This may be due to common genetic risks for autoimmune syndromes among all of these disorders. Or, it may be that gluten sensitivity results in intestinal dysfunction, exposing the immune system to undigested food materials and infectious organisms that lead to other autoimmune diseases.

In a study looking at ninety-two people with immune thyroid disorders, ninety people with non-immune thyroid disorders and 256 normal people, 4.3 percent of the immune thyroid group had gluten-related antibodies. This was compared to only 1.1 percent of the non-immune thyroid group and 0.4 percent of the normal group.[279] These findings, indeed, support an autoimmune link between the two conditions of gluten sensitivity and autoimmune thyroid disease.

Studies Support the Link

Along the lines of polyglandular syndrome, a study examining 370 children and adolescents with type I diabetes were screened for autoimmune thyroid antibodies and for gluten-related antibodies. In these children, who were followed over a period of several years, 11.4 percent developed thyroid antibodies and 3.2 percent developed gluten-related antibodies. Interestingly, in those children who developed gluten antibodies and thyroid antibodies, the gluten antibodies developed first, in most cases.[280]. This could mean that gluten sensitivity induced thyroid immune disease by causing disruption to the intestinal lining in some children.

Damage to the Thyroid Occurs Before Symptoms Develop

In another pediatric study, 573 consecutive children were examined in a hospital setting. The gluten-sensitive children were then evaluated with thyroid antibody testing and thyroid blood testing. Out of the gluten-sensitive children, 26.2 percent had thyroid antibodies, but only two-thirds of this group had blood testing showing hypothyroidism.[281] This means that thyroid antibodies circulate in many gluten-sensitive children long before they develop thyroid symptoms.

Prevention Is Key When It Comes to Thyroid Disease

In this same pediatric study, a gluten-free diet was implemented in the gluten-sensitive group, and follow-up testing of the thyroid antibodies and thyroid replacement dosages were performed. The researchers unfortunately found no effect on thyroid disease or treatment with a gluten-free diet.[11] In an adult study of fifty-two gluten-sensitive patients with immune thyroid disease, similar findings were reported. Thyroid antibodies increased with age, and they increased despite a gluten-free diet.[4] In one small study looking at five patients with autoimmune thyroid disease and gluten sensitivity, a gluten-free diet did allow a reduction in the thyroid medication dosage but no other benefits.[282].

And When It Comes To Prevention, Gluten Avoidance Is Critical

From this information, two things are clear. First, gluten sensitivity is increased in patients with autoimmune thyroid disease, and thyroid disease is increased in patients with gluten sensitivity. Secondly, once both conditions are present, a gluten-free diet will help gluten symptoms and the risk of developing other serious diseases, but it does not eliminate thyroid dysfunction. It may be that in order to prevent thyroid disease in gluten-sensitive patients, avoiding gluten before the onset of thyroid antibodies may be the key.

If You're Sensitive to Gluten Please Get Your Thyroid Evaluated

As a general guideline, any patient with gluten sensitivity should be evaluated for thyroid dysfunction such as Grave's disease or Hashimoto's disease. Likewise, any patient with thyroid disorder should be tested for gluten sensitivity. Some researchers strongly suggest testing any first-degree family member for gluten sensitivity if they suffer from autoimmune thyroid disease or type I diabetes.[283] All of this information supports a common immune mechanism between gluten sensitivity and immune thyroid disease.

Another Reason Early Diagnosis of Gluten Sensitivity Is Important

If gluten exposure in gluten-sensitive patients triggers the development of autoimmune thyroid disease, making a diagnosis of gluten intolerance early is very important. If thyroid disease is already present, diagnosing gluten sensitivity, of course, is still important. At the very least, gluten-containing diets in gluten-intolerant patients can hinder the absorption of thyroid medication, thus making it difficult to treat the thyroid disorder.[284].

Screening Is Easy

As far as testing, studies investigating gluten intolerance and immune thyroid disease show that blood antibody testing for gluten is a good screening tool. Both antibodies for transglutaminase (tTG-Ab) and endomysial tissue (EM-Ab) are useful in detecting early gluten sensitivity in these thyroid patients.[285] One study demonstrated that anti-gliadin antibodies had high sensitivity in identifying Grave's disease patients with gluten sensitivity.[286] Overall, routine blood testing is adequate and intestinal biopsy is not required. If blood testing is questionable, a gluten elimination diet is the next screening measure for assessment.

Summary

Now that you have been adequately supplied with the evidence, you realize that diagnosing gluten sensitivity is very important in relationship to immune thyroid diseases. What is most disturbing is that, according to current scientific studies, once thyroid disease has developed, treating the gluten sensitivity has little effect on the thyroid disorder other than helping intestinal absorption of thyroid medication.

Because gluten can trigger immune disorders like type I diabetes, dermatitis herpetiformis, rheumatoid arthritis and others, it seems obvious that gluten can also be the root cause of thyroid disease through immune mechanisms. It is important to diagnose gluten sensitivity before immune thyroid disease ever develops, to have a potential effect on curbing the need for thyroid treatment.

Existing Thyroid Disease Can Lead to Further Autoimmune Diseases

If Grave's disease or Hashimoto's disease has already developed, certainly a gluten-free diet for gluten sensitivity is necessary to prevent the many other health complications that can develop. But it is also important so that thyroid medication can be absorbed effectively from the digestive tract. Because thyroid disease increases with age, and because it is higher in the gluten-intolerant population, periodic thyroid testing is recommended in all gluten-sensitive patients over time.

If you have thyroid disease, or have a family member who does, you should be evaluated not only for your thyroid gland function but also for gluten sensitivity. And the sooner, the better. Delaying the diagnosis of gluten sensitivity only places your health at greater risk.

Fourteen

Osteoporosis

Overview

Osteoporosis and its lesser known predecessor, osteopenia, affect millions of Americans and account for a significant degree of disability. In this chapter, you will learn how gluten causes these conditions and how it does so through multiple mechanisms. Gluten's affecting the absorption of needed nutrients, triggering of immune dysfunction and causing hormonal imbalances are some of the important pathways that can lead to bone loss as people age, when they have gluten sensitivity.

Forty-Four Million People Affected in the U.S. Alone

Currently, statistics show that ten million people in the U.S. alone suffer from osteoporosis, and an additional thirty-four million have osteopenia. Literally, osteopenia means "a deficiency of bone" and osteoporosis means "porous bone." The density of bone material is what determines whether you have osteopenia or osteoporosis.

Standards for what healthy bone density should be are well-established through tests on millions of people. If bone density is reduced to a mild to moderate degree, this is termed osteopenia.[287] If bone density is moderate to severely reduced, it is defined as osteoporosis. Gradations of severity are determined by how far one's bone density is from normal.

Caucasian and Asian Women Are at Greater Risk

Women are twice as affected by osteoporosis and osteopenia as men, but men, indeed, suffer from osteoporosis as well. Both osteopenia and osteoporosis increase with age, and some races are affected more than others. Caucasian and Asian races are affected greater than black or Hispanic races in general. While these disorders have been prevalent for some time, the increasing age of the population is causing the frequency of the condition to rise significantly.[288]

As a result, pharmaceutical companies have cashed in on developing new medications that are used to treat these disorders.[289] Not only, in this chapter, will we highlight gluten's role in osteopenia and osteoporosis, but we will also demonstrate serious concerns about the use of these medications.

Is Gluten Sensitivity a Root Cause of Osteoporosis?

Bone health in particular is affected by diet and lifestyle, and these conditions can be changed to improve your health. Through several mechanisms, gluten can be a root cause of these conditions. It is our intent to make sure that you are aware of all of them and how common gluten sensitivity is in relationship to bone disorders. First, let's take a look at what you might have been told already concerning osteoporosis and osteopenia.

What Your Doctor Likely Told You About Osteoporosis

Medically, osteoporosis and osteopenia share the same risk factors and the same causation. As far as risks, certainly, being female and becoming older increase your chances of having these disorders. There is no way to change these parameters. In addition, both have a higher occurrence within families supporting a genetic risk. Again, not much you can do about that either. But several dietary and lifestyle factors do influence the occurrence of osteoporosis and osteopenia.

Your Bones Are Constantly Remodeling Themselves

Bones are constantly changing at every stage of life. You may have thought that bones stop growing after you reach adulthood, but that is not the case. Your bones are constantly undergoing a process called remodeling. Remodeling occurs as a balance between bone growth and bone destruction mold the bone into its strongest condition. For instance, if you decided to take up mountain climbing, there may be different stress points on your skeleton compared to your prior activities. Certain bones, and locations in those bones, need to strengthen while other areas may need less support. Bone remodeling allows your bones to adapt to your level of activity as you age.[290]

After age thirty-five, we begin destroying more bone than we build. This can be very slow, or it can be accelerated, depending on your risk factors. People with larger frames have a larger "bone bank" and are less likely to develop osteoporosis or osteopenia compared to someone with a thin frame. Other risk factors also include alcohol use, tobacco use, excessive caffeine intake and use of certain medications. In particular, steroids and certain types of anti-depressants, called SSRIs, can cause a more rapid loss of bone.[291]

Your Bones Like You to Be Active

Because our bones respond to activity, exercise helps promote good bone strength and density, whereas a sedentary lifestyle can cause bone loss to occur more rapidly. This is why daily exercise is a good, preventative measure against developing osteoporosis. Diet is also a major factor in protecting you from osteoporosis or accelerating its development. The most important nutrients include calcium and vitamin D.

Have Your Vitamin D Levels Checked

Vitamin D is a very important nutrient for our bodies. While we can produce large amounts of vitamin D through our skin from sunlight exposure, recent evidence supports that sunscreen, civilized lifestyles and locations away from the equator have made this a limited source for most of us. Therefore, a large part of this nutrient is obtained orally, in fortified milk, certain fish like mackerel and salmon, orange juice and a few other food sources. Vitamin D is needed to absorb calcium from our diet into our body, so it can build strong bones. Without enough vitamin D, calcium is likely to be low.[292]

Calcium and phosphorus are the necessary minerals to create new bone formation. Various hormones, such as calcitonin, thyroxin, cortisol, estrogen and others, guide bone remodeling, but calcium, phosphorous and vitamin D are crucial for this balance to be effective.[293] As a result, dietary deficiencies of either vitamin D or calcium can be a cause of osteoporosis and osteopenia. Anything that affects the digestive tract, hindering absorption of these micronutrients, places one at risk.

Bone Loss Occurs Silently

Regarding symptoms, a big problem with osteoporosis, and with osteopenia in particular, is that symptoms are absent during the early period of bone loss. A fracture of the spine, hip or wrist may be the first indication that these conditions are present. Certainly, fractures are painful and slow to heal because normal bone remodeling is affected. Other symptoms can include stooped posture, loss of overall height and generalized bone pain or back pain.[294] However, since symptoms coincide with significant bone loss, waiting for symptoms is not recommended. Testing allows earlier diagnosis and a much better chance at effective intervention.

Have Your Bone Density Evaluated

The diagnosis of osteopenia or osteoporosis is made by measuring the actual density of your bones and comparing it to normal. Radiology tests that are common include DEXA scans (dual energy x-ray absortiometry), ultrasounds and quantitative CT imaging. Generally, these examinations are recommended for women over age sixty-five, postmenopausal women with at least one risk factor, women with spine abnormalities, women in early menopause, women on steroids and women with endocrine disorders affecting hormone levels.[295]

While lifestyle and dietary treatments are the safest and best ways to treat osteoporosis, the use of medications is abundant in treating this condition. Initially, oral estrogens were used, but they have been found to increase breast and uterine cancers in many women. Other estrogen creams or medications, like Evista, that mimic estrogen's effect on bones, are being used with a presumptively safer profile.

Medications for Osteoporosis Have Some Pitfalls

Most common, these days, is the use of biphosphonates.[296] These drugs, like Fosamax and Boniva, keep existing bone from being destroyed; thus, the density of the bone is better. But the bone has become denser with older, brittle bone, not newly formed bone.[297] If you have been diagnosed with osteoporosis, there is a good chance you have been prescribed one of these medications. We will discuss some of their potential negative side effects later in this chapter.

Diet Plays a Role in Osteoporosis

Overall, osteopenia and osteoporosis are well-known conditions in aging individuals. While some risk factors are unchangeable, other known factors affecting osteoporosis offer great potential to prevent these conditions and avoid unnecessary treatments. Diet happens to be a significant factor that has the power to prevent these disorders, and this is where gluten sensitivity plays a significant role. Let's look at some of the ways in which gluten can lead to these unfortunate bone conditions.

Dorothy's Osteoporosis Miracle

Dorothy was diagnosed with severe osteoporosis well before being diagnosed with gluten intolerance in her sixties. In addition to her regular regimen of care, which included gentle exercise and good dietary intake of minerals and calcium, she also began a gluten-free diet. Symptomatically, she felt better, describing herself as "stronger." More importantly, her repeat bone density scan, performed two years later, showed an improvement, which is quite uncommon.

Her doctor at the time was quite perplexed. Most of the time, serial bone density scans, at best, hopefully show stability with adequate treatment, but in Dorothy's case, gluten elimination seemed to provide additional benefit. How did this happen and by what mechanism? Read on!

What You Need to Know About Osteoporosis and Osteopenia

As you can see from the above discussion, any disorder that affects the intestinal lining has the potential to disrupt vitamin D and calcium absorption, thus secondarily affecting bone health. And, medically, if a diagnosis of celiac disease or other intestinal disorder is known, it will routinely be addressed. However, despite this knowledge, we rarely see a routine assessment for gluten sensitivity in our patients who present with osteopenia or osteoporosis. Several times, we have successfully been able to improve our patients' bone health by eliminating gluten from their diets and implementing better dietary and lifestyle changes.

Because gluten affects the body in so many different ways in relationship to osteoporosis, this section will be divided into the different mechanisms of how gluten causes poor bone health. In addition, the ill effects of many osteoporosis medications are underappreciated, and we want you to be aware of those serious risks to your health. By the end of the chapter, you will understand why anyone with osteopenia, osteoporosis or risks for either condition should be tested for gluten sensitivity.

Mechanism #1: Gluten's Effects on Vitamin D and Calcium

Bones need calcium to stay healthy, since calcium is a basic nutrient for new bone formation. Insufficient calcium causes reduced new-bone growth and results in weaker bones. Calcium needs vitamin D in order to be fully absorbed from our diets. Insufficient vitamin D secondarily causes low calcium levels, which then cause weakened bones.

Let's go one step further. Vitamin D needs an intact intestinal lining in order to be absorbed properly itself and facilitate calcium absorption throughout the body. A damaged intestinal lining affects bone health through this mechanism, which is where gluten sensitivity comes into play.

Gluten Sensitivity Affects Your Ability to Absorb Vitamin D and Calcium

Interestingly, the ability of the intestinal lining to absorb vitamin D and calcium is affected early in gluten sensitivity. If you recall, the intestinal lining has small, finger-like projections, called villi, that allow an increased surface area for absorbing nutrients. Vitamin D is actually absorbed most effectively at the ends of these villi.

When gluten sensitivity is present, the tips of the villi are the first area affected, and vitamin D absorption from the diet is impaired early in the process. That means that long before a person may have gluten-related symptoms, vitamin D (and therefore calcium) is having difficulty getting absorbed into the body.

The other nutrient that is also absorbed from the ends of the villi is lactose, which is a sugar carbohydrate in milk products. Gluten-sensitive patients are often lactose intolerant as well because of this phenomenon. Two things can result from this. First, if lactose intolerance is known, then milk products are reduced or avoided. This is one source of vitamin D. Secondly, if lactose intolerance is not known, continued dietary intake of lactose can result in diarrhea. Diarrhea speeds the food material through the intestines, allowing less time for nutrient absorption.

Study Reveals That Forty Percent of Osteoporotic Women Have Gluten Sensitivity

In a study examining thirty-three patients with osteoporosis, all under fifty-five years of age, thirteen were found to be gluten-sensitive. This is forty percent of young osteoporosis patients! Once they were placed on a gluten-free diet, all demonstrated an increase in both calcium and vitamin D levels without any other dietary changes. The authors, of course, recommended that all patients with osteoporosis be evaluated for gluten sensitivity.[298] An excellent idea, in our opinion.

Gluten-Sensitive Children Already Show Calcium Deficiencies

Children are not immune to this process either. Another researcher examined thirty-four gluten-sensitive children who were untreated, twenty-eight who were gluten-sensitive and on a gluten-free diet for a year, and sixty-four normal, unaffected children. Out of the three groups, 17.6 percent of the untreated group had low calcium levels whereas only 3.6 percent of the treated group showed this finding.

The Same Children Also Show Decreased Bone Density

In addition, bone density testing was performed in these children. While the treated group and normal children had equal bone density values, the untreated group's bone density was significantly lower.[299] These children had no bone symptoms and, likewise, would have never been evaluated for poor bone health. This stresses the need for early diagnosis and intervention. Even in the elderly, unexplained low calcium should prompt an assessment for gluten sensitivity since standard measures of treating osteoporosis and osteopenia can be ineffective if gluten is the root cause.[300]

Achieving Normal Vitamin D Levels Should Be a Goal

It is worth mentioning that the prevalence of vitamin D deficiency among all individuals is underappreciated as well. While vitamin D can be produced by our skin in large amounts when exposed to sunshine and ultraviolet light, the current use of sunscreen, the limited exposure to midday sun and the fact that many people live away from equatorial regions have resulted in a heavier reliance on oral methods of obtaining vitamin D. Unfortunately, foods rich in vitamin D, like milk, orange juice and salmon, make up a small portion of most diets, and oral supplements provided by health professionals appear to provide amounts of vitamin D that are too low to address a deficiency condition.[301]

In order to achieve optimal vitamin D levels in the bloodstream, daily supplements should be in the range of 3000 IU, rather than 800 IU. This dose has been routinely studied without risk of toxicity.[302] By keeping vitamin D levels in the normal range, calcium will be maximally absorbed to meet the needs of your bone structure. Not only is the ability to absorb vitamin D and calcium important, but so is the proper intake.

Mechanism #2: Gluten's Effect on the Immune System

As noted in many other affiliated diseases, gluten causes many health problems through immune system disruptions. To review, there are three main immune problems that can occur with gluten sensitivity. First, because gluten sensitivity develops in part due to a genetic risk, people with gluten sensitivity have HLA genes that regulate the immune system and make them vulnerable to gluten sensitivity. These same genes can also make the same person susceptible to other autoimmune disorders.

Secondly, when antibodies are made against gluten or its related enzymes in an individual, these antibodies may attack normal body tissues because the tissues look similar to gluten or the enzyme's structure. This type of autoimmune development is called "mimicry," since the tissue's structure mimics the structure of gluten.

Lastly, exposure to gluten in a patient with gluten sensitivity can result in damage to the intestinal lining. This results in a leakiness that allows poorly digested food particles and disease-causing organisms access to our bodies. These truly are foreign to our immune systems and can result in an immune response that normally should not occur.

Your Own Immune System May Be Damaging Your Bones

In osteopenia and osteoporosis, there is now evidence that immune mechanisms related to gluten exist. In gluten sensitivity, one of the antibodies that can develop is against the tissue transglutaminase or tTG. This is the enzyme that helps digest gluten and often serves as the focus of an immune attack once it's attached to the gluten proteins. Interestingly, bone also has its own transaminases that are responsible for the formation and resorption of bone. It has been shown that anti-tTG antibodies from blood samples of gluten-sensitive patients cross-react with bone's transaminases more than fifty percent of the time. Tests also demonstrate that this cross-reactivity and total antibody levels decrease once these individuals are placed on a gluten-free diet.[303]

Therefore, the attack that is originally launched against gluten and its protein complexes gets "confused" and also attacks similar structures in bones and cartilage, resulting in their destruction. This, in turn, prevents the normal bone process from occurring, which leads to osteopenia and osteoporosis. Other researchers also have made the comment that the link between gluten sensitivity and osteoporosis is not simply a dietary issue of calcium and vitamin D. Immune system proteins affect bone formation and resorption. As a result, the only long-term option of treatment is avoiding gluten completely.[304]

The Attack Is Silent yet Progressive

What is concerning is that immune mechanisms related to gluten sensitivity start early in life and may be asymptomatic and silent for decades. Even if calcium and vitamin D levels are normal, gluten can still be causing bone weakening by triggering autoimmune attacks on the bone. One report described evaluating forty-one children with gluten sensitivity who had been diagnosed at least one year prior. Of these, forty-nine percent had decreased bone mineral density of their tibial (shin) bones on radiology scans. In the children who had been on a gluten-free diet, this figure was twenty-six percent while those not on a gluten-free diet totaled sixty-eight percent.[305] The fact that twenty-six percent still had reduced bone density despite diet treatment suggests that gluten mechanisms were present well before diagnosis and that they affected normal bone growth.

Once Again, Early Diagnosis Is the Key

Another study examined 165 adults who had been diagnosed with gluten sensitivity. Twenty-five percent of these patients had suffered fractures as a result of osteoporosis, compared to eight percent in an age-matched control group. In this twenty-five-percent group, eighty percent of the individuals had fractures prior to their confirmed diagnosis of gluten sensitivity.[306] This stresses the point of making an early diagnosis.

Mechanism #3: Gluten's Effect on Hormones

While vitamin D is labeled a vitamin, it indeed has many hormonal effects. However, since vitamin D was covered above, we will not discuss it again in this section in relationship to gluten. Instead, we will focus on the two other hormone systems that are influenced by gluten sensitivity.

The largest is through the adrenal system and the other is through thyroid function.

Stressed Adrenal Glands Can Cause Osteoporosis

If you recall from the earlier chapter on adrenal function, gluten can cause chronic stress to one's body, resulting in adrenal exhaustion. Whether it is from dietary factors, infections, cancer or mental factors, the adrenal glands can become secondarily stressed. Under these conditions, the adrenals produce greater stress hormone, called cortisol.[307]

Cortisol is similar to the drug prednisone, and prednisone is known to cause osteoporosis and osteopenia. While a history of chronic prednisone use is an indication for early screening for osteoporosis, the same recommendations are not made for chronic stress, which can have the same effects created through an exhausted adrenal system.

Weakened Adrenal Glands Make Less Estrogen, Which Affects Bone Density

Additionally, when chronic stress from gluten sensitivity stimulates the adrenal gland to produce cortisol, the adrenal gland selectively makes cortisol, neglecting the production of other hormones, including estrogen.[308] That means two things. First, reduced levels of estrogen affect bone remodeling and bone health, accelerating bone loss. Secondly, a reduction in estrogen production can cause early menopause, which is a risk factor for osteoporosis as well. As gluten causes continued inflammation and immune-system activation, the adrenal glands attempt to balance this stress with cortisol as long as they can. This is a common mechanism of how gluten causes osteopenia and osteoporosis.

Men Are Not Immune to This Stressor

For men, low testosterone has been identified as a risk factor for osteoporosis.[309] In the same way that gluten causes a reduction in estrogen production, gluten also causes a decrease in testosterone production.

With the chronic stress of gluten sensitivity, the adrenals curb testosterone production by selectively making cortisol instead.[310] Again, this places men at a similar risk through these hormonal changes, invoked by gluten.

Study Proves That Gluten-Free Diet Improves Bone Density

If you wonder to what extent gluten can cause these hormonal changes in osteoporosis, let us give you an example from a study conducted in eighty-six patients with gluten sensitivity. In the study group, forty percent had osteopenia and twenty-six percent had osteoporosis. All of these individuals were initially untreated for their gluten sensitivity.

Post-Menopausal Women Show Improvement on Gluten-Free Diet

After being placed on a gluten-free diet for several weeks, significant improvements in their bone mineral density occurred uniformly. What is noteworthy is that even post-menopausal women had significant improvement in bone density by eliminating gluten from their diet.[311] Did eliminating dietary gluten increase the production of estrogen in these women? That is a possible mechanism.

Hyperthyroidism Linked to Bone Loss

The other mechanism through which gluten causes osteopenia and osteoporosis hormonally is through thyroid dysfunction. As mentioned in the last chapter, hyperthyroidism or excessive thyroid replacement causes an increase in metabolic rate. This causes a more rapid loss of bone since new bone formation is unable to keep up with bone destruction. As a result, bones become weak and brittle. Gluten induces thyroid dysfunction through immune mechanisms in gluten-sensitive individuals, but the hormonal effect through excessive thyroid hormone production affects bone health.

The thyroid gland also produces another hormone, called calcitonin. This hormone slows down bone loss, but when deficient, bone destruction proceeds unchecked.[312] Gluten can cause damage to the thyroid gland through autoimmune attack, and this can result in a drop in calcitonin. This thyroid hormone is not as potent as other hormones in the body that affect bone remodeling, but calcitonin still has a beneficial effect on promoting strong bones.

Normalizing Bone Density Associated With Early Diagnosis

The above mechanisms are what we know today as major hormonal influences in osteopenia and osteoporosis caused by gluten sensitivity. There very well may be others. One researcher has demonstrated that out of thirty children and adolescents with gluten sensitivity, a gluten-free diet had a better chance of normalizing bone if instituted prior to puberty.[313] This alludes to possibly some other hormonal factors yet to be realized. Regardless, hormonal effects caused by gluten in gluten-sensitive individuals are significant as a cause of poor bone health.

A Word About Osteoporosis Medications

In the last five years, an explosion of prescriptions has been written for osteoporosis medications. Specifically, Fosamax has been a market leader for years, and now, Boniva has entered the market. Both Fosamax (Merck) and Boniva (Roche) are biphosphonates, and they both improve bone density by slowing down the destruction of old, brittle bone. Neither enhances new bone formation. As a result, the increase in bone density is only due to accumulation of weaker, established bone.[314]

Medications Linked to Formation of Abnormal Bone

More concerning in the last several months is the increase in lawsuits being filed regarding jawbone necrosis. Jaw necrosis refers to an accelerated destruction of the bone material in jawbones, resulting in serious deformities and dysfunction. The biphosphonates are associated with this condition. Also, stomach pain, stomach ulcers, muscle and joint pains, and bony aches are all associated with these medications.[315]

Because pharmaceutical companies have powerful lobbyist groups, they have a loud voice when it comes to "greasing the wheels" of drug approval. Despite our serious health care financial crunch, these drug industries continue to make huge profits. There is not much profit in simply promoting vitamin D, calcium and a dietary avoidance of gluten.[316] In situations such as this, you really have to step back and use your common sense.

For instance, recent ads market Boniva subtly through actress Sally Fields. She mentions the benefits of Boniva while reading her journal or as part of a group of women fighting osteoporosis. At no time does Fields state that she is being paid by Roche to promote the product. Likewise, the ad does not list the side effects of the drug because Fields is the spokesperson, not the company itself.[317] Both are clearly misleading in terms of the information provided to the consumer. Misleading advertisements should be red flags that cause you to question a company's true mission.

Osteoporosis Is Treatable Naturally

We have had tremendous success in our clinic by focusing on lifestyle, exercise and diet in both women and men who have osteopenia and osteoporosis. As you have seen, a significant portion of osteoporosis patients have gluten sensitivity, and the effects on bone density begin even in childhood. Be sure to pay attention to these very treatable risk factors and then consider medications only if absolutely necessary. Chances are, you will be able to avoid toxic medications like the biphosphonates.

Summary

It is apparent that gluten sensitivity is a significant factor in triggering osteopenia and osteoporosis in many people. Ranges have varied, but larger studies suggest that as many as forty percent of all osteoporosis patients have gluten sensitivity.[318] Given that twenty-eight million people are affected by overt osteoporosis, over eleven million people could therefore be helped by identifying gluten as the root cause.

Many People Can Be Helped

There has not been any large study to date looking at osteopenia. Based on the number of patients we see in our clinic, anecdotally, we suspect that the number of people with osteopenia is even greater than that of people with overt osteoporosis.

Many Children Are at Risk

One of the most concerning findings has been the presence of poor bone health in children with gluten sensitivity, which is grossly underestimated in our society. While gluten elimination in these children can restore normal bone density, studies have shown that even children who have been on gluten-free diets for three years continue to have reduced-sized skeletal bones.[319] We cannot stress enough how important it is to have children who are at risk for gluten sensitivity evaluated early. Early diagnosis and treatment of gluten sensitivity is important to their long-term health, for reducing other autoimmune diseases and promoting healthy bone formation.

You Can Regain Bone Density

For older patients with osteopenia and osteoporosis, identifying gluten sensitivity can be the key to returning bone density back to normal. In a trial of twenty-eight patients known to have gluten sensitivity, bone density was assessed over a five-year period after the patients were placed on a gluten-free diet. Bone mineral density increased in all patients and stabilized after one year of treatment. Over the ensuing four years, no decline in bone density was noted as long as the patients maintained their gluten abstinence.[320]

If you are one of the millions suffering from osteopenia or osteo-porosis, you should be evaluated for gluten sensitivity. This is the only way to determine if the treatment you are prescribed is likely to be effective over time. Again, you must get to the root cause in order to establish the most effective treatment.

SECTION FOUR

Other Gluten-Related Disorders Including Depression, Weight Gain, Fibromyalgia and Memory Loss

In the preceding section, we discussed some of the common health conditions that often have gluten as a root cause. In this section, we will now review some disorders that are not quite as prevalent among the population but still are commonly caused by gluten sensitivity.

In each case, the same mechanisms of causation, which involve immune system dysfunction, disruption of the intestinal lining and nutritional effects, are likely to be the main pathways by which gluten affects health. By now, you should have a good understanding of each of these mechanisms. While the way in which gluten causes these disorders will be highlighted, detailed descriptions will be skipped for the sake of not being too repetitious.

The Same Condition Can Have Different Root Causes in Different People

Including disorders within this section is not to imply that these conditions have a lesser importance. Fibromyalgia, depression and weight gain are very common health conditions that are listed in this section but, likewise, have a wide array of causes, of which gluten sensitivity is only one. Skin conditions and hepatitis are not as common, but have a higher chance of being gluten-related. Therefore, this section contains health conditions that are, overall, less common, or the percentage of them caused by gluten intolerance makes up a smaller figure. Neither should minimize the importance of seeking gluten sensitivity as a root cause, as you will see.

Many Common Health Problems Share Gluten as Their Root Cause

The most notable finding in this section is the sheer number of health disorders that share gluten sensitivity as a potential mechanism of cause. This highlights gluten's effect on our body's digestive and immune systems, and highlights the importance of diet and nutrition. We really are what we eat!

Fifteen

Celiac Hepatitis

A relatively recent term, "celiac hepatitis" refers to a number of conditions wherein the liver is affected by gluten sensitivity. Celiac hepatitis does not simply mean that you have celiac disease, as any form of gluten sensitivity places one at risk for liver dysfunction. Liver changes can be mild, with abnormal blood testing and no symptoms, or the changes can be severe, with cirrhosis and liver failure. Predominantly, liver dysfunction in gluten sensitivity is felt to be related to auto-immune mechanisms usually through genetic risk of autoimmune dysfunction, intestinal leakage with exposure to foreign proteins and infections, or antibody mimicry attacking the liver.

Sixteen Percent of Patients With Autoimmune Hepatitis Are Gluten-Sensitive

As a result, autoimmune hepatitis is the most common form of celiac hepatitis. This is a disorder of young children and adults, with women and girls being affected most commonly. Medical professionals cite medications, infections and genetic risk as the main causes, failing to mention gluten sensitivity as a root cause the majority of the time.[321]

Despite sixteen percent of patients with autoimmune liver disease having gluten sensitivity, routine evaluation for this disorder is not prescribed.[322] In our clinic, rarely do we evaluate a patient with liver dysfunction who has already been assessed for gluten sensitivity.

Symptoms Vary But Worsen With Time

Symptoms of celiac hepatitis can be vague at times. Fatigue may be the only symptom. Other symptoms can include lightheadedness, abdominal discomfort, joint pains, skin itchiness, nausea and vomiting. If liver dysfunction is more significant, anemia and a yellowing of the skin, called jaundice, can develop. When severe liver dysfunction occurs, confusion and cirrhosis can develop, eventually resulting in liver failure. A percentage of these patients go on to have liver transplants.[323]

Gluten and Liver Disease

Several studies have assessed the occurrence of liver dysfunction in gluten sensitivity. Most of the time, symptoms are either mild or absent, and the most common abnormal finding is elevation of liver enzymes during routine blood testing, rather than symptoms. Liver enzymes are part of a normal blood chemistry panel with annual physical examinations, so detecting these abnormalities is not uncommon. What is uncommon is the subsequent investigation for gluten sensitivity.

Forty Percent of Patients with Gluten Sensitivity Show Elevated Liver Enzymes

In forty percent of people with gluten sensitivity, elevated liver enzymes are found during routine blood testing. In addition, all of these individuals respond to a gluten-free diet with normalization of liver enzymes within weeks to months.[324] These findings have been repeatedly verified.[325] It is therefore strongly recommended that all individuals with elevated liver enzymes be evaluated for gluten sensitivity.

The Liver Responds Beautifully to a Gluten-Free Diet

Amongst our many reasons for writing this book, here is another example. Frustratingly, we usually find that patients who have elevated liver enzymes without severe symptoms are almost always told to just wait and see what happens at their next annual physical. The idea of waiting a year or more while gluten reactions continue to irreversibly damage the body is a practice we hope to change by increasing the medical profession's awareness of gluten intolerance.

Gluten Sensitivity and Liver Disease Are Ten Times More Common Than in the Normal Population

In looking at the more severe end of the spectrum, a higher percentage of end-stage liver disease patients have gluten sensitivity. In one study, 488 patients with advanced liver dysfunction were tested for gluten-related antibodies. Three percent of these patients had celiac disease, compared to only 0.6 percent of the control group that was tested.[326] In other studies, patients with gluten sensitivity and chronic, severe liver disease were ten times more common when compared to the normal population.[327]

Gluten Sensitivity Precedes Liver Disease

Various liver dysfunctions that account for Celiac hepatitis can include mild liver tissue damage, autoimmune hepatitis, gall bladder disease and different forms of cirrhosis.[328] It is interesting to note that in more than two-thirds of people with concurrent liver disease and gluten sensitivity, gluten sensitivity preceded the diagnosis of liver dysfunction.[329] Researchers, as a result, suspect that genetic factors, duration of gluten exposure and age of exposure to gluten all affect the development of celiac hepatitis in these individuals.[330]

Celiac Hepatitis and Response to Gluten Elimination

In assessing response to dietary changes with a gluten-free diet, mixed results have been found, but trends clearly have surfaced from the studies performed. The rule appears to be that treating gluten sensitivity earlier results in a more favorable response to dietary changes. In people with gluten sensitivity and elevated liver enzymes on blood tests only, the response seems to be universally beneficial.[331] All patients respond well once gluten is eliminated from their diet.

Once Again, Early Diagnosis and Elimination of Gluten Are the Keys

However, in patients with autoimmune hepatitis or more chronic liver disease, the benefits are not as profound. In these people, there is a noted reduction in liver antibody levels and gluten-related antibody levels, but the liver dysfunction does not typically revert back to normal. Additional therapy, such as immunosuppressive medications, is still required to treat the liver condition.[332] The degree of reversibility of liver dysfunction with a gluten-free diet is postulated to correlate to the timing and duration of gluten exposure in gluten-sensitive individuals.[333]

Complications of Celiac Hepatitis

Because celiac hepatitis is linked most commonly to autoimmune hepatitis or autoimmune gall bladder dysfunction, complications involve other immune system disorders. If you have read through the preceding chapters of this book, you will recognize several of these conditions as being also closely linked to gluten sensitivity in general.

Complications Prove Gluten's Causative Role

These complications include vitamin B12 deficiency, rheumatoid arthritis, type I diabetes, Hashimoto's thyroiditis and anemia.[334] If adequate research had not already been completed demonstrating the relationship between gluten and liver dysfunction, this list of complications should certainly trigger suspicion that gluten was involved in the cause of liver dysfunction, since they all share gluten as a common cause.

The most severe complication is, of course liver, failure and/or cirrhosis. Cirrhosis is best thought of as severe scarring of the liver, resulting from repeated inflammation. In the case of celiac hepatitis, this inflammation and cirrhosis are unrelated to alcohol, though alcohol can accelerate the process. The immune attack on the liver, induced by gluten sensitivity, eventually leads to scarring of the liver and an inability to function. In these individuals, liver transplant may be the only option.

Summary

The take-home point in celiac hepatitis is similar to that of other gluten-related health conditions. Be tested for gluten sensitivity early! Evidence of liver disorders in association with gluten sensitivity supports that the longer gluten intolerance exists, the more likely it is that irreversible liver damage can occur. Also, once an immune attack on the liver starts, the less likely it is that a beneficial response to a gluten free-diet will be seen.

Many People Have Elevated Liver Enzymes— Find Out if You Do

The largest group of people that currently could be helped by early testing is those with elevated liver enzymes in their blood without severe symptoms. These enzyme elevations should be seen on routine annual medical exams and provide a great clue that gluten sensitivity is present. Again, forty percent of all gluten-sensitive patients have elevated liver enzymes! These individuals are likely to respond to a gluten-free diet and avoid the long-term complications of celiac hepatitis.

Celiac hepatitis is underappreciated, and even routine medical advice fails to suggest gluten sensitivity testing in patients with evidence of liver dysfunction. Be sure to have annual blood tests that include liver enzymes and ask for a copy of the report. If liver enzyme elevation is present, you need to be checked for gluten sensitivity.

And, as previously mentioned in our discussions of other disorders, if you are at risk for gluten sensitivity because of concurrent disorders or a family history of gluten or autoimmune disorders, please be tested early. Waiting can result in irreversible immune conditions and damage your health. Celiac hepatitis is a good example of this. Because it affects predominantly young individuals, the point of early diagnosis cannot be stressed too much.

Sixteen

Depression and Gluten Sensitivity

Eric's New Life

Eric O. was a forty-nine-year-old attorney who had left his profession due to his poor health and depression. He came into the clinic after seeing our commercial. Throughout his entire life, he'd had several debilitating symptoms. He suffered from chronic headaches three times per week, for which he used aspirin or Advil. He suffered from "ADD" symptoms, noting that he couldn't focus and his mind constantly wandered. However, his worst symptom was unrelenting depression.

He was not only unhappy, but came across to others as being angry. He'd had to receive anger management counseling once as a result of an outburst. Doctors had prescribed many medications, from antidepressants to lithium. His diagnoses ranged from depression to bipolar disease. He felt hopeless, depressed and on the border of suicidal.

Eric had gone through a divorce eight years prior and had basically stopped doing much ever since. He had lost most of his

261

friends and had no desire to meet new people. He stated that he had to fight himself to even get out of bed in the morning, even after twelve hours of sleep. He had absolutely no motivation, which made living life almost impossible.

After one week on the modified elimination diet, Eric felt less tired and was intrigued by the change. Now, barely six weeks into the program, Eric is doing outstandingly well. He has enjoyed a thirty-pound loss of fat and a ten-pound weight gain of muscle. He has dropped from a fifty-inch waist to a forty-three-inch waist. He hasn't suffered a single headache since he eliminated gluten from his diet. He also describes incredible mental clarity that he wishes he'd had earlier, during his years of education and law practice.

But the best change is his outlook on life. The hopelessness, depression and suicidal thoughts are gone. He is happy and is making new friends while enjoying what he calls a "natural high" associated with just feeling good physically.

Overview

Being an extremely common health disorder, depression affects more than twelve million people in the United States alone. In addition, depression is, without discrimination, affecting all ages and races across the world. Typically, depression begins in one's early twenties, but it certainly can occur at any age and be a lifelong struggle. Though women are reported to be affected almost twice as commonly as men, many feel that this statistic is skewed because women are more likely to seek medical attention for depression than men.[335]

Gluten Sensitivity Causes Depression and Other Mood Problems

Gluten's relationship to depression, and, to a lesser extent, to other mood problems such as anxiety, has been a recently recognized association.

There has been some debate regarding cause and effect related to depression and disease. Is depression a secondary reaction to having an illness, or is the illness actually causing depression to occur? Studies now support the latter, and this is consistent with our experience. Physical illness can affect one's mind, one's mood and one's emotional response, and scientific evidence is indeed showing that gluten sensitivity can be a root cause of depression.

Through this chapter, you will understand what symptoms occur with depression as well as common beliefs about the causes, complications and risk factors surrounding depressive states. More importantly, you will also be able to understand how gluten sensitivity causes depression and when to be concerned that gluten is a potential cause.

The Basics of Depression

Depression is an extremely common health condition and it affects quality of life for many people. Symptoms can include a variety of complaints such as apathy, feelings of hopelessness, sad emotions, unexplained crying spells, erratic sleep patterns, fatigue, irritability, lack of libido and shifts in one's weight.[336] Depression can alter many different parameters of your daily functions as your mood motivates, guides, supports and balances many aspects of your life.

The Concept of a Chemical Imbalance Is Not Supported by Research

Specifically, serotonin is a major substance that seems to be deficient, and this has led to many drug treatments for depression that increase serotonin. While the concept of a chemical imbalance in the brain is widely promoted as the cause of depression, scientific studies do not fully support this theory. Recently, when antidepressant medications were tested against placebos, there were no significant differences in outcome regarding how the patients' symptoms responded.[337]

Antidepressants Are Dangerous and Ineffective

Because antidepressant drugs do not treat the root cause of the problem, and considering the life-threatening consequences that side effects of these antidepressants can create, we are adamantly opposed to their use. Depression is a symptom that can create mental changes, but that does not automatically translate into the fact that depression is caused by a mental problem. Depression is another symptom, and just like other symptoms already discussed in this book, there exists a root cause to this symptom. Yes, there can be environmental causes, including stressful life events such as loss of job, loss of a loved one or catastrophic illnesses, that can contribute to depression.[338] But as we discussed earlier, these are stresses on the body that create physiological changes resulting in bodily malfunctions. These malfunctions eventually manifests in symptoms.

Depression Is a Symptom
for Which the Root Cause Must Be Discovered

For some people, symptoms may be headaches or stomach problems, and for others, the symptom may be depression. The root cause of the problem is important to discover because it will lead to permanent recovery from the condition. Routinely, gluten and other dietary factors are not mentioned as causes of depression despite our extensive clinical experience demonstrating the contrary.

Other than the above causes of depression, chronic illnesses can certainly place you at risk for developing depression as well.[339] Chronic disorders, such as gluten sensitivity, can have depression as an inherent symptom unrelated to other symptoms or associated mental stress. While distinguishing depression as a reaction or a symptom in some situations can be difficult, evidence in gluten sensitivity supports that depression is indeed a symptom and not a secondary phenomenon.

Depression Comes With Other Health Risks

Having depression is a risk for even bigger complications above and beyond poor quality of life. Other complications can include abuse of alcohol and/or drugs, social conflicts with relationships, vocational problems at work or school, or even suicide. This causes serious problems for a depressed person, but the costs to our society are also high as depressed people have other health conditions more commonly and are much less productive in general.

There Are Natural Treatments That Avoid Dangerous Drug Side Effects

Additionally, the amount of prescription medications prescribed for depression is enormous, and these medications are riddled with side effects. Side effects can even include suicide and violent behavior. Identifying other natural approaches to the treatment of depression is therefore important, as is eliminating the true, underlying cause.

Her Lifelong Depression and Anxiety Were Eradicated

B.R. was a fifty-six-year-old woman who had suffered from chronic depression since her youth. "When you look at pictures that were taken of me as a child, it's obvious that something was wrong—I never looked happy," She said.

With the depression came anxiety, which she described as constant, and she had particular difficulty socially as a result. After her first child, she had postpartum depression that was severe, and after her second child, she was not only depressed but also very achy and tired.

She was suspicious that food was causing some problems

and experimented with dietary changes and vitamins but without much success. When she came to see us, she was excited about the HealthNOW Method's getting to the root cause of her problems. She was convinced that some foods could be a component of her problem, and it turns out that she was correct.

The functional tests that examined her digestive, adrenal and liver functions revealed an intestinal infection, adrenal fatigue and gluten sensitivity. Eradicating the infection, treating the adrenals and removing gluten from her diet dramatically improved her depression and anxiety, and she was significantly more comfortable in social situations. She was ecstatic about the changes and she now describes herself as being more relaxed moment to moment, with improved ability to focus and concentrate. Eliminating gluten as the root cause made a tremendous impact in a lifelong battle with depression.

Gluten Sensitivity and Depression— Cause and Effect

Many researchers have now demonstrated that gluten exposure in gluten-sensitive individuals can cause depression. One good study evaluated sixteen newly diagnosed gluten-sensitive people and performed assessments to determine if depression was present. Compared to normal individuals, the patients with gluten sensitivity scored much higher for having depression. What is important also is that the depression was unrelated to abdominal complaints or other symptoms.[340] This supports that the depression was not a secondary phenomenon of simply having an illness.

Gluten-Sensitive Patients Show a Higher Incidence of Depression

Another study out of Sweden assessed forty-two people with known gluten sensitivity, and of this group, eight had depression and/or anxiety.[341] Even though the sample was small, the percent affected was nineteen percent, which is significantly higher than a normal population, which averages four to five percent.[342] The authors' opinion, based on the study, was that depression may be severe in individuals with gluten sensitivity.[343]

Children With Gluten Sensitivity Are Not Immune to Depression

As mentioned earlier, depression most commonly begins after age twenty, but childhood depression also occurs. The findings in children with gluten intolerance are disturbing in this regard. Research evaluating twenty-nine children and adolescents with gluten sensitivity conducted assessments for depression and behavior disturbances. Compared to twenty-nine other children without gluten intolerance, thirty-one percent of the affected children had depression compared to seven percent of the control group. Additionally, twenty-eight percent had disruptive behavior problems compared to three percent of the healthy group. These researchers also noted that depression was the presenting symptom for many of these children, who eventually were diagnosed as gluten-sensitive.[344]

How Does Gluten Cause Depression?

So, depression is more common in gluten sensitivity, and depression is caused by gluten intolerance rather than being a secondary symptom of having gluten sensitivity. But how does gluten cause depression? One theory is related to the previously mentioned changes in serotonin affected by gluten intolerance. One study examined nine adolescents with depression and gluten sensitivity. In this group, levels of tryptophan were lower than those in normal adolescents. Tryptophan is a required amino acid (a digestive product of proteins in our diet) needed to make serotonin. These nine children were placed on a gluten-free diet, and within three months, their depression had resolved without medication.[345]

Malabsorption of Nutrients Is One Mechanism

This suggests that gluten somehow causes a reduction in serotonin by reducing the body's ability to absorb tryptophan from its diet. One theory is that gluten in sensitive individuals causes this through intestinal effects on the digestive lining. Inability to absorb necessary vitamins and amino acids is impaired because of the intestinal inflammation triggered by gluten.

Removing gluten from the diet thus corrects this problem over several weeks, and amino acid levels, and subsequently serotonin, return to normal, eliminating depressive symptoms. In particular, gluten researchers recommend that if a person is depressed, gluten antibody testing should be performed. Gluten-sensitive people with depression will often respond well to gluten-free diets.[346]

Gluten's Attack on the Nervous System Is a Second Mechanism

Other authors suspect that some people with depression who also suffer gluten intolerance are affected by autoimmune attacks on the nervous system. This, in essence, would cause similar changes in serotonin and neurochemistry.[347]

Brains of Children With Gluten Sensitivity Show Inflammation

Children with gluten sensitivity have been noted to show MRI-scan evidence of brain inflammation. In looking at seventy-five children with gluten sensitivity who were already on diet treatment, twenty percent had evidence of abnormalities on their brain MRI scans, supporting inflammation. Compared to the children who had normal MRI scans, the only difference noted was the length of gluten exposure. In other words, the chance of brain changes increased with the duration of gluten in their diet.[348] Early testing and treatment, once again, cannot be stressed enough.

Summary

Depression's being a mental illness is not as objectively evaluated as other medical conditions, like high blood pressure or diabetes, but regardless, it is a real and common health disorder that affects millions. In individuals with gluten sensitivity, it appears that somewhere between twenty and thirty percent are affected by depression, which is significantly higher than estimates of the normal population, which are around five percent. While you might suspect that this increase in percentage is secondary to having an illness like gluten intolerance, studies show that this is unrelated to typical complaints associated with gluten sensitivity.

Gluten-Free Diets Help Depression in Children and Adults

Mechanisms by which gluten can cause depression likely stem from malabsorption of necessary vitamins and amino acids from the diet, immune inflammation of brain tissue, or both processes simultaneously. It is clear that some individuals will respond well to gluten elimination from the diet. As always, the most important thing is considering gluten as a root cause, testing for gluten sensitivity and implementing a gluten-free diet as soon as possible. For both children and adults, this remains an important point that we wanted to stress.

Seventeen

Obesity, Weight Gain and Gluten

Angies's Weight Loss Success

Angie was a young woman with many problems. Being twenty-five pounds overweight was definitely one of them. She was frustrated by not being able to lose the weight and was never sure if the fatigue, bloating and severe stomachaches were related to the weight gain or not. She was literally at the end of her rope when she first came to see us.

We not only found her to be gluten-sensitive but further diagnosed the presence of several infectious organisms in her body. Over the course of several months, Angie lost the twenty-five pounds that had been plaguing her for so long. She couldn't believe how easily it came off. Her weight remained stable, and she could eat anything she wanted as long as she remained off gluten. Her fatigue and digestive complaints fully resolved as well. Her motto became, "No gluten = feel great!"

Overview

Contrary to classic medical opinion, gluten intolerance is not associated with weight loss the majority of the time. In fact, it is simply the opposite. Gluten-sensitive patients are overweight approximately forty percent of the time due to various direct and indirect factors.[349] Because of the misperception that most individuals suffer weight loss when they have gluten sensitivity, a greater number of people go undiagnosed. This perception needs to change.

Sixty-Six Percent of Adults and Eighteen Percent of Children Are Overweight or Obese

As you are aware, obesity has been an increasing problem for America for decades, and in the past decade, childhood obesity is also becoming an epidemic. Let's consider some astounding statistics. According to the Centers for Disease Control, sixty-six percent of all adults over the age of twenty are overweight or obese. Thirty-two percent are overtly obese. For children, eighteen percent are categorized as overweight.[350]

Gluten Is the Culprit in Many People's Obesity

These numbers are incredible! Even if gluten sensitivity were the cause of being overweight or obese in one percent of cases, the number of people affected would still be hundreds of thousands. By our assessment, gluten sensitivity is a root cause of being overweight much greater than one percent of the time.

The first steps are to appreciate the scope of the problem, and then to understand the mechanisms by which obesity and weight gain develop when intolerant to gluten. Some are primary and some are secondary. By making you, as well as the medical community, aware of this as a cause, our hope is that gluten sensitivity will be diagnosed earlier and more accurately, and that greater emphasis on our diets will be universally accepted as an intervention for many medical conditions.

The Basics of being Overweight or Obese

Generally speaking, accepted medical knowledge about weight gain and obesity considers genetics, age and gender to be primary risk factors. Metabolism slows as we age, so unless caloric intake declines concurrently, weight gain increases as we get older. Women are affected more commonly that men and obesity, in particular, is more common within families, which suggests a genetic component. Dietary patterns and learned behaviors that favor weight gain can be the main causes within families, however, rather than genes, so not all overweight individuals have genetic predisposition. Environment can also play a role.[351]

Who is considered overweight and who is considered obese? Medically, clinicians use a formula called the body mass index or BMI. BMI figures in your height and weight and then calculates a number for an assessment of weight category. A BMI less than twenty-five is normal; a BMI from twenty-five to thirty is overweight; and a BMI greater than thirty is obese.

The Waistline Tells the Tale

As another means to a guideline, percent of weight over your ideal body weight or your waistline circumference can be used as an estimate. Obesity is considered present if you are twenty percent over your ideal weight. Likewise, for women with waistlines greater than thirty-five inches and men with waistlines greater than forty inches, excessive weight or obesity is likely present.[352]

Many Factors Come Into Play

Many factors contribute to weight gain and obesity, including poor diet choices, lack of adequate activity, some medications that have weight gain side effects and other medical conditions. Specifically, adrenal dysfunction, low thyroid states, arthritis (by limiting activity) and diabetes all cause weight gain in many individuals.

Treatments Abound But Few Work

Treatments are targeted at dietary changes, behavior modification and increasing activity. Medications for weight loss that suppress fat absorption from the intestine or that increase satiety, reducing hunger, are commonly used, but all have unpleasant side effects. More and more, obese patients are actually turning to complicated abdominal surgery to either reduce stomach size or bypass intestinal absorption areas to effectively reduce weight.[353]

Obesity Causes Other Serious Health Conditions

As our country sees the number of overweight individuals gradually increasing, other, secondary health issues are increasing as well. These include high blood pressure, heart disease, stroke, high cholesterol, sleep apnea, arthritis, diabetes and several others. Even cancers like colon cancer, breast cancer and prostate cancer (three of the most common cancers) are complications of obesity.[354] This is not simply a social epidemic but a true health epidemic in our country, and an increased awareness and change in behavior is mandatory in order to make a significant impact.

Gluten Sensitivity and Obesity

A large study looking at 371 children with gluten sensitivity demonstrated that only five percent were underweight, despite most medical texts describing weight loss as being a key feature of the diagnosis. Actually, thirty-nine percent were either overweight or obese out of this group.[355] This has been substantiated in other studies as well. Another, examining forty-seven adolescents, demonstrated that fifty-one percent, who were not adhering to a gluten-free diet, suffered from being overweight or obese.[356]

Another Reason Why Gluten Sensitivity Is Missed

If current diagnostic criteria for evaluating people for gluten intolerance include the stereotype of being underweight, many symptomatic individuals will never be checked for gluten sensitivity.

How and Why the Weight Gain Occurs

If diarrhea is a common symptom of gluten sensitivity as well as malabsorption, then why is weight gain so common? The answer to this question lies in the stress of having gluten intolerance. As outlined earlier in the book, gluten sensitivity is a chronic health stress on the body affecting many organs, including the immune system and digestive system. Our hormonal system (specifically the adrenal glands) increases stress hormone (cortisol) production, which causes disturbances in our metabolism and weight.[357] Cortisol, like prednisone, causes weight gain around the abdomen, makes it harder to use glucose from the diet, and increases fatigue through poor sleep mechanisms. All of these result in weight gain.

Other mechanisms of causation include a higher chance of having reduced thyroid function in gluten intolerance. Thyroid hormone stimulates our metabolic rate, and when it is low as a result of gluten sensitivity, a slower metabolism means a reduced ability to use the calories we digest. The end result is that these calories are stored as fat, increasing our weight over time.

If Your Cells Are Starving, Your Metabolism Slows and Weight Gain Results

Lastly, the malabsorption associated with gluten intolerance results in less nutrients being absorbed by the cells. The cells are essentially "starving." The body has a built-in mechanism to thwart starvation and does so by dramatically decreasing its metabolic rate. Much as we see with thyroid malfunction, this reduced ability of the body to burn what it has consumed results in weight gain, often despite a moderate calorie intake.

Obesity Solved

C.T. came into our clinic in 2006 after having multiple complaints for more than twenty years. While being overweight was not her primary complaint, she was more than twenty percent over her ideal weight. Her main symptoms instead included back and hip pain, for which she had been to many chiropractors without long-term benefit. Also, she was incredibly exhausted.

Through elimination of gluten from her diet, she not only had resolution of her back and hip pain, but also lost thirty-five pounds in the process. Her energy level was also restored to normal. In many patients who suffer weight gain, the stress of the added weight can result in joint stress and pain. This, indeed, may have been the case with C.T., since her weight loss was quite dramatic, but it's also important to consider the anti-inflammatory effects that are re-initiated once gluten is removed from the diet. We see many patients whose achy joints resolve once they remove gluten from their diet.

The Vicious Cycle of Poor Food Choices and Feeling Ill

Being a chronic health condition, gluten sensitivity can result in poor dietary choices in general. If you are suffering from abdominal complaints, fatigue, poor sleep, joint aches, etc., food choices have been shown to be less than optimal when symptoms are present. In fact, under any chronic stress condition, most will choose a higher caloric, high-fatty-content meal.[358] Of course, this will often worsen your complaints since you are not aware of the gluten sensitivity, and the cycle perpetuates itself over and over again. Many patients whom we have treated for gluten sensitivity have had tremendous weight loss in the months after gluten elimination in the diet was started.

Don't Get Discouraged—It May Take Some Time

Because of adrenal gland effects and cortisol production, elimination of gluten from the diet may not immediately resolve a weight problem. The chronic stress of gluten sensitivity took a long time to cause adrenal exhaustion, and, therefore, can take some time to improve. In formal studies assessing weight-loss response in gluten sensitivity, one demonstrated an obese five-year-old who had a favorable response to a gluten-free diet. The only symptoms prior to diagnosis were obesity, intermittent abdominal pain and a family history of gluten sensitivity.[359]

Other studies have suggested that a gluten-free diet itself can trigger weight gain,[360] but many factors are at play here, including ongoing adrenal dysfunction, possible concurrent intestinal infections and food choices when avoiding gluten in the diet. Many patients are so excited to find all the gluten-free "goodies" on the market that they forget to take into account the extra calories they are consuming.

A Proper Treatment Plan

The only true resolution to gluten sensitivity and weight gain is to eliminate gluten from the diet, allow the adrenal glands to recover, make healthy dietary choices and treat any concurrent health conditions. In our clinic, uniformly, we see a dramatic improvement, including weight normalization, within several weeks to months in the majority of our patients.

Summary

Treating individuals with medications and surgery to correct their weight problems truly is targeting the symptoms and not the cause; plus, side effects from these treatments can be profound. More than any of the other conditions covered in this book, obesity and weight gain are effects of dietary and lifestyle choices. Age, genetic risk and gender play parts, but being involved in your diet and activity choices is the most effective and rewarding therapy when dealing with weight gain.

Through effects on the immune system, the hormonal system and the digestive system, gluten sensitivity commonly causes obesity and weight gain as well. While a study has yet to be performed that identifies an exact percentage, there is no question, from our experience, that gluten sensitivity causes weight gain in a significant number of people. If you have no other identified cause for weight gain, be tested for gluten intolerance. Not only can you get back to your ideal weight, but you also can live healthier in the process.

Eighteen

Fibromyalgia and Gluten Sensitivity

One of the purposes behind what we do is not only to help our patients, but to educate them so that they can, in turn, help others.

Sharon Helps Her Sister Regain Health

Sharon has been a patient for many years. She checks in occasionally, just to get information about the latest breakthroughs in clinical nutrition and to continue her good health. Recently, she came in and shared the story of her sister.

Sharon's sister basically had all the same symptoms Sharon had suffered from before coming to see us. Her sister had chronic stomach problems of pain and constipation. They had been with her since the fourth grade. She suffered from joint, muscle fatigue and pain that was just excruciating. She lived on ibuprofen, which only took the edge off her pain. She had been diagnosed with chronic fatigue and Epstein-Barr virus, but she had not received any help for her symptoms.

As so many patients experience, Sharon's sister had been told that she was depressed and that much of the problem was likely in her head. Sharon told me that talking to her sister was like reliving her past. Their symptoms were identical and their viewpoints on life were similar as well. Specifically, her sister stated that while she wasn't suicidal, it was difficult to contemplate continuing life the way she felt. The pain and fatigue were so debilitating that life didn't seem worth living.

Due to a family event, the sisters were brought together. They lived in different states and so rarely got to see one another. Once Sharon laid eyes on her sister and they talked about her health, Sharon gave her a sisterly diagnosis. She informed her sister that she was likely gluten-sensitive and that she must stop eating gluten immediately. Her sister had trouble believing that her lifelong complaints could be tied to a food, but was open to getting a lab test.

Her antibody test for gluten was positive. Within two days of eliminating gluten from her diet, Sharon's sister called her with the amazing news. She hadn't needed any ibuprofen, which she normally consumed six times a day for pain. Still in disbelief, she told Sharon that it must have been all in her head. She waited a week, because she was enjoying the dramatic cessation of pain, and then she tempted fate by eating a hot dog with the bun. The pain returned with a vengeance. She needed no further convincing and made plans to take further lab tests to rule out any infections that might be present.

But the best part was when Sharon's sister thanked her for proving that it wasn't all in her head and for restoring her will to live.

Overview

If you are a sufferer of fibromyalgia, then you understand the frustrations of this disorder. Frequent, unrelenting pain, stiffness, fatigue, lack of sleep and depression are just some of the more common symptoms, yet, to date, the cause of this prevalent condition is stated in the literature as being unknown. This is another area wherein symptomatic treatment is the primary focus of attention despite some hard evidence that dietary factors indeed play a role.

Much Success Is Seen in Fibromyalgia With a Gluten-Free Diet

Anecdotally, we have witnessed over and over again the resolution of the classic muscle aches and tender points in response to gluten elimination. Adrenal fatigue, poor blood sugar control and hidden infections round out the most frequent root causes of this condition that we find. Among our patients who have enjoyed this response, there is no question as to the link between fibromyalgia and gluten sensitivity.

More People Have Fibromyalgia than Type I Diabetes

In the United States, between four and eight million people suffer from fibromyalgia, which is roughly two percent of the population. Of these individuals, ninety percent are women.[361] This figure may be skewed because of the tendency of men to delay medical evaluation for fibromyalgia-type symptoms. Regardless, the number of people dealing with daily symptoms from this disorder exceed the number of type I diabetics in our country.

Little Research Has Been Done on Fibromyalgia

With its frequency, you would anticipate abundant research into its causation, but, because of the nature of fibromyalgia's symptoms and the lack of objective lab or exam abnormalities, these endeavors have been limited. Additionally, some physicians fail to consider this as a real health disorder, even today.

For those who have fibromyalgia complaints, there is little question as to its realness. Multiple therapies have been tried, including medica-tions, physical treatments and dietary manipulations, with varying success. In this chapter, we would like to present our view, from clinical experience, of what can be a root cause of this condition in a significant number of people.

The Basics of Fibromyalgia

In individuals who have fibromyalgia, symptoms are actually multiple. Most commonly, widespread pain in musculoskeletal areas are promi-nent and typically involve certain areas. These areas include the back of the head, upper back and neck, upper chest, hips, knees and elbows. In addition, areas in these regions have tender spots that usually overlie where muscle tendons or ligaments attach to bony surfaces. In fact, the criteria used for diagnosis is the presence of at least eleven of these tender spots and a duration of symptoms for at least three months.[362]

Multiple Symptoms Are Present

Other symptoms include fatigue with sleep disruption, irritable bowel symptoms, headaches, jaw pain, depression, tingling, numbness and diffi-culty concentrating. Controversy exists over the sleep issues in that some clinicians see sleep disturbances as a primary cause of fibromyalgia symp-toms and others see fibromyalgia as resulting in disrupted sleep. Either way, studies have supported that sleep quality in patients with fibromyalgia is affected by being lighter than normal individuals' deep sleep.[363]

Multiple Causes Are Posed

While standard medicine does not define a known cause, a theory of central sensitization exists, which holds that people with fibromyalgia are overly sensitive to all forms of stimulation (touch, movement, sound, etc.). Possible mechanisms of cause are thought to be multiple. Consid-erations for causes include genetics, concurrent infections, hormonal imbalances, mental stress, inadequate sleep, preceding injuries and dysfunction of muscle metabolism. Fibromyalgia has been shown to be more common within family relatives, and age of onset is between early to middle age for both women and men. Concurrent conditions that may increase the development of fibromyalgia include sleep disorders, rheumatoid arthritis and irritable bowel syndrome.[364]

Treatment Is Symptomatic in Nature

Symptomatic treatment is, unfortunately, the standard when helping fibromyalgia patients. Pain medications are used to treat the pain associated with the condition, and various drugs are offered to help reduce pain and promote better sleep. The categories of drugs prescribed include muscle relaxants for stiffness, sleep medications and the drug Lyrica, which is a recently approved medication used for fibromyalgia pain.

In addition to medications, other therapies are utilized such as massage, chiropractic care and acupuncture. All of these treatments can be beneficial in selected people, but often, the relief is temporary, requiring frequent reassessment. This is the nature of symptomatic treatment since the underlying cause is not being addressed.[365]

Dietary Causes Have Been Examined

Dietary manipulations have also been tried with some success. One study examined the response of a group of fibromyalgia patients to the elimination of MSG (monosodium glutamate) and aspartame in their diets. In the four patient studies, all had a beneficial response in their fibromyalgia symptoms. The authors felt as though these chemicals were excitotoxins that made the body hypersensitive; thus, their elimination resolved the fibromyalgia complaints.[366]

Other investigations have looked at vegan and vegetarian diets. These studies have shown some varying responses that have been likely due to other variables within the vegan and vegetarian guidelines of what was eaten. One study did support that eighteen patients with fibromyalgia had beneficial responses to a strict vegan dietary regimen over a three-month period.[367] Others that looked at a vegetarian diet failed to show any significant benefit at all.[368]

Diet Does Play a Role

Conclusions about the current medical beliefs among clinicians support that fibromyalgia is caused by a multitude of factors, and in a significant number, diet plays a role. When looking at four to eight million people in the United States alone, it is evident that diet should be a greater focus of our attention in treating this condition than is currently present.

Fibromyalgia and Gluten Sensitivity

Large review studies examining gluten sensitivity in patients with fibromyalgia have supported a higher frequency in this population. In a survey study of over 1,000 gluten-sensitive individuals of varying ages, nine percent had fibromyalgia as well.[369] This is much higher than the two percent in the normal population. Our experience would support even higher figures, which are likely due to the large number of gluten-sensitive people who go undiagnosed each year.

Seventy-Three Percent of Fibromyalgia Sufferers Had Concurrent IBS

To get a better handle on this number, it may be more accurate to look at the number of people who suffer abdominal complaints, like irritable bowel syndrome, with fibromyalgia symptoms. These statistics are staggering. In one research endeavor, an investigator found, in 123 patients with fibromyalgia, that seventy-three percent suffered from irritable bowel syndrome.[370] In another study, seventy percent of the fibromyalgia patients sampled had irritable bowel syndrome.[371]

IBS Is Highly Correlated to Gluten Sensitivity

As we showed in the prior chapter on irritable bowel syndrome, a high percentage of these patients have undiagnosed gluten sensitivity. It is safe to assume that many of these patients with both fibromyalgia and irritable bowel syndrome indeed suffer from gluten intolerance.

Gluten-Sensitive Patients Have Higher Incidences of Fibromyalgia and IBS

In a review of many different studies of gluten sensitivity, it was noted that people with celiac disease or gluten sensitivity often have fibromyalgia and irritable bowel syndrome complaints together. The authors identified some of these patients as having secondary infections of the intestinal tract, and that their symptoms all responded well to antibiotic treatments.[372]

Secondary Infections Need to Be Treated

We often find that our patients with gluten sensitivity suffer the same problem. Even after eliminating gluten from their diets, secondary infections of the intestines, like H. pylori, parasites or other pathogenic organisms, require treatment before a full response is seen. The chronic effects on the immune system and the decline in adrenal and hormonal function allow a greater susceptibility to these infections. These add insult to the already present injury that gluten is causing.

Fibromyalgia and Chronic Fatigue Left Her Miserable

C.V. had been diagnosed with fibromyalgia for many years prior to coming into our office. Like many fibromyalgia patients, she had chronic fatigue as well. Most of her joint pains were constant and chronic, and no matter what she tried, nothing worked for long.

We diagnosed her as being gluten-sensitive. Through dietary elimination of gluten, she initially lost twenty pounds and had improvements in her joint complaints and energy level. Her subsequent tests also showed a parasitic infection in her intestine (not uncommon with chronic gluten sensitivity), and treatment of this eventually led to resolution of all joint and muscular symptoms.

C.V. is quite pleased now and would never venture away from her gluten-free diet. She is one of the many success stories we have seen wherein gluten has been identified as a root cause.

The Immune System and Adrenal Glands Are Parts of the Picture

Other likely mechanisms of causation between gluten and fibromyalgia include autoimmune attack of muscular and joint-related tissues in the body, similar to mechanisms described in arthritis syndromes. Also, adrenal exhaustion causing hormonal changes affect the ability of musculoskeletal tissues of the body to maintain themselves in a healthy state. With adrenal exhaustion, natural steroids, like cortisol, become depleted and no longer control the inflammation that occurs with use of the body in its daily routines. This persistent inflammation can lead to the pain described in fibromyalgia.

Though the number of people who have fibromyalgia and gluten sensitivity is not known precisely, the figure is significant. More importantly, in a condition that is widely held as not having a known cause, identifying gluten sensitivity as a root cause is incredibly important. Not only can it avoid unnecessary treatments with medications and therapies, but it can allow resolution of complaints and restore health.

Summary

Fibromyalgia is a common health disorder that has advanced significantly in frequency in the last three decades, and it affects significant numbers of people. It causes loss of function, depression, impaired social relations and a reduced quality of life. And, despite its prevalence, the underlying cause, for many people, remains elusive.

Gluten Is Often a Cause

From our experience, a great number of patients with fibromyalgia are gluten-sensitive, and elimination of gluten in their diets results in dramatic improvements in their lives. Scientific literature supports this as well, although it is very unlikely that your clinician has explored gluten sensitivity as the cause.

Evaluate Adrenal Function and Gluten Sensitivity

For the price of your quality of life and the costs associated with symptomatic treatments, you owe it to yourself to be tested for gluten sensitivity and adrenal fatigue. Getting to the root of the problem will be much more satisfying than simply appeasing your symptoms.

Nineteen

Skin Disorders and Gluten Sensitivity

Overview

The spectrum over which gluten sensitivity manifests as health disorders is amazing. Many bodily systems can be affected, as you've seen, and none is more interesting than disorders of the skin. It has long been known that dermatitis herpetiformis (DH), a severe skin rash, has been linked to gluten sensitivity, and as further discoveries have allowed further insight, the mechanism by which gluten sensitivity and DH coexist has been well defined. Additionally, there are other skin disorders associated with gluten intolerance that are less well-known. Each of these will be considered in this chapter.

Skin Conditions Are Very Common in Gluten-Sensitive Patients

By far, DH is the most common and, usually, the most severe skin condition linked to gluten sensitivity. While prevalence statistics have not been formally assessed in the United States, prevalence in Europe has been defined as one case in every 2,000 people.[373] Likewise, reports indicate that twenty-five percent of celiac disease patients suffer DH at some time.[374] This makes dermatitis herpetiformis a common manifestation of gluten sensitivity.

Other skin conditions, such as psoriasis, eczema, acne, dry skin and palmoplantar pustulosis (a type of psoriasis appearing on the palms and the soles), have also been reported in association with gluten sensitivity. Excluding dermatitis herpetiformis, rough estimates state that nearly ten percent of all patients with gluten sensitivity have skin disorders at some time or another.[375] Therefore, being aware that gluten intolerance can trigger skin conditions can be very important if you are struggling from a lack of response to treatment. It may be that avoiding gluten is your answer to addressing the main underlying cause.

The Basics of Dermatitis Herpetiformis and Other Skin Conditions

Dermatitis herpetiformis (DH) is an active skin disorder that presents with blisters on the skin in symmetrical areas over the body. The areas typically affected include the elbows, knees, buttocks, lower back and back of the head. The blisters are usually inflamed and red, and severe itching and burning can be present. Many times, patients may have the burning and itching before a rash ever appears.[376] We actually have had several patients suffering in this fashion for years without a rash ever being present.

Gluten Antibodies Deposit Themselves Within the Skin

The cause of DH is quite interesting. All cases of DH are due to gluten sensitivity. Essentially, gluten triggers an immune reaction within the body, and the antibodies produced then circulate through the bloodstream and are deposited within the skin. Specifically, IgA antibodies triggered by gluten exposure lodge between the epidermal layer (outermost layer of skin) and the other dermal layers of the skin.[377] This then induces an inflammatory reaction, which causes the severe rash, the itching and the burning pain. For reasons that are not clear, anti-inflammatory medications like ibuprofen may actually worsen the condition.[378]

A Gluten-Free Diet Is the Simple Solution

Treatment for DH includes a medication called Dapsone, which halts the inflammatory reaction, and institution of a gluten-free diet. Avoidance of gluten is effective at keeping DH in remission and can actually be the sole treatment if the rash is not too severe.[379] The purpose of Dapsone is to quiet the rash and pain as soon as possible while allowing the avoidance of gluten to resolve the underlying problem.

Drugs Don't Prove Useful

Actually, side-by-side trials, testing whether a gluten-free diet plus Dapsone versus a gluten-free diet alone was more effective, have been performed. In one study, seventy-two patients with DH were split into two groups for this purpose. Over eighteen months, the gluten-free diet plus Dapsone treatment experienced an eighty-nine-percent remission rate, but similarly, the gluten-free diet alone treatment yielded an eighty-seven-percent remission rate. Both were comparable in effect, given enough time for a response.[380]

Eczema, Psoriasis, Acne and Dry Skin

Though less well-appreciated, gluten sensitivity, as mentioned, is associated with eczema, psoriasis, acne, dry skin and palmoplantar pustulosis (PPP). PPP can be associated with Sjogren's syndrome, which is an immune condition manifested by dry eyes, dry mouth and arthritic pains. Sjogren's was discussed earlier in relationship to gluten in the arthritis chapter of this book.

In PPP, pustules (that are not infected) form between the layers of the skin, similar to DH. However, the affected areas are only on the palms of the hands and soles of the feet. Twenty-four percent of these patients have positive anti-gliadin antibodies, which are antibodies against gluten's protein components. Like other gluten-related skin conditions, this also successfully responds to avoidance of gluten.[381]

Jeff Had Been Suffering Since Age Two— He's Now Forty-Seven

Jeff is a high-powered businessman in the field of real estate. When he came into the office he promised us a monument built in our honor if we could do anything for his lifelong eczema. As early as age two, Jeff was completely covered with skin that appeared burnt and peeling. His allergies were so bad that he was anaphylactic. The condition truly was life-threatening.

The severity of the allergies improved somewhat with age but he still suffered, and between the eczema and allergies, he claims, there is no drug or topical cream he hasn't tried in his four-decade-long search for relief. He saw experts in the allergies field and hosts of dermatologists and spent many thousands of dollars on doctor visits and treatments. But he still suffered.

It has been several years since Jeff began our program and it was great to catch up with him recently and discover that he is still doing well. He's on absolutely no medications and has no eczema or allergy symptoms—except when he cheats on his diet.

As you've probably guessed we found that Jeff was gluten-sensitive. His adrenal glands were also quite fatigued. Within a few months of getting off gluten and following our program his eczema was dramatically improved. It continued to improve and, after close to a year, was completely gone.

He states that there was no coincidence involved in removing gluten from his diet and his relief from the eczema and allergies; he knows this because the symptoms will return when he has a dietary indiscretion. Within hours to two days after consuming any gluten his eczema will return. Similarly a chronic loss of sleep for several days will result in symptoms.

Jeff is Italian and, of course, enjoyed many a gluten-laden pasta meal before discovering his gluten sensitivity. After many long decades of searching for relief, he sums up his experience as follows: "Who would have EVER thought it was gluten?"

What Is known About Gluten Sensitivity and Skin Disorders

Other than what has been described already about gluten-related antibodies being deposited in the skin in dermatitis herpetiformis and palmoplantar pustulosis, other mechanisms by which gluten sensitivity causes skin problems exist. For instance, dry skin and acne can both result from nutritional deficiencies related to gluten intolerance. Specifically, vitamin A and E deficiencies, along with poor fatty acid absorption, can result in poor skin health. As gluten causes intestinal inflammation and disruption of the digestive lining, these important vitamins and nutrients cannot be adequately absorbed from the diet.[382]

A Reaction to Gluten Associated With Skin and Joint Inflammation

Other skin disorders, such as eczema and psoriasis, likely have immune system causes in relation to gluten sensitivity. One important research study took 114 patients with psoriasis and arthritis and identified five as having celiac disease by biopsy of the small intestine. Instead of looking at these five patients, the study evaluated the remaining 109 individuals. What they found was that a high number had anti-gliadin IgA antibodies in their blood, and the higher the antibody level, the greater the inflammation of the skin and joints.[383] This supports the association of psoriasis in gluten-sensitive patients who do not meet celiac disease criteria. It also supports an immune system mechanism of cause.

Sixty-Nine Percent of Gluten-Sensitive Children Have Skin Disorders

The same skin disorders associated with gluten intolerance in adults occurs in children. In an assessment of fifty-five children with gluten sensitivity, the most common skin disorder was dry skin, which affected about sixty-nine percent.[384] The remainder had a constellation of eczema, psoriasis or DH. Of children and adults who suffer from DH, only ten percent have classic gluten-related symptoms otherwise. That means that ninety percent of all DH patients would be "silent" gluten-sensitive patients if it were not for the skin disorder. Again, all patients with dermatitis herpetiformis have gluten sensitivity by definition.[385]

Skin Disease Responds Favorably to Gluten-Free Diet

While nutritional deficiencies caused by gluten and direct immune reactions against gluten account for many cases of skin disease, indirect immune mechanisms also exist. As previously mentioned in other chapters, the disruption of the integrity of the intestinal lining by gluten can allow other foreign particles to gain access to our bodies and trigger immune reactions. In a rare skin condition called cutaneous leucoclastic vasculitis, a severe rash occurs as immune complexes against non-gluten proteins are deposited in the skin. The reason why this is felt to be gluten-related is that all patients respond immediately to a gluten-free diet. Therefore, the authors propose that the mechanism of cause is gluten's causing a damaged intestinal lining, or a leaky lining, which, in turn, allows foreign particles to cross.[386]

Essentially, the same mechanisms by which gluten causes many health disorders apply to skin disorders as well. Gluten elimination effectively treats skin problems in all patients, whether it is dry skin, eczema, psoriasis or DH. The challenge is identifying gluten as the root cause so directed treatment can be encouraged.

Summary

Your skin is actually the largest organ system of your body, and as you now know, it also can be affected commonly by gluten in your diet. Gluten sensitivity can cause a variety of skin conditions, and it causes them through immune and nutritional mechanisms as it does in other disorders of the body. Of the skin disorders, the most noteworthy is dermatitis herpetiformis, which can cause severe blistering of the skin with intense itching and pain. This, as well as all the other skin problems, responds well to elimination of gluten in the diet.

   While dermatitis herpetiformis (DH) is usually recognized as a gluten condition once the rash appears, identifying the earlier stages of DH may be difficult. Likewise, other skin conditions, like eczema and psoriasis, may not prompt a routine assessment for gluten sensitivity as the association is not known. Because these disorders can be caused by gluten, it is important that you and your clinician be aware of the role gluten can have in your rash or skin problem.

Twenty

Gluten Sensitivity and Memory Loss

Overview

With the advancement in age of the baby boomers, many health disorders have increased in prevalence, but two of the most rapidly growing disorders are dementia and memory loss. This chapter will address memory loss in relation to gluten sensitivity, but it is important to realize that memory loss and gluten intolerance affect not only the elderly but younger adults as well. Gluten-induced memory loss occurs for reasons that will be described below, but it is a rarity that clinicians identify this symptom with gluten sensitivity if classic digestive symptoms are absent. For this reason, we wanted to bring this to your attention.

Alzheimer's Affects Millions and Is Very Costly

Statistics for memory loss itself are hard to come by, but the majority of those with memory loss are diagnosed as having Alzheimer's disease. The prevalence of Alzheimer's disease affects at least 1.5 percent of the population and a total of 5.2 million Americans. Its estimated impact via both direct and indirect costs to us as a nation is $148 billion!

Alzheimer's disease is also the seventh-leading cause of death.[387] While this is an underestimation of all those who suffer memory dysfunction (since not everyone who complains of memory loss has Alzheimer's disease), the figures provide a dramatic portrayal of the significance of these disorders.

High Percentage of People With Poor Memory Are Gluten-Sensitive

Of the population affected by impaired memory function, a significant percentage is affected by gluten sensitivity. Some research has demonstrated brain abnormalities in patients with gluten sensitivity that correlates with poor memory function; also, beneficial responses to gluten elimination have been demonstrated if intervention occurs early. These are the important points that we will stress as you read this chapter.

The Basics of Memory Loss

As stated, not everyone who has memory loss suffers from Alzheimer's disease, although this is the most common disorder of memory. Clinicians now separate memory loss into mild cognitive impairment (MCI) and other conditions such as Alzheimer's disease, amnesia from brain trauma, dementia from hardening of the arteries, etc.

Statistically, twelve percent of everyone over the age of seventy has mild cognitive impairment, and half of these people will go on to have Alzheimer's dementia. In other words, if you have mild cognitive impairment or memory loss, your risk for developing Alzheimer's dementia is quadrupled compared to the normal population.[388]

Multiple Factors Affect Memory

Memory loss can be due to many factors. Certainly, memory loss develops more commonly as you age, but you do not necessarily have to be older to have this problem. For many, genetic factors play a significant role in the risk of developing memory decline. If you have an immediate family memory with Alzheimer's disease, your chances of developing it as well are greater than ten percent. Alzheimer's falls into a category of memory loss caused by a premature degeneration (or aging) of the brain. Other degenerative conditions that affect memory also exist, but none are well-understood in terms of cause.

Most causes of memory loss are attributed to four categories of disease. These categories are degenerative, trauma-related, vascular and emotional. Memory loss from emotional causes includes depression. This was discussed in the earlier chapter on depression as it relates to gluten sensitivity. Vascular causes refer to damage caused to the brain by strokes or small blood vessel injury. Blood vessels can become damaged from high blood pressure and atherosclerosis over time.

Thyroid Problems and Vitamin B12 Are Implicated

Other conditions that are less common include a deficiency of vitamin B12 as well as low thyroid disorders.[389] These latter two conditions were also discussed earlier due to their relationship to gluten sensitivity.

If thyroid function is normal and B12 levels are adequate, treatment for memory problems is often focused on two areas. First, treatments are used to slow down the process of memory loss. Because brain inflammation at a cellular level has been identified, medications such as antioxidants and anti-inflammatories are often given. Secondly, other treatments try to enhance a person's memory chemically, with medications such as Aricept or Exelon.[390] These may offer some benefit in symptom severity, but they have some serious side effects, and none have been shown to delay the progression of memory loss over time.

Memory Loss and Gluten Sensitivity

Given that we have already discussed other conditions of brain dysfunction in relation to gluten, it is not surprising that gluten can affect memory as well. Chapters that discussed attention deficit disorder and depression have been detailed already. Overall, gluten sensitivity and neurological problems are quite common, with seven percent of gluten-sensitive patients having memory loss, neuropathy or other brain-related symptoms.[391]

Nervous System Disorders Succumb to Gluten-Free Diet

Some gluten-sensitive patients have rare nervous system disorders such as Amyotrophic Lateral Sclerosis (ALS), also known as Lou Gehrig's disease,[392] and others can even have seizures.[393] Neither of these is common, but of the few known cases, they have responded remarkably well to gluten elimination. Because the occurrence of general memory loss is more prevalent than these other neurologic conditions, we will focus on this disorder primarily.

To demonstrate the association between gluten sensitivity and memory loss, researchers evaluated thirteen patients with severe cognitive decline who had been diagnosed with gluten sensitivity within the previous two years. Common symptoms included poor memory, confusion, personality changes and trouble with calculations. In the lab results, all demonstrated abnormalities on their brain MRI scans, and a significant proportion also had other neurological symptoms. Because of these other neurologic findings, the authors concluded that gluten sensitivity likely had a relationship to the memory loss.[394]

In another study, 160 patients with gluten sensitivity were examined for neurological symptoms. Of these patients, thirteen had some type of neurological complaint, including three who had memory dysfunction. Once these patients started a gluten-free diet, seven of the thirteen had resolution of their neurological symptoms. In data analysis, it was further found that those who responded had been known to have gluten sensitivity for less than six months. Also, in the majority, neurological symptoms preceded any other gluten-related complaints.[395]

Gluten Antibodies Are Known to Damage Brain Tissue

Gluten-related mechanisms that cause memory dysfunction are most likely two-fold. First and most commonly, antibodies made against gluten or related proteins can damage brain tissue. This,, in turn causes various neurological symptoms including memory loss.

Vitamin B12, Often Deficient With Gluten Sensitivity, Is Necessary for Memory

Research has shown that patients with neurological symptoms have elevated gluten-related antibodies. These antibodies have been shown to be present in gluten-sensitive patients regardless of whether digestive symptoms were present or not.[396] Other mechanisms may involve nutritional deficiencies due to gluten's effect of damaging the intestinal lining. Decreased vitamin B12 absorption from the diet is often present in gluten sensitivity if the intestinal lining is affected. Vitamin B12 is a necessary nutrient for memory to function well, and its depletion is a known cause of memory loss.[397]

Gluten Causes Abnormal Blood Flow to the Brain

To support gluten's involvement as a root cause in memory dysfunction, two additional studies have examined the blood flow to the brain in patients who are sensitive to gluten. In one, thirty-four gluten-sensitive patients were examined with sixteen on a gluten-free diet and eighteen eating regular, gluten-containing diets. Overall, seventy-one percent of the patients had abnormalities in blood flow to the frontal parts of the brain, and the patients who had ingested gluten during the study had the greatest areas of damage.[398]

Adhering to a Gluten-Free Diet Normalizes Blood Flow to the Brain

In the other study, thirty patients with gluten sensitivity were examined by blood flow scans. Fifteen were on a gluten-free diet while the remaining fifteen were not. Results showed that seventy-three percent of the patients on the unrestricted diet had blood flow abnormalities to the brain, while only seven percent of the patients on the gluten-free diet had these findings.[399]

Restriction of Blood Flow Followed by Normalization Causes Damage

In studies that have examined stroke and heart attack events, one of the causes of injury to an organ can be what is called "reperfusion." Reperfusion is where there is an increase in blood flow in an area that has had previous blood flow restriction. For example, in a patient who has had a recent stroke, an artery to the brain tissue is clogged suddenly. As soon as the tissue fails to receive blood flow, the lack of oxygen and nutrients begin to cause damage to the cells in that area of the brain. If enough time goes by (usually a few hours), the damage is irreversible. If blood flow is then re-established after this period of time, the reperfusion can cause big problems because the tissues' structure is no longer healthy and intact. This can result in microscopic or even large areas of bleeding.

Your Brain Appreciates It When You Don't Cheat on Your Diet

Instead of the lack of blood flow causing a smaller area of injury, the subsequent return of blood flow to a damaged area of tissue can make the injury even larger. This, presumptively, can also happen when a person with blood flow limitations from gluten sensitivity no longer eats a gluten-containing diet. Reperfusion of blood flow to the area occurs as the gluten-induced inflammation resolves, and this, then, causes further injury. The goal is to therefore identify gluten sensitivity and avoid gluten before these blood flow changes begin to occur.

Keep Your Memory Sharp on a Gluten-Free Diet

Putting together all of these findings, gluten is found to be a root cause of memory loss in a significant number of people, and most of the time, gluten triggers the immune system to damage parts of the brain, limiting blood flow as a result. In order for our memories to work well, our brains need good circulation of blood to supply them with vital nutrients and oxygen. Identifying gluten as a cause early and eliminating it from the diet in sensitive individuals can help a large number of people with memory dysfunction.

Summary

The ability to remember and to think logically is crucial to our day-to-day functioning, and the increase in memory disorders is a tremendous concern for each of us as it pertains to ourselves, our families and our society as a whole. While many causes of Alzheimer's disease and other memory conditions are not known, a significant number of people with memory dysfunction suffer from gluten intolerance. Studies support gluten's role in causing memory and cognitive difficulties, and it also supports findings showing brain injury from including it in our diet.

Truly, it would be a tragedy to miss diagnosing gluten as the root cause of one's memory disorder. Based on the evidence presented in this chapter, memory and many other neurological disorders can be the result of gluten sensitivity. If this pertains to you or your family, consider gluten sensitivity testing. And, consider it sooner rather than later, as evidence supports that delayed diagnosis can cause irreversible injury. Taking this first step could make a huge impact on your health.

SECTION FIVE

Finding and Eliminating the Cause

We have now discussed a tremendous amount of information about gluten sensitivity and how it affects the body in diverse ways. From the digestive tract to just about every other bodily system, gluten has the potential to cause many symptoms and health disorders in sensitive individuals.

"Silent" Gluten Sensitivity Causes Harm

We have intentionally stressed the importance of being tested for gluten sensitivity if you are at risk, regardless of whether symptoms exist or not. So many "silent" gluten-sensitive patients are unaware of the harm they are doing to their bodies. Undetected, silent gluten sensitivity poses serious risks for developing irreversible immune disorders and health problems. Additionally, many people, even though seemingly silent, notice a marked improvement in their health once gluten is taken out of their diets.

Criteria for Diagnosis Is Antiquated

In this section, we will discuss the diagnostic tests available for gluten disorders. This is a problematic area because for decades, the health field has focused solely on celiac disease as the standard for gluten sensitivity. This has led to criteria for diagnosis that no longer apply, given recent information. We will identify this discrepancy as we discuss our approach to detecting gluten as a potential root cause.

The Gold Standard Is Symptomatic Improvement on a Gluten-Free Diet

In our experience, and from scientific literature, the true gold-standard test for symptomatic patients is the resolution of symptoms and the improvement of function by eliminating gluten from the diet. In asymptomatic patients, we rely on diagnostic tests for screening, but we often also use gluten elimination from the diet to screen for hidden symptoms.

Sometimes We Don't Know How Good We Can Feel

"Hidden symptoms" refers to complaints or symptoms that patients don't realize are present until they eliminate gluten from their diets. Patients will often tell us that they thought a symptom was just "who they were" rather than a reversible complaint. As a result, patients may suddenly experience a significant boost in energy and vitality, which highlights an underlying fatigue that was previously accepted as normal. They truly didn't think it was possible to feel that good.

Screening for Early Detection Makes Good Sense

The entire book, up to this point, has shown that gluten sensitivity can be the cause of many serious health problems, and it also can cause many unrecognized complaints. Therefore, we strongly urge that screening for gluten sensitivity is absolutely necessary to allow for early detection and for avoidance of these many health disorders.

A Dietary Change Is Not Difficult When Good Health Is the Result

One misconception is that eliminating gluten from the diet can be incredibly burdensome. We have not found this to be the case. In our experience, symptomatic patients and many silent gluten-sensitive individuals feel incredibly healthier once they become gluten-free. A gluten-free diet is also healthier in other aspects by nature of the increase in fruits, vegetables and other macronutrients that goes along with removing simple carbohydrates from your diet. Because some clinicians cannot fathom a gluten-free diet for themselves, they are unable to recommend it to their patients. We will discuss these aspects of diet in Chapter 22.

What if Symptoms Persist After Going Gluten-Free?

We will also briefly cover an important concept that we often find in our clinic. After eliminating gluten from our gluten-sensitive patients, several have continued to exhibit complaints due to the presence of nutritional deficiencies, secondary infections, secondary food allergies and adrenal exhaustion. This is important to realize as these conditions need special care and attention to regain one's full health. Remember, the effects of gluten on the body have been occurring for months, if not years, and therefore, many secondary health problems can develop during that time. Part of our diagnostic investigation is to search for these factors as well.

What's a Mother to Do?

You may remember the earlier case study of A., a seventeen-year-old high school student suffering from chronic stomachaches and migraines. When he came to see us in the beginning of his senior year, he was in danger of not graduating, despite being extremely bright, simply due to the quantity of school he was missing due to his ailments.

Halfway into the second week on the modified elimination diet, he was feeling better and having less headaches. His lab test revealed a positive test for gluten sensitivity. When he occasionally stumbled onto a little gluten, the results were intensely painful for him and a multi-day migraine ensued.

Several months later, his mother spoke to his pediatrician, to update him on the true source of her son's chronic stomachaches and headaches. Upon relating the entire story to her doctor, he stated that the only way to know if A. had celiac disease definitively was to put him back on gluten for a minimum of one to two months and then perform a biopsy of his intestine. A.'s mother was amazed at the recommendation, given her son's intense sensitivity to gluten. Needless to say, she declined to put her son through the trial of gluten and a follow-up biopsy.

When Doctors Disagree

There have been many such instances as A.'s. When we diagnose patients with gluten sensitivity, they have marked changes in their health and witness for themselves what gluten ingestion causes. Yet, they are often told by their own physicians or gastroenterologists one of two things:

1. They need to start eating gluten for a couple of months and take a biopsy to be sure.
2. Their biopsies are negative, so there's no reason for them to avoid gluten in their diets.

By now, you understand the effects that gluten has on your health. It is important to understand these mechanisms, but it is also important to understand the realities of diagnostic testing and gluten-free diets. Understanding these topics will avoid any confusion when you undergo testing or have treatment discussions with your health practitioner.

Education Is the Answer

Our goal is to educate patients and clinicians alike so that a lack of understanding and knowledge does not lead to delays in accurate diagnosis or needless suffering for those with gluten sensitivity.

Twenty-One

Diagnosing Gluten Sensitivity: Are You or Aren't You?

As science has learned how gluten affects the body and the immune system, diagnostic testing has also rapidly evolved. Today, there are several blood tests that were not available two decades ago.

Lab Tests Have Limitations

Advances have mostly occurred in being able to detect specific antibodies. While these antibody tests are very important, they also have limitations of which you will need to be aware. In this chapter, we will discuss all the available tests as they pertain to gluten sensitivity and what information you are likely to receive from other clinicians. Additionally, we will demonstrate the shortcomings of these tests and some fallacies in common practice among clinicians when assessing the presence of gluten sensitivity.

Celiac Disease Is but a Small Fraction of the Gluten Sensitivity Category

Before we start, there is an important concept that must be stressed. For many decades, celiac disease was felt to be the only health disorder related to gluten sensitivity. It was not until recently that an abundance of information revealed multiple health disorders related to gluten sensitivity that are distinct from celiac disease. Celiac disease is defined as a type of gluten intolerance that damages the small intestine and causes villous atrophy. If you recall, small intestine villi are the small, finger-like projections that help us absorb nutrients from our diets. In celiac disease, these villi are severely damaged and shrink. This is labeled "villous atrophy."

A Biopsy Is Not Accurate for Gluten Sensitivity

Because celiac disease was thought to be the only gluten disorder, the definitive diagnosis of celiac disease has been an intestinal biopsy to show villous atrophy. What we now realize is that celiac disease represents a fraction of all gluten-related disorders. Despite this, many clinicians believe that a biopsy must be performed to diagnose gluten sensitivity, and if it's negative, they believe that this effectively rules out a gluten disorder. This is absolutely not true!

A Little Tutorial on Your Immune System

As a matter of explanation, we want to talk about the immune system in relation to gluten and the digestive tract. The immune system makes five different classes of antibodies, which are IgG, IgA, IgM, IgE and IgD. Of these, we will only consider IgG, IgM and IgA, as these are the key antibodies that cause gluten-related disorders. IgA is primarily produced along the intestinal lining and represents an important part of our bodies' defense systems against foreign bacteria, viruses and parasites that may come from our diets. If someone is sensitive to gluten, the immune system works overtime to attack gluten as it attempts to enter the bloodstream from the intestines. IgA antibodies are produced in high numbers in the intestinal lining as a defense barrier.

IgA antibodies against gluten are often more sensitive at detecting gluten sensitivity than IgG antibodies because gluten affects the intestinal lining most of the time in gluten sensitivity. However, because IgA production is in overdrive, depletion of IgA levels in gluten-sensitive patients commonly occurs over time. Actually, IgA deficiency is fifteen times more common in gluten-sensitive patients than in normal individuals.[400] When IgA deficiency is present, then antibody tests that only check for IgA levels of antibodies may be falsely negative. IgG levels, however, are not depleted and are a more accurate test of gluten intolerance in people with low IgA levels.

Gluten Sensitivity Can and Does Exist Without Celiac Disease

As we discuss various diagnostic tests, be sure to keep the above items in perspective. Celiac disease is a type of gluten intolerance with severe intestinal damage. Other forms of gluten sensitivity can coexist with celiac disease, or gluten sensitivity can exist without it. Our goal is to identify all forms of gluten sensitivity so that appropriate treatment can be instituted. Also, when choosing gluten antibody testing, be sure to check both IgA and IgG levels to reduce false negative results.

Common Tests to Diagnose Gluten Sensitivity

While many tests exist that screen for other disorders, this section will cover only those specific to gluten sensitivity. For example, a colonoscopy may be performed for abdominal complaints looking for colon cancer, ulcerative colitis or other colon conditions. A CT scan or MRI of the abdomen may be performed to look for bowel perforations, infections or masses. If a person has gluten sensitivity affecting other parts of the body, a multitude of tests may be performed. Migraines or memory loss may prompt MRI brain scans. Joint pains can evoke many unrelated blood tests and x-rays. It is beyond the scope of this book for us to discuss all of these exams.

Instead, we will cover the tests specifically performed when gluten sensitivity is suspected. These are not in any particular order. We will then discuss, in detail, our own specific approach, once you have a better understanding of the tests available. We will also cover additional testing at the conclusion that pertains to nutritional deficiencies, concurrent food allergies and concurrent infections.

Blood Testing

GENETIC BLOOD TESTS—genetic blood studies assess an individual's capacity to carry one of the HLA genes that is associated with gluten sensitivity. Studies support that ninety percent of patients with gluten sensitivity carry the HLA DQ2 gene, and others may carry the HLA DQ8 gene commonly.[401] These tests are not performed as commonly now as other antibody tests, which are more accurate and have thus replaced them.

However, genetic screens can be helpful in individuals who are at risk of having gluten sensitivity. For example, in relatives and children of gluten-sensitive individuals with negative blood antibody tests, HLA patterns can indicate future risk. If both HLA DQ2 and HLA DQ8 are absent, the risk of being gluten-intolerant is minimal and it would negate the need for future testing for the individual. If positive, continued periodic screening and a gluten-free diet would be indicated.

The other area of benefit in genetic testing is for children. The ease of testing by simply swabbing the inside of the mouth makes this less invasive for a small child. This may be a reasonable screening test in children at risk for gluten sensitivity.

ANTI-GLIADIN ANTIBODIES—if you recall, gluten is composed of two major proteins, gliadin and glutenin. Gliadin is the component that triggers the immune reactions in sensitive people, and therefore, many people with gluten sensitivity have antibodies to this protein.

Testing for anti-gliadin antibodies (AGA) is a simple blood test, but studies have shown that it is less sensitive for detecting celiac disease compared to other antibodies, which will be discussed later. The confusion, as stated earlier, is that the ability of AGA to detect gluten intolerance has been defined in conjunction with a positive intestinal biopsy. While this may be a standard for celiac disease, we now know that this is an inaccurate standard for gluten sensitivity. In fact, AGA may be the best current diagnostic test when considering all gluten-related disorders.

In testing for AGA, antibodies of both the IgG and IgA classes are checked since low total levels of IgA may be present.[402] As described above, if a person has low total IgA levels, antibody tests for IgA may be falsely negative.

ANTI-ENDOMYSIAL ANTIBODIES—unlike anti-gliadin antibodies, anti-endomysial antibodies (EM antibodies) are auto-antibodies. What do we mean by this? Gliadin is a gluten protein, so, therefore, when the immune system attacks it, is not attacking "self" tissues but, instead, a foreign food protein. In contrast, as gliadin is absorbed through the intestinal lining, it attaches to the smooth muscle cells of the intestinal wall. EM antibodies are directed against proteins of these smooth muscle cells, and, therefore, EM antibodies are directed against "self" tissue. This defines them as auto-antibodies.

Because EM antibodies attack the smooth muscle of the small intestine, these antibodies correlate better with damage to the intestine wall. Studies have supported an accuracy rate of approximately ninety percent for celiac disease. Actually, in one study, EM antibodies were present in 100 percent of individuals when total villous atrophy was present.[403] However, EM antibodies are ineffective in detecting individuals with silent or subclinical gluten sensitivity.[404] If minor involvement of the intestinal lining occurs or if no intestinal involvement is present, EM antibodies are much less accurate.

As with anti-gliadin antibodies, EM antibody testing should evaluate IgG and IgA forms of antibodies for the same reason as described above. If a gluten-sensitive patient is IgA-deficient, IgA EM antibodies may be falsely negative even for celiac disease.

ANTI-TISSUE TRANSGLUTAMINASE ANTIBODIES—similar to anti-endomysial antibodies, anti-tissue transglutaminase antibodies (tTG antibodies) are also auto-antibodies directed against "self" tissue. After gliadin crosses the intestinal lining, a special enzyme called tissue trans-glutaminase binds to gliadin and takes off a portion of the protein. This portion is called glutamine. tTG antibodies are antibodies that are directed against the complex of gliadin attached to tissue transglutam-inase. Because tissue transglutaminase is a "self" enzyme, tTG antibodies are also auto-antibodies.

Also, like anti-endomysial antibodies, tTG antibodies are ninety-percent accurate in celiac disease[405] because they represent immune system attack at the level of the intestinal lining. Gluten sensitivity that involves minor intestinal injury or no villous atrophy will be less likely detected by tTG antibodies.[406] Therefore, tTG antibodies correlate best with villous atrophy, as several studies have supported, and a negative tTG antibody test (or EM antibody test, for that matter) does not rule out gluten sensitivity when intestinal involvement is minimal or absent.

While some researchers support tTG antibodies as being a sensitive test for identifying celiac disease,[407] it is less sensitive for gluten sensi-tivity in a broader sense. This makes logical sense given the location of where this enzyme acts on gliadin. Disorders related to gluten sensitivity that do not involve the intestinal tract would be unlikely to trigger tTG antibody response from the immune system.

DEAMINATED GLIADIN ANTIBODIES—after tissue transglutaminase detaches the glutamine portion from gliadin, the remaining gliadin protein is termed a "deaminated" gliadin. The immune system can make specific antibodies against several different parts of the gliadin protein, and a deaminated gliadin can provoke different antibodies to be produced, compared to an intact gliadin protein.

As a result, newer antibody tests detect antibodies made against deaminated gliadin selectively. In studies looking again at celiac disease patients only, deaminated gliadin antibodies had an accuracy rate of approximately eighty-five percent, making it comparable to EMA and tTG antibody tests.[408]

The ability of deaminated gliadin antibodies to detect gluten sensi-tivity outside of celiac disease is not known. In celiac disease patients with IgA deficiency, the IgG test for deaminated gliadin antibodies was as effective as tTG tests.[409] Because testing for deaminated gliadin antibodies offers little advantage over tTG and EMA antibody tests, it is usually not commonly ordered. It may be an effective tool in screening for gluten sensitivity but, to date, these studies have not been performed.

TOTAL SERUM IGA LEVEL—low total levels of IgA antibodies are rarely found in the normal population, with one out of every 600 people having this condition,[410] but in gluten sensitivity, low IgA levels are more common. This reflects the increased IgA antibody production in the intestine, to fight off gluten as it attempts to enter our bodies.

If a low level of IgA is present, then certainly, IgG varieties of the antibody tests described above will be more accurate in diagnosing gluten-related conditions. In general, total IgA levels are not ordered often since IgG antibody tests are usually ordered concurrently. Therefore, defining a low IgA level adds little information in making a diagnosis. There is a general theory, however, that a lower IgA level suggests greater inflammation of the intestinal lining and greater chronicity of disease. A low IgA level may provide some insight into duration of disease.

Saliva Testing

SALIVA ANTIBODY TESTING—while serum antibody testing has been shown in some studies to be more accurate than saliva testing in gluten-sensitive patients,[411] IgM and IgA antibodies are also made in the saliva, allowing a less-invasive way of screening for gluten sensitivity.

The difficulty is that these saliva tests have yet to be tested against patients' responses to a gluten-free diet in large populations. The saliva tests are therefore not as widely accepted in the medical community. However, our clinical experience shows the tests to be very accurate when correlated with clinical changes that occur with a gluten-free diet. There are research projects currently underway to show the validity of saliva testing, and it is our belief that saliva testing, in the future, may become one of the best screening tests because of its ease and low cost.

Fecal Testing

FECAL ANTI-GLIADIN ANTIBODIES—as you may recall, the immune system begins its line of defense against gluten in sensitive individuals at the intestinal lining by producing IgA antibodies. In keeping with this information, it is predicted that IgA levels against gliadin in the stool may be a more sensitive reflection of gluten intolerance compared to blood testing.

One researcher has conducted extensive research in this area and reports that 100 percent of celiac disease patients have fecal anti-gliadin antibodies (fAGA) and over seventy percent of those with gluten sensitivity have fAGA. This research has yet to be independently duplicated by other research studies, but if the current research holds true, then someday, fecal testing may prove to be one of the best and most reliable methods of testing for gluten sensitivity.

Scopes and Biopsies

UPPER ESOPHAGOGASTRODUODENOSCOPY (EGD)—despite the advent of less-invasive blood, saliva and fecal tests, there are several clinicians who feel as though a small intestinal biopsy is required before instituting a gluten-free diet.[412] These clinicians may not have distinguished between celiac disease and the bigger category of disease that falls under gluten sensitivity, or they may not be aware of the broad effects that gluten can have on our health.

As research supports, celiac disease represents a fraction of all gluten-related health disorders. Additionally, there exists a misconception by a few that a gluten-free diet is a major inconvenience as a treatment. This lends some clinicians to support biopsies for "proof" before committing one to what they feel is a very restrictive diet. In actuality, being gluten-free is quite easy and very healthy. Better understanding of this among clinicians may also change an insistence on small-intestinal biopsies.

EGD is administered to a person while he or she is in a lightly sedated state. A flexible tube with a light and a tiny camera at the end of the scope is slowly inserted through the mouth and navigated through the esophagus and stomach, and into the upper portion of the small intestine. The small intestine is vast, and EGD only assesses the first five feet or so of the small intestine. This causes some significant limitation in terms of finding pathology in many cases.

In addition to directly visualizing the intestinal lining, EGD can biopsy portions of the intestinal wall for evaluation. Small pinchers take little pieces of tissue that can be examined later under a microscope. Specifically, in gluten disorders, findings sought include villous atrophy and inflammation of the intestinal wall.

Unfortunately, contrary to some people's beliefs, a negative biopsy does not rule out gluten sensitivity. In fact, it does not even rule out celiac disease 100 percent of the time. Because EGD samples only a portion of the small intestine, and because the area of intestinal lining chosen for biopsy may not be involved with inflammation, a biopsy can be falsely negative, even when celiac disease is present. The small intestine is twenty-one feet long, with a surface area the size of a tennis court. With that picture in mind, one can appreciate that a biopsy, even in celiac disease, may fail to make an accurate diagnosis.

Secondary Tests—Looking For "Hidden" Infections

While we will not go into great detail about these examinations and diagnostic tests, we do want to stress (and hopefully have already proven to you) that having gluten sensitivity for a prolonged time can cause secondary health problems. Chronic stimulation and attack of the immune system makes the body vulnerable to other infections, which we see commonly. Evaluating for the presence of parasites, amoebas, bacteria, etc. is critical for not only regaining one's health, but for the successful healing of a damaged small intestine.

Evaluating for Food Allergies and Nutritional Deficiencies

Also, nutritional deficiencies as a result of intestinal inflammation are significant problems for many with gluten sensitivity. Calcium, magnesium, vitamin B12 and iron are just a few of these that are commonly seen. Concurrent food allergies, such as lactose intolerance, can also develop secondary to being sensitive to gluten. Lastly, adrenal exhaustion must be considered in many patients with longstanding, gluten-related disorders, as we discussed in the chapter on adrenal disorders.

The most common scenario we see involves a patient suffering for many years with gluten sensitivity. We are able to make the diagnosis and proceed to eliminate gluten from the diet. Improvements occur, but all symptoms are not completely resolved. Secondary testing then reveals one or more of these other health problems that require further attention until complete restoration of health can be achieved. The following are some examples of these types of investigations.

Secondary Testing Procedures
Following a Gluten Sensitivity Diagnosis

- Vitamin levels, including vitamin B12, vitamin B6, vitamin D, calcium, magnesium, phosphorus and others
- Fecal testing for parasitic, amoeba or bacterial infections
- Blood, breath or fecal tests for intestinal infections such as H. pylori
- Saliva tests for adrenal exhaustion
- Modified elimination diets to determine food allergies and intolerances
- Blood hormonal assessments of thyroid, reproductive and adrenal functions
- Bone density scans for osteoporosis and osteopenia detection
- Screening for toxins such as mercury and lead exposure
- Clinical assessment for ongoing neurological or physical stress

Our Approach Is to Identify the Root Cause

We have helped numerous people who have suffered for years with gluten sensitivity but have not been accurately diagnosed previously.

Many of our success stories utilizing the HealthNOW Method are included in the preceding chapters, and you are undoubtedly aware now of the scope of gluten-related health disorders. The bottom line is that there is no perfect blood test or biopsy protocol to define 100 percent of those with gluten sensitivity. At least, not yet. Therefore, you have to consider the limitations of these tests as you undergo evaluation.

Our approach to a person in poor health is first to identify the symptoms and to which bodily system these symptoms are related. The next step is to find what stressor may be affecting this bodily system and remove it. Stressors can include toxins, foods, infections, malnutrition, physical stress, emotional stress and others. Because our bodies are so resilient, once we eliminate the stressors, our bodies have an amazing ability to heal over time.

Just to Reiterate: Intestinal Biopsies Do Not Diagnose Gluten Sensitivity!

We have already covered the misconception that an intestinal biopsy is the true gold standard for making a diagnosis of gluten intolerance. While it has a high yield for diagnosing celiac disease, it falls well short of making an accurate diagnosis of gluten sensitivity. There is blood testing of various antibodies which has enabled many patients with celiac disease and gluten sensitivity to receive an accurate diagnosis without a biopsy.

Investigators in the *New England Journal of Medicine* have supported that biopsies are not necessary in celiac disease if blood testing is positive.[413] However, in a group of celiac disease patients with positive biopsies, fifteen percent had negative blood tests supporting limitations in blood testing as well.[414] Even in celiac disease, lesser degrees of villous atrophy and intestinal inflammation decrease the chance that blood tests will be positive.

Screening Is for Everyone

Our algorithm for diagnostic testing in gluten sensitivity is to screen everyone. It is our belief that gluten sensitivity testing should be part of an annual health examination. Given the impact this dietary substance can have on multiple areas of the body, why shouldn't we screen for gluten sensitivity? As a means of prevention of further illnesses and a lower quality of life, the benefits in costs alone would outweigh the costs of screening.

The Lab Test Is Easy

How do we test everyone? Generally, everyone is tested with a saliva and blood evaluation of anti-gliadin antibodies (IgG and IgA) as well as anti-tissue transglutaminase antibodies (IgG and IgA). In small children, we will consider an oral swab for genetic screening for HLA patterns.

A Trial on a Hypoallergenic Diet

At the same time, we place all patients on a modified elimination diet (MED), for ten days, that eliminates gluten and other common food allergens, such as cow's milk, corn and soy products, while invoking a good balance of healthy foods, such as lean protein, vegetables and fruits. By assessing the response to the MED and the results of the diagnostic tests, we will receive a highly accurate assessment of gluten intolerance.

Neglecting to Diagnose a Food Reaction Can Prevent a Patient's Recovery

The question may be asked: Why do we treat patients with symptoms as well as patients with no symptoms the same? For instance, a first-degree relative of a patient with gluten sensitivity may feel fine, so why place him or her on the MED? The answer lies in our experience. Even in asymptomatic patients, we have found that seventy percent have an improvement in their health in the short period of time they are on the MED. They had symptoms of which they were not aware, or, most commonly, their body had simply adapted to the effects that gluten had been causing.

Does Eliminating Gluten From Your Diet Improve Your Symptoms?

For us, the gold standard for diagnosing gluten sensitivity is not an intestinal biopsy or a blood test. It is a beneficial response to complete elimination of gluten from the diet. We have hundreds of patients who have benefited from this diagnostic approach of getting to the root cause. Rather than putting someone through an endoscopic procedure and biopsy unnecessarily, better accuracy of diagnosis is obtained by gluten elimination from the diet.

Screening Can Eliminate So Much Needless Suffering

Regarding serial testing of children and family members who are at risk for gluten sensitivity, we recommend screening early to avoid the complications associated with undiagnosed gluten health disorders. In a recent study of 171 relatives of celiac disease patients, all of whom were negative for antibody blood testing, six later became positive on subsequent testing. Conversion to a positive test occurred as early as six months in some, but more than three years later in others. Five of these six patients were asymptomatic.[415] This stresses the needs for serial screening in anyone who is at risk for gluten sensitivity. For children of gluten-sensitive parents, we recommend gluten elimination from the diet automatically.

Going Gluten-Free Does Not Have to Be Difficult

In the next chapter, we will discuss the modified elimination diet in greater detail and discuss gluten-free diets. Many clinicians seem to be fearful of placing a person on a gluten-free diet for the rest of his or her life, but the reason for this, in light of one's health, is not justified. By providing the abundance of information now available on gluten and its potential impact on your body's health, we sincerely hope to raise awareness of the difference between gluten sensitivity and celiac disease. We also hope to enhance the ability of those suffering to finally find gluten as the real cause of their problem.

Twenty-Two

The Truth
About Being Gluten-free

Eighteen Years of Anxiety Was Debilitating

L. was a lovely, forty-nine-year-old woman, with a ready smile, whose seemingly calm, pleasant exterior belied an eighteen-year problem with severe anxiety. She had sought out psychotherapists to no avail. L. also complained of being about twenty pounds overweight and suffered from migraines and fatigue. But it was her debilitating anxiety that was ruining her life.

Her gluten sensitivity test was borderline high and her adrenal glands were under stress in formal testing. Over the course of her first two weeks on the HealthNOW program, while instituting the modified elimination diet, she felt much better and lost seven pounds. During the first month of care, she felt much improved and continued to lose weight.

Her daughter was getting married, and she had some concerns about how she would do with her anxiety. The wedding occurred six weeks after she began the program, and she was amazed by how well she felt and how little anxiety occurred. After two months, she felt like a new person. Her anxiety of eighteen years was completely gone!

Unfortunately, she felt so much better that she became lax about her gluten avoidance. Six weeks later, she returned for a visit, complaining of anxiety, indigestion, vertigo and fatigue. Realizing that reintroduction of gluten had occurred, we quickly recommended eliminating it once again. Two weeks later, she was again doing well and was convinced that gluten was indeed the link to her anxiety.

Let's Clear Up Any Misconceptions

We have referenced a gluten-free diet throughout the book, and indeed, it is the only effective treatment for gluten sensitivity. Not only will we define gluten-free living, but we also will discuss the truthful facts about eliminating gluten from your diet. Unfortunately, misconceptions abound regarding the limitations of avoiding gluten. It is important to understand exactly what is accurate and what is not.

Once Certain Diseases Have Been Triggered, There Is No Turning Back

Once you have been diagnosed as gluten-sensitive, you will need to remain gluten-free to avoid recurrence of gluten-related symptoms and the development of irreversible health conditions. If your body cannot tolerate gluten, exposure to gluten even in small amounts can lead to conditions such as diabetes, thyroid dysfunction, rheumatoid arthritis and others that will likely not resolve by simply eliminating gluten again. Once these conditions develop, they are ever-present. This is why we encourage early diagnosis and a lifelong commitment to being gluten-free.

Why Is a Gluten-Free Diet a Healthy Diet?

What is underappreciated is that there are many additional health benefits gained by converting to a gluten-free diet if done properly. We are big proponents of good nutrition, and the foods allowed on a gluten-free diet actually promote healthy eating. All you have to do is look around at our society and see the effects of poor dietary habits. Highly processed foods, high caloric intake, foods with high fat content and quick-fix carbohydrates all have resulted in a meteoric rise in obesity rates. While the intent of a gluten-free diet is to prevent gluten-induced health disorders, other benefits for your health will result as well.

Gluten-Free Living

What Can't I Eat?

Gluten, as you are now aware, is a protein found in wheat, rye and barley. It is also in less commonly known cereals such as spelt, kamut, couscous, bulgur, farina, matzo, seitan, semolina, triticale and graham flour. These are the cereals that must be avoided in order to maintain a gluten-free diet. Until you actually pay attention to these foods in your diet, you may not appreciate how ubiquitous they have become in our society.

Many other processed food products can have gluten as a result of added wheat starch or other, more hidden ingredients. For example, soy sauce and processed meats are some examples that contain gluten within their ingredient lists. It is important to become knowledgeable about what foods often have gluten and which ones don't. Increasingly, labels require statements as to whether a product is gluten-free or not. This has been helpful, but hazards still exist when dining out. This is why gluten awareness in your diet is essential.

Accidental gluten ingestion is common because of hidden

gluten in many foods. Creamed vegetables typically contain gluten, as do malted foods. Thickeners, sauces and marinades are other common foods that contain gluten. Anything that contains wheat starch (which is a common additive) contains gluten. Be sure to check labels and ask dining establishments about your food options if you are at all unsure about the content.

What Can I Eat?

Bread and pasta products that are gluten-free include those made with rice, corn, potato and soy, most commonly. Other, less-common grains that are safe include amaranth, quinoa, sorghum, millet and buckwheat, while other gluten-free products include an array of seeds, nuts and beans, which are also safe to eat. They include flax, garfava beans, tapioca and nut flours.

Guide to Avoiding Foods Containing Gluten

Grains and Starches

Gluten is present in many grains and starches, as shown in the following table:

Contains Gluten		Gluten-Free	
Wheat	Kamut	Amaranth	Beans
Wheat germ	Matzo	Rice	Flax
Wheat grass	Seitan	Corn	Garfava
Rye	Semolina	Soy	Sorghum
Barley	Spelt	Potato	Millet
Bulgur	Triticale	Quinoa	Buckwheat
Couscous	Oats*	Tapioca	Arrowroot
Farina	Oat bran*	Tef	Nut flours
Graham flour	Oat fiber*		

controversial due to contamination

Foods that often contain Gluten

Malt, typically from barley or corn	Marinades	Sausages (some)
Breading	Meat Balls	Self-basting Poultry
Broth	Meat Loaf	Soup Bases
Coating Mixes	Meat substitutes (Tofurky and others)	Soy-based veggie burgers
Communion Wafers	Monosodium glutamate	Soy sauce
Crab cakes	Pastas	Stuffings
Croutons	Processed Meats	Tamari
Hydrolyzed vegetable protein—willl say "wheat"	Rice Dream-processed w/ barley	Textured vegetable protein
Imitation Bacon	Roux—a sauce base	Thickeners
Imitation Seafood	Sauces	Vital wheat gluten found in imitation meats

Alcohols

Beer is made from grains and thereby contains gluten. Most other alcohols such as scotch, rye and vodka, while made from grains that are glutinous, are distilled, which removes the gluten, thereby making them safe to consume. Do keep in mind that alcohol, when mixed with gluten in food, seems to magnify the reaction and therefore should be avoided. Further, many patients who have celiac disease or who are gluten-intolerant have intestinal infections that create a poor reaction to alcohol.

Always Read the Label

The key to understanding the gluten-free diet is to become a good ingredient label reader. Foods with labels that list the following ingredients are questionable and should NOT be consumed unless you can verify they do not contain or are not derived from prohibited grains. Remember, you need to be gluten-free, not just wheat-free. Also, many products say that they are gluten-free while having ingredients such as oats, hemp, wheat grass, malt or starch, which may contain gluten and cause intolerant persons to react negatively. Don't be fooled and compromise your health—always read the ingredient list carefully. If in doubt, write to the company online. Most companies are very forthcoming with such information.

- Bran
- Brown rice syrup (frequently made from barley)
- Caramel color (infrequently made from barley)
- Dextrin (usually corn but may be derived from wheat)
- Dry roasted nuts (processing agents may contain wheat)
- Flour or cereal products
- Hydrolyzed vegetable protein (HVP), vegetable protein, hydrolyzed plant protein (HPP), hydrolyzed soy protein or textured vegetable protein (TVP) (read label; it will say "wheat")
- Malt or malt flavoring (usually made from barley)
- Malt vinegar
- Modified food starch of modified starch (read label; it will say "wheat")
- Starch (source should be labeled)
- Soy sauce or soy sauce solids (wheat-free soy sauce is available)
- Ricola cough drops
- Emergen-C in raspberry and mixed berry flavors only; the other flavors are fine

Pasta, Beer—It's All Available Gluten-Free

Many gluten-free pastas and even beer products now exist. Food products will be developed according to consumers' needs, so as the awareness of gluten sensitivity increases, these foods will continue to expand. We have been diagnosing gluten sensitivity for fifteen years, and the release of new, gluten-free products has, thankfully, skyrocketed in the past few years. The need to create gluten-free products has been addressed by some larger companies recently, including General Mills and Anheiser-Busch.

Real Food Is Naturally Gluten-Free

So far, we have identified breads, pastas and cereals mostly. But one of the greatest advantages of a gluten-free diet is that all animal protein, nuts, seeds, fresh vegetables and fruits are naturally gluten-free. These harbor vitamins and minerals (both known and unknown) that are essential for our health. In choosing to eat less processed, "real" foods, it is much easier to avoid accidental gluten contamination while simultaneously improving the type of nutrition you consume. Much of the American diet is composed of highly processed foods, breaded products and simple sugars, all of which are poor choices for our bodies to function well.

Simple Carbohydrates Aren't Good For You Anyway

Simple carbohydrates and sugars are problems by themselves. These foods cause rapid absorption of glucose into our bodies, which raises our blood glucose levels immediately. Our tissues then either utilize or store this glucose and the levels in our blood streams drop as rapidly as they rose. This roller coaster is detrimental to our bodies' normal metabolisms and causes cravings for more sugar as the levels suddenly drop.

Fruits and Vegetables Provide Healthful Complex Carbohydrates

By choosing complex carbohydrates such as vegetables and fruits, absorption evolves more slowly, thus eliminating the rapid rise and fall of glucose in the blood. This eliminates cravings and makes us feel more balanced and energized.

Properly Done, a Gluten-Free Diet Is a Very Healthy Diet

There are some restrictions in foods with gluten-free living, but those restrictions can facilitate making healthier choices in your diet. By selecting natural foods that are gluten-free, you receive vitamins, minerals and nutrients that promote better long-term health. The majority of our patients who now enjoy gluten-free living would not consider reverting because of how dramatically better they feel.

How Much Gluten Is Too Much?

Debates have considered what may be an amount of gluten that could be tolerable by a person who is gluten-sensitive. One study that examined forty-nine biopsy-proven celiac disease patients showed that dosages of less than fifty milligrams a day were tolerable based on intestinal examinations.[416] But again, these were only a select type of gluten-intolerant individuals, celiac disease patients, and not the entire spectrum of individuals with gluten sensitivity. Another study found that one milligram of gluten (or one-sixtieth of a teaspoon of wheat flour) was enough to prevent intestinal healing.[417]

The Smallest Amounts Are Still Problematic

In quantifying gluten, flours made from wheat, barley or rye have approximately 300 milligrams of gluten per teaspoon. One teaspoon is five milliliters in volume. So, any food containing one milliliter of flour (which is not very much) has sixty milligrams of gluten present. This is the reason why contamination is a concern. This amount of gluten contamination can occur in households that use the same appliances and utensils for gluten-containing and gluten-free meal preparations. Therefore, additional precautions must be used if this is the case.

So, what is the actual answer to safe gluten doses? The answer appears to be very individualized. Researchers can detect intestinal changes at fifty milligrams of gluten per day, but in lesser dosages, it remains an unanswered question, whether we are able to detect ill effects in other parts of the body. This is a bigger concern, as gluten has the potential to affect many systems in our bodies and limit good health.

Because gluten can cause so many health problems outside of the digestive system, we cannot be certain that lower doses are not harmful. Whether it is from a communion wafer once a week or a crouton that gets into the salad, small amounts of gluten can trigger reactions in sensitive individuals.

Basically, If You See Gluten Coming, Cross the Street!

We recommend complete avoidance of gluten as a result. Converting to a gluten-free diet is the goal to ensure optimal health, and by choosing to eat more fresh fruits, vegetables and other complex carbohydrates, you will receive other health benefits beyond gluten elimination. Non-celiac gluten disorders, such as neurological illnesses, have been described with doses much lower than fifty milligrams of gluten a day. For sensitive individuals, tiny amounts of gluten in the diet can still cause an immune reaction.[418] Converting to a gluten-free lifestyle and embracing a healthy diet is the clearly safe choice.

Vitamin Considerations: Do You Need to Supplement Your Diet?

Prior to instituting a gluten-free diet, many individuals who are gluten-sensitive have vitamin and mineral deficiencies. As gluten causes inflammation of the intestinal lining and damage to villi, the ability to absorb these micronutrients becomes diminished. Some vitamins and minerals are affected more than others, and therefore, replenishment of these nutrients is important.

Vitamin B12 Deficiencies Are Extremely Common in Gluten-Sensitive Patients

For example, vitamin B12 can be impaired long-term as a result of gluten sensitivity, even after a gluten-free diet is started. The enzyme required in the intestine to absorb vitamin B12 can be permanently affected by immune attack, so longstanding replacement of vitamin B12 in some people may be needed.

B Vitamin and Mineral Status Should Also Be Evaluated for Deficiency

Other common vitamins and minerals that are deficient with gluten sensitivity include thiamine, riboflavin, vitamin B6, vitamin D, calcium, magnesium, iron, zinc and selenium. In order to improve health as quickly as possible, adding supplements of these micronutrients should be considered along with a gluten-free diet. Providing supplements without eliminating gluten won't result in improvement because the offending agent (gluten) has not been removed.

As Healing Takes Place, Absorption of Nutrients Improves

Once a gluten-sensitive individual eliminates gluten in his or her diet, the intestinal wall can begin to heal. This then allows nutrients to gradually replenish tissues of the body so optimal health can be regained. One of the biggest misconceptions about gluten-free diets is that they cause multiple vitamin deficiencies as a result of the restriction of certain foods. Micronutrients such vitamin B6, vitamin B12, iron, folate and calcium have been described as being potentially low while on a gluten-free diet. Some studies describe these deficiencies in people on gluten-free diets, but it appears to be more a reflection of their poor choice of foods rather than the avoidance of wheat, barley and rye products.[419]

Your Healthy Diet in a Nutshell

In actuality, making healthy choices of fruits, vegetables, lean proteins and healthy fats that do not contain gluten give your body a much greater balance of vitamins and minerals than the typical gluten-containing diet. We are still learning about the many micronutrients that exist within fruits and vegetables, so natural food sources are likely more comprehensive in providing all the nutrients that your body needs. Mankind existed thousands of years before wheat and other cereal products were introduced into the standard diet. Eliminating gluten in your diet is not a cause of vitamin deficiency. Indeed, avoiding gluten can only improve your health.

Supplementation Is a Good Idea

For our patients who begin gluten-free diets, we generally recommend a high-quality, daily multivitamin and mineral supplement. Specifically, vitamin D, vitamin B12, other B-complex vitamins, calcium, magnesium, iron and folate are the main focuses. Vitamin B12 can be difficult to absorb in a damaged intestine, so B12 injections are the quickest way to build up this very important vitamin. If injections aren't available, find a sublingual form of B12 that you can dissolve under your tongue. The potential effects of chronic gluten sensitivity on the digestive system, bone and joint health, and the immune system can cause particular levels of these micronutrients to fall. Supplementation allows optimal ability of one to start healing from the long-term effects of gluten on the body. If additional deficiencies are found beyond these micronutrients, a supplementation program will be tailored to address them.

Periodically Assessing Nutrient Status Is a Good Idea

Supplementation combined with good dietary choices is something we monitor over time. As part of our annual assessment of gluten-sensitive patients, we routinely check vitamin status. This has been recommended by top researchers in the field.[420]

If micronutrient deficiencies are found, we first reassess if the person is truly avoiding gluten completely in their diet. Secondly, we re-examine their food choices and supplement consumption. If neither of these provides a reason for continued deficiency, laboratory testing to evaluate any presence of infection or diminished detoxification ability will commence. In this manner, we ensure that the body has all possible stressors isolated that could interfere with its ability to heal itself and maintain good health.

Failing to Stay Gluten-Free: How Serious Is It to "Fall off the Wagon"?

As mentioned, once you are found to have gluten sensitivity, you must always remain gluten-free in order to avoid recurrence of symptoms. Gluten sensitivity is not like an infection that resolves after treatment. It is a permanent feature, similar to the color of your eyes or the shape of your face. Even if you stay off gluten for forty years, the moment it is reintroduced into your system, your body will react negatively.

It's Your Choice—We're Just Trying to Help You Make an Informed Choice

Like many lifestyle changes, leading a gluten-free life is a decision and a choice. It is important to understand that what we eat does affect our health. If a person feels better once off gluten, then he will have an easier time committing to a gluten-free diet. In other words, there is a positive reward immediately for making the dietary change.

But for people who are identified as being gluten-sensitive by testing and have no obvious symptoms, the lack of positive feedback makes compliance more difficult. Compared to symptomatic people, asymptomatic people fail to adhere to a gluten-free diet much more often.[421]

Even people found to have symptoms with gluten sensitivity show noncompliance with a gluten-free diet about thirty percent of the time.[422] Sometimes, this is a result of poor planning or a lack of commitment to their health, but other times, it is due to accidental gluten ingestion. The increased number of processed foods and the frequency by which we dine away from home makes accidental gluten ingestion more common.

What About Oats?

As an aside, we do want to make a comment about oats. While oats themselves do not contain gluten, contamination during the collection and processing of oats with other grains has resulted in significant gluten content in the final product. Therefore, oats are only considered safe if obtained from certain manufacturers that guarantee gluten-free quality. Currently, known manufacturers of "safe" oat products include gluten-freeoats.com, creamhillestates.com and bobsredmill.com.

Awareness Among Food Manufacturers Is Increasing

In the last decade, a significant increase in gluten awareness in food products has developed. In Europe and a few non-European countries, dietary guidelines require food products to be labeled according to the gluten content. In this country, in order to be labeled gluten-free, certain criteria also must now be met.

Gluten-free beers now are much more common and even General Mills has removed barley malt from their Rice Chex cereal to make it gluten-free. This increase in store products being promoted as gluten-free will lead to greater menu choices in restaurants as well. Many restaurant chains now have gluten information for their meals online, for viewing before going to the restaurant. Like many changes in life, it takes planning and preparation until new habits become second-nature.

The Benefits of Being Gluten-Free

Unlike many clinicians, we walk the walk of a gluten-free lifestyle ourselves, so we personally experience the benefits of healthier living as a result of our dietary choices. In addition to choosing to be gluten-free, we also make choices to eat healthy with fresh fruits and vegetables as well as lean proteins and healthy fats.

What Does Your "Care and Feeding Manual" Say?

Your body didn't come with a care and feeding manual, but one of our goals as clinicians is to provide one to each patient so that they feel in control of how to create the level of health they desire. Gluten is a food protein that is detrimental to many people's health if included in their diet and may definitely be on the "not recommended" list in your care and feeding manual.

Your Body Is Unique—Get to Know It

People differ in terms of their sensitivity to foods. Many cannot tolerate the standard American diet of processed foods, simple carbohydrates, sugar and high fat content. These foods cause stress to the body that leads to secondary infections, adrenal exhaustion and malnutrition. Similarly, gluten can cause these same problems in sensitive individuals, in addition to many other health disorders. A significant part of accepting the need to eliminate gluten in your diet is realizing that this sensitivity exists for you.

Once you accept that you are at risk for gluten-related disorders and commit to a gluten-free diet, you will not only enjoy being free of gluten-related symptoms, but you will also enjoy other healthy effects of a good diet. Too little emphasis is placed on diet today. Our bodies have tremendous potential to heal themselves if we simply identify and remove the stressors while providing it with good nutrition and care. These stressors are what we define as the root causes of your symptoms, and gluten is one such root cause that is extremely common.

Twenty-Three

Concluding Thoughts for You, Our Readers

Our Purpose

In writing this book, our purpose has been to bring gluten sensitivity to the forefront not only for the public but also for medical clinicians worldwide. For too long, gluten in the diet has been minimized as a cause of many complaints, to the detriment of many people's quality of life. Misperceptions about this dietary protein have allowed symptoms and ill effects in the body to continue while a simple remedy is available.

Let's Focus on the Root Cause

The HealthNOW Method focuses on getting to the root cause. It targets the underlying stressor that creates symptoms and seeks to eliminate this stressor, to allow the recuperative abilities of the body to engage. In contrast, too many clinicians today fail to seek the root cause, and in so doing, never achieve a goal of true health for their patients. Instead, symptoms are masked with medications or treatments, but the root cause is allowed to continue.

Gluten-Related Disorders
Have Been Ignored Too Long

This has been abundantly apparent in gluten-related disorders. Despite the tremendous scientific literature and medical research information available, the majority of clinicians view gluten sensitivity as being synonymous with celiac disease only. While celiac disease is a common manifestation of gluten sensitivity, it is not the only gluten-related disorder by far. Failing to recognize this fact not only leads to misidentifying the root cause, but it also leads to unnecessary treatments that carry side effects and costs.

Let's All Work Together to Increase Awareness

By increasing the awareness of all the disorders gluten intolerance can create, appropriate treatments can be implemented. The added benefit to this approach is lowered healthcare costs by eliminating needless treatments and unnecessary testing, and by invoking preventative measures earlier. The first step is to encourage clinicians, and subsequently patients, to use more accurate terminology. Let "celiac disease" refer to the type of gluten intolerance that causes villous atrophy with inflammation of the intestinal lining, and other gluten disorders shall be referred to as "gluten sensitivities." In this manner, we can begin to understand and act in accordance with how gluten causes illness.

As you can now understand, gluten can result in a wide array of health disorders. Osteoporosis, arthritis, thyroid disease, migraines, depression, IBS, skin disorders, liver inflammation, clumsiness and diabetes are just a few of the more common health conditions caused by gluten in the diet. And while gluten may not be the most common cause of these conditions, it is by no means rare. Most of these conditions have gluten as a cause at least five percent of the time, if not higher.

Mask Your Symptoms or Treat the Root Cause—Your Choice

Do you think it is healthier to seek gluten as the cause and eliminate it from the diet, or is it healthier to ignore dietary causes and temporarily eliminate symptoms with medications? Assuming that symptoms resolve in both cases and no side effects occur from the medication, damage to your health is still ongoing if the offending agent remains present.

Symptoms are the body's way of alerting us that something is wrong. By masking symptoms with treatments that fail to address the root cause, we can do more harm than good because it gives us a false impression that things are now ok. Usually, this is not the case.

Our Approach to Health: The HealthNOW Method

Our approach to health is uniquely focused on getting to the root cause of symptoms. One of the many joys of what we do for a living is experiencing the human body's amazing ability to heal itself. We have often dubbed ourselves "stress detectors and removers" as, ultimately, it seems that once that job is accomplished, the body is then unencumbered enough to do what it does so innately well, which is heal itself.

Repeatedly, in our patients, we find that various stressors are causing their problem or problems to occur. These stressors include dietary substances like gluten but also many others, including infections, toxins, emotional stressors, poor sleep, malnutrition due to a poor diet or malabsorption, etc. Our attention is focused on isolating these stressors and removing them. Once eliminated, the body can then recuperate on its own, and optimal health and functioning is restored.

It's an Approach That Makes Sense

This is a logical and practical approach to health. The function of our bodies is to stay healthy, not to invite disease and illness. If something upsets the healthy balance of a body, mechanisms within the body are able to correct the problem, unless the stress becomes overwhelming. The body can become overwhelmed because a stressor is too powerful, or it may occur because the stressor has existed for too long a period of time. Either way, the stressor is the underlying problem.

An Example of the HealthNOW Method at Work

Recently, one of our patients, E., drove this point home as she described her experience after two and a half months on the program. She is now a forty-two-year-old woman who was about forty pounds overweight when she came to see us. Her friends could never understand why she had a weight problem, considering her diet and exercise regimen.

E. herself was becoming increasingly frustrated as she only saw the scale go in the opposite direction, despite her best intentions. She'd used to be a size six or eight but had become a size twelve. Prior to seeing us, she had experienced some success in losing weight with a nutritionist. But when the weight started to come back, she couldn't figure out what she was doing wrong. E. also suffered from bloating, gassiness, PMS and fatigue.

As you can probably guess, we found E. to be gluten-intolerant. Additionally, her adrenal glands were stressed and malfunctioning; she had low B12; and she had a high body fat content of thirty-one percent. After adhering to our modified elimination diet, her digestion improved. During the first month on the program, she saw little change, but after the first month, she saw a five-pound drop in her weight. She also noticed an improvement in energy and a big difference in her PMS and fatigue.

On her last clinic visit, just months after being on the HealthNOW Method, she had lost a total of twenty-three pounds. She described it as "a switch being flipped" and her metabolism being "allowed to kick in." She was still eating well and exercising almost daily, but the difference was the elimination of gluten in her diet and a healthy change in diet and lifestyle.

What happened here? Why the dramatic turnaround in all her symptoms? The right stressors were identified and eliminated. E. is just one of many who now understand what healthy changes make her body function effectively.

How Would the Traditional Medical Approach Proceed?

In most clinicians' offices today, this approach is not what is practiced. Instead of seeking a stressor, signs of pathology or disease are sought. For example, a person is diagnosed with low thyroid function. Blood tests are ordered that define the low thyroid state, and, possibly, a scan of the thyroid gland is ordered to look for any pathology. If negative, medication replacement of thyroid hormone is given and a follow-up appointment is scheduled to ensure that the drug therapy is working. No root cause is sought. No search for an underlying stressor is conducted.

How Does the HealthNOW Approach Differ?

Our approach is different. The same person in our office would likewise be diagnosed through blood tests to define low thyroid function, but then, causes of this would be sought. The thyroid gland does not just suddenly give out without a reason. What dietary causes might be present? What lifestyle problems might be at play? Is there an infection or autoimmune reaction resulting in this bodily stress?

We Are Relentless in Seeking Out the Root Cause

By logically addressing each potential stress area, an underlying cause is often found. Once eliminated, the body can then heal itself and thyroid function can be restored (without adding another medication to the list). Which method targets true health? The answer seems obvious to us.

What Do We Do When All Traditional Lab Tests Are Negative?

Tests like MRI scans and x-rays are snapshots of parts of the body. They can certainly be helpful when looking for pathology or disease effects, but they are of little use when looking for body malfunction before

pathology is visible. Infections, cancers, hormonal imbalances, malnutrition and many other health problems exist months and even years
before pathology can ever be seen. This stage, prior to disease, is called
a "period of malfunction." Most traditional diagnostic tests fail to show
functional problems, as they were only created to detect disease.

Functional Testing Is the Answer

Functional testing is more sensitive and best used when looking for the
root cause of one's symptoms because it is designed to detect malfunction. These tests include such things as assessments of food reaction,
blood tests that identify malfunction of a system (like the liver, heart or
adrenals), and tests for the presence of infections. Finding these conditions before pathology occurs is ideal because it will more than likely
result in reversibility once the stressor is eliminated. This is the case with
gluten. Ultimately, the goal is to identify a stressor before it has created
a disease or pathology.

Gluten Is a Facet of Poor Health That Shouldn't Be Missed

In pursuing our standard approach to health and symptoms, we have
found that gluten is a common thread amongst the complaints of many
people. Eliminating gluten has resulted in better health for so many of our
patients and it has been a causative agent in a much wider variety of symptoms than we ever anticipated. Having witnessed this, we felt compelled to
educate others about how common gluten-related health conditions are.
Rather than being misled and unnecessarily medicated, elimination of
gluten can restore health and quality of life for many people.

Moving Forward

Where should we go from here? From our perspective, healthcare in
general needs a major shift in its focus. In the U.S., we spend far too

much on pharmaceuticals and diagnostic testing and pay too little attention to preventative measures and lifestyle. As a country, we are all guilty of going into a physician's office for a "quick fix." You have a complaint, you make a doctor's appointment, you get a prescription and you feel better for a while. But is this really a good approach to health?

Immune disorders are increasing. Adult obesity and childhood obesity are escalating at a dangerous rate. Chronic fatigue, fibromyalgia and depression are incredibly common. Heart disease, cancer and diabetes continue to be the top killers of our society. Testing and medication for these conditions are not the ultimate answers. Preventative measures and the elimination of stressors to our bodies is what we should be targeting. Diet, lifestyle, exercise and a practical approach to health are not only more cost-effective, but are more effective overall.

Why Are Diet and Nutrition Not Stressed More in Medicine?

Do you ever wonder why dietary measures are not a larger part of your medical visits? What about nutrition? Sure, these receive lip service as a means to improve health, but how much of your medical visits entail discussions about what you should eat and how you should live? In the standard fifteen-minute office visit, our guess is that one or two minutes, on average, cover diet, lifestyle and preventative measures of health. Greater time is allotted to discussion of tests, discussions of pathology and instructions on medication use and side effects. Why is this? Because we want a quick fix and not a long-term approach to health, and because medicine focuses on disease instead of health.

Unfortunately, another reason for these habits is financial. Pharmaceutical companies have large marketing budgets and powerful lobbyist groups that encourage this behavior. Likewise, the increasing threat of lawsuits for medical malpractice has led physicians to rely on diagnostic tests as a means to protect themselves from these risks. In a courtroom, positive or negative tests are objective evidence that support a physician's decision. A subjective response to a change in diet or lifestyle is not as powerful and more prone to interpretation and manipulation. These two powerful factors have influenced how healthcare is approached today.

We Must Change the Face of Healthcare

In order to get back on track, we must demand a shift from a disease-focused system to a health-focused system. We have to accept that ill health did not develop overnight and that restoration of health may take time. In developing a healthcare system that actually promotes health, it is critical to focus on a good diet, a healthy lifestyle and the avoidance of bad health behaviors. As long as we continue to mask symptoms with medications instead of targeting the root causes, the ability to improve the public's health will remain poor. We should get to a point where medication and surgeries are the exceptions and not the norm.

With a Little Effort We Could Enjoy Much Better Health

Currently, in other countries, such as Italy, all children are screened for gluten sensitivity. Because of its frequent ability to be a root cause of so many health disorders, we believe that this should be standard practice worldwide. Just imagine if five percent of all the disorders mentioned in this book could be effectively treated by eliminating gluten from the diet. How much cost savings in medication prescriptions, diagnostic testing and physician office visits would be realized? How much better would the overall quality of life be for those millions of people?

Test Yourself, Test Your Family and Tell Your Friends

It is without question that everyone who has a first-degree relative with gluten sensitivity should be tested for gluten intolerance. This is partic-ularly important in children as growth rates and concurrent neurological and immunologic disorders can be prevented by earlier identification. Persons with a high prevalence of immune disorders in their families should also be screened because of gluten's common presence as a cause of many immune health problems. For us, this is a starting point in identifying gluten sensitivity as a root cause. Hopefully, as we move into the future, gluten sensitivity screening will be part of an annual examination for all individuals.

Parting Words

In summary, we hope that this book has opened your eyes to the common problems associated with gluten sensitivity. In detailing each set of symptoms as well as each common disorder associated with gluten sensitivity, we wish to increase widespread awareness of the effects of this dietary protein. What we have found in our clinical practice has, indeed, been supported by ample medical research. Yet, a minority of clinicians appreciates this, and even fewer have changed their practice styles to incorporate this knowledge into patient care.

Diet and lifestyle are powerful determinants of good health. Simply that our health care culture has failed to place these aspects in high priority should not mean that we ignore their importance. By considering gluten as a root cause, we begin to take a step in the right direction, toward true health and symptom-based healthcare.

For the many who are gluten-sensitive, eliminating gluten in their diets provides the necessary means to allow their bodies the power to heal themselves. It is in this fashion that we should begin to look at health in general, and in so doing, we can finally get to the root of the problem instead of simply masking the symptoms.

—To your good health!
Drs. Vikki and Richard Petersen

ENDNOTES

1. James Braly and Ron Hoggan, *Dangerous Grains* (New York: Penguin Putnam, Inc, 2002), 36-47.
2. S. Helms, "Celiac Disease and Gluten Associated Diseases," *Alternative Medicine Review* 10 (2005): 172-92.
3. Celiac Sprue Association, "A Brief History of Celiac Disease," Celiac Sprue Association, http://www.csaceliacs.org/CD.php (accessed February, 25, 2008).
4. Joseph Murray, MD, "The Widening Spectrum of Celiac Disease," *American Journal of Clinical Nutrition* 69 (1999): 354-65.
5. Aristo Vodjani, PhD, "Medical Diagrams," TheGlutenSyndrome.net, http://www.glutensensitivity.net/VojdaniDiagrams. htm (accessed February 25, 2008).
6. Giuseppe Gobbi, "Coeliac disease, epilepsy, and cerebral calcifications," *Brain and Development* 27 (2005): 189-200.
7. Russell Blaylock, MD, *Excitotoxins: The Taste That Kills* (Santa Fe, NM: Health Press, 1997), 59-91.
8. Braly, *Dangerous Grains*, 36-47.

9. New Hall Mill, "The Evolution of Wheat-Introduction," New Hall Mill, http://www.newhallmill.org.uk/wht-evol.htm (accessed February 28, 2008).

10. Kilmer McCully, "The Significance of Wheat in the Dakota Territory, Human Evolution, Civilization, and Degenerative Diseases," *Perspectives in Biology and Medicine* 44 (2001): 52-61.

11. New Hall Mill, "The Evolution of Wheat-Introduction."

12. Gary Vocke, "Wheat: Background," United States Department of Agriculture Economic Research Service, http://www.ers.usda.gov/ Briefing/Wheat/consumption.htm (accessed February 28, 2008).

13. Parris Kidd, "Autism, an Extreme Challenge to Integrative Medicine. Part II: Medical Management," *Alternative Medicine Review* 7 (2002): 472-99.

14. George J. Armelagos, "Take Two Beers and Call Me in 1,600 Years," *Natural History* May (2000): 1-5.

15. McCully, "The Significance of Wheat in the Dakota Territory," 52-61.

16. Melissa Smith, *Going Against the Grain: How Reducing and Avoiding Grains Can Revitalize* (New York: McGraw-Hill Professional, 2002), 3-107.

17. C. Feigherty, "Coeliac Disease," *British Medical Journal* 319 (1999): 236-239.

18. New Hall Mill, "The Evolution of Wheat-Introduction."

19. Stanley Cauvain, *Bread Making* (Cambridge: Woodhead Publishing, 2003), 1-589.

20. New Hall Mill, "The Evolution of Wheat-Introduction."

21. Ibid.

22. D. Kamin, "The Iceberg Cometh: Establishing the Prevalence of Celiac Disease in the United States and Finland," *Gastroenterology* 126 (2004): 359-361.

23. Kenneth Fine, MD, "Early Diagnosis of Gluten Sensitivity: Before the Villi are Gone," Celiac.com, http://www.celiac.com/articles/759/1/Early-Diagnosis-of-

Gluten-Sensitivity-Before-the-Villi-are-Gone-by-By-Kenneth-Fine-MD/Page1.html.

24. Cauvain, *Bread Making*, 1-589.
25. P. Green, "Mechanisms Underlying Celiac Disease and Its Neurologic Manifestations," *Cellular and Molecular Life Sciences* 62 (2005) 791–799.
26. Celiac Sprue Association, "A Brief History of Celiac Disease."
27. New Hall Mill, "The Evolution of Wheat-Introduction."
28. Vodjani, "Medical Diagrams."
29. Suda Kumagai, et al, "Improvement of Digestibility, Reduction in Allergenicity, and Induction of Oral Tolerance of Wheat Gliadin by Deamidation," *Bioscience, Biotechnology, and Biochemistry* 71 (2007): 977-85.
30. Fine, "Early Diagnosis of Gluten Sensitivity."
31. Aristo Vojdani, PhD, et al, "Infections, Toxic Chemicals and Dietary Peptides Binding to Lymphocyte Receptors and Tissue Enzymes Are Major Instigators of Autoimmunity in Autism," *International Journal of Immunopathology and Pharmacology* 16 (2003): 189-99.
32. G. Oderta, "Thyroid Autoimmunity in Childhood Celiac Disease," *Journal of Pediatric Gastroenterology and Nutrition* 35 (2002): 704–705.
33. Vodjani, "Medical Diagrams."
34. Fine, "Early Diagnosis of Gluten Sensitivity."
35. Vodjani, "Medical Diagrams."
36. Jeffrey Bland, "Understanding the Origins and Applying Advanced Nutritional Strategies for Autoimmune Diseases," *Synthesis Seminar Audio Download* March 2006, http://www.jeffreybland.com (accessed March 8, 2008).
37. Alan Lucas, et al, "Primary Prevention by Nutrition Intervention in Infancy And Childhood," *Nestle Nutrition Workshop Series Pediatric Program* 57 (2005): 1-108.
38. Lucas, "Primary Prevention," 1-108.
39. Ibid.
40. Ibid.

41. S. Guandalini, "The Influence of Gluten: Weaning Recommendations for Healthy Children and Children at Risk for Celiac Disease," *Nestle Nutrition Workshop Series Pediatric Program* 60 (2007): 139-51.

42. Jill M. Norris, MPH, PhD, et al, "Risk of Celiac Disease Autoimmunity and Timing of Gluten Introduction in the Diet of Infants at Increased Risk of Disease," *JAMA* 293 (2005) 2343-51.

43. Guandalini, "The Influence of Gluten," 139-51.

44. Hilde K. Brekke, et al, "Breastfeeding and Introduction of Solid Foods in Swedish Infants: The All Babies in Southeast Sweden Study," *British Journal of Nutrition* 94 (2005): 377–82.

45. V. Kumar, "Predictive Value of Serology Testing in Celiac Disease," Enabling Support Foundation, http://www.enabling.org/ia/celiac/ predic.html (accessed March 8, 2008).

46. M. Hadjivassiliou, "Gluten Sensitivity as a Neurological Illness," *Journal of Neurology, Neurosurgery, and Psychiatry* 72 (2002): 560-3.

47. Bland, *Synthesis Seminar Audio Download* March 2006.

48. Tarcision Not, "Thyroid Disease: Celiac Disease Is Linked to Autoimmune Thyroid Disease," *Digestive Diseases and Sciences* 45 (2000): 403-6.

49. Jeffrey Bland, "Duration of Exposure to Gluten and the Risk of Autoimmune Disorders in Patients with Celiac Disease. SIGEP Study Group for Autoimmune Disorders in Celiac Disease," *Gastroenterology* 117 (1999):297-303.

50. Murray, "The Widening Spectrum of Celiac Disease," 354-65.

51. Giovanna Zonomi, et al, "In Celiac Disease, a Subset of Autoantibodies Against Transglutaminase Binds Toll-like Receptor 4 and Induces Activation of Monocytes," *Clinical Immunology* 119 (2006): S25.

52. Vodjani, "Medical Diagrams."

53. Ibid.

54. Aristo Vodjani PhD, MT, Thomas O'Bryan, DC, CCN, DACBN, "The Immunology of Gluten Sensitivity Beyond the Intestinal Tract," TheGlutenSyndrome.net, http://www.glutensensitivity.net/Vojdani_Immun_Glut_SenAug07 -1.pdf (accessed March 8, 2008).

55. Sanjay Bhadada, et al, "Does Every Short Stature Child Need Screening for Celiac Disease?" *Journal of Gastroenterology and Hepatology* 23 (2008): 353-6.

56. M. Arbuckle, "Development of Autoantibodies Before the Clinical Onset of SLE," *New England Journal of Medicine* 349 (2003):1526-33.

57. Blaylock, *Excitotoxins: The Taste That Kills*, 59-91.

58. Murray, "The Widening Spectrum of Celiac Disease," 354-65.

59. Douglas Drossman, et al, "U.S. Householder Survey of Functional Gastrointestinal Disorders," *Digestive Diseases and Sciences* 38 (1993):1569-80.

60. Fine, "Early Diagnosis of Gluten Sensitivity."

61. Kamin, "The Iceberg Cometh," 359-361.

62. K. Juuti-Uusitalo, et al, "Gluten Affects Epithelial Differentiation-associated Genes in Small Intestinal Mucosa of Coeliac Patients," *Clinical and Experimental Immunology* 150 (2007): 294-305.

63. R. Bascom, et al, "Immunoglobulin A Deficiency," eMedicine, http://www.emedicine.com/Med/topic1159.htm (accessed March 15, 2008).

64. Ibid.

65. Murray, "The Widening Spectrum of Celiac Disease," 354-65.

66. Harold Pruessner, MD, "Detecting Celiac Disease in Your Patients," *American Family Physician®* 57 (1998), *http://www.aafp.org/afp/980 301ap/pruessn.html.*

67. Gerald Holtmann, et al, "Mental Stress and Gastric Acid Secretion," *Digestive Disease and Science* 35 (1990): 998-1007.

68. CE Taylor, et al, "Control of Diarrheal Diseases," *Annual Review of Public Health* 10 (1989): 221-44.

69. P. Usai, et al, "Effect of Gluten-free Diet and Co-morbidity of Irritable Bowel Syndrome-type Symptoms on Health-related Quality of Life in Adult Coeliac Patients," *Digestive and Liver Disease* 39 (2007): 824-8.

70. C. Hallert, et al, "Evidence of Poor Vitamin Status in Coeliac Patients on a Gluten Free Diet for 10 Years," *Alimentary Pharmacology & Therapeutics* 16 (2002): 1333-9.

71. R. Avery, "Severe Vitamin K Deficiency Induced by Occult Celiac Disease BR96-026," *American Journal of Hematology* 53 (1996): 55.

72. S. Popat, et al, "Genome Screening of Coeliac Disease," *Journal of Medical Genetics* 39 (2002): 328-31.

73. J. Gass, et al, "Combination Enzyme Therapy for Gastric Digestion of Dietary Gluten in Patients With Celiac Sprue," *Gastroenterology* 133 (2007): 472-80.

74. Kamin, "The Iceberg Cometh," 359-361.

75. M. Hadjivassiliou, "Gluten Ataxia in Perspective: Epidemiology, Genetic Susceptibility and Clinical Characteristics," *Brain* 126 (2003): 685-91.

76. M. Hadjivassiliou, et al, "Neuromuscular Disorder as a Presenting Feature of Coeliac Disease," *Journal of Neurology, Neurosurgery, and Psychiatry* 63 (1997): 770-5.

77. Green, "Mechanisms Underlying Celiac Disease," 791-9.

78. M. Hadjivassiliou, et al, "The Humoral Response in the Pathogenesis of Gluten Ataxia," *Neurology* 58 (2002): 1221-6.

79. Hadjivassiliou, "Gluten Ataxia," 685-91.

80. M. Hadjivassiliou, "Headache and CNS White Matter Abnormalities Associated With Gluten Sensitivity," *Neurology* 56 (2001): 385-8.

81. Ibid.

82. Hadjivassiliou, "Gluten Ataxia," 685-91.

83. Green, "Mechanisms Underlying Celiac Disease," 791-9.

84. Vodjani, "The Immunology of Gluten Sensitivity Beyond the Intestinal Tract."

85. D. Cakir, et al, "Subclinical Neurological Abnormalities in Children With Celiac Disease Receiving a Gluten-free Diet," *Journal of Pediatric Gastroenterology and Nutrition* 45 (2007): 366-9.

86. M. Hadjivassiliou, et al, "Neuropathy Associated With Gluten Sensitivity," *Journal of Neurology, Neurosurgery, and Psychiatry* 77 (2006): 1262-6.

87. A. Cristofolini, et al, "The Prevalence of Headache in a Population of Health Care Workers and the Effects on Productivity Costs," *La Medicina del Lavoro* 99 (2008): 8-15.

88. N. Zelnick, "Range of Neurologic Disorders in Patients With Celiac Disease," *Pediatrics* 113 (2004): 1672-6.

89. Hadjivassiliou, "Headache," 385-8.

90. J. Pascual, et al, "A Woman With Daily Headaches," *The Journal of Headache and Pain* 6 (2005): 91-2.

91. P. Collin, "Celiac Disease, Brain Atrophy, and Dementia," *Neurology* 41 (1991): 372-5.

92. Ibid.

93. Hadjivassiliou, "Gluten Ataxia," 685-91.

94. M. Takahashi, et al, "Behavioral and Pharmacological Studies on Gluten Exorphin A5, a Newly Isolated Bioactive Food Protein Fragment in Mice," *Japanese Journal of Pharmacology* 84 (2000): 259-65.

95. AM Knivsberg, et al, "A Randomized Controlled Study of Dietary Intervention in Autistic Syndromes," *Nutritional Neuroscience* 5 (2002):251-61.

96. Cakir, ""Subclinical Neurological Abnormalities," 366-9.

97. Giuseppe Gobbi, "Coeliac disease, Epilepsy, and Cerebral Calcifications," *Brain and Development* 27 (2005): 189-200.

98. M. Kieslich, "Brain White-Matter Lesions in Celiac Disease: A Prospective Study of 75 Diet-Treated Patients," *Pediatrics* 108 (2001): e21.

99. PA Pynnönen, et al, "Gluten-free Diet May Alleviate Depressive and Behavioural Symptoms in Adolescents With Coeliac

Disease: A Prospective Follow-up Case-series Study," *BMC Psychiatry* 17 (2005): 1-14.

100. G. Addolorado, "Regional Cerebral Hypoperfusion in Patients with Celiac Disease," *The American Journal of Medicine* 116 (2004): 312-7.

101. Pynnönen, "Gluten-free Diet," 1-14.

102. Zelnick, "Range of Neurologic Disorders," 1672-6.

103. BioHealth Diagnostics, "Chronic Stress Response™ Chart," BioHealth Diagnostics, http://www.biodia.com/TechnicalCharts/ChronicStressChart.pd f (accessed March 27, 2008).

104. Ibid.

105. BioHealth Diagnostics, "Steroidal Hormone Principle Pathways," BioHealth Diagnostics, http://www.biodia.com/TechnicalCharts/ SteroidalHormonechart.pdf (accessed March 28, 2008).

106. BioHealth Diagnostics, "HPA-HPT Axes," BioHealth Diagnostics http://www.biodia.com/TechnicalCharts/HPA-HPT AxesChart.pdf (accessed March 28, 2008).

107. Ibid.

108. WJ Gunn, et al, "Epidemiology of Chronic Fatigue Syndrome: The Centers for Disease Control Study," *CIBA Foundation Symposium* 173 (1993): 83-101.

109. AJ Cleave, et al, "Low Dose Hhydrocortisone in Chronic Fatigue Syndrome: A Randomized Crossover Trial," *Lancet* 353 (1999): 455-8.

110. GJ Canaris, et al, "The Colorado Thyroid Disease Prevalence Study," *Archives of Internal Medicine* 160 (2000): 526-34.

111. C. Sategna-Guldetti, et al, "Prevalence of Thyroid Disorders in Untreated Adult Celiac Disease Patients and Effects of Gluten Withdrawal: An Italian Multicenter Study," *The American Journal of Gastroenterology* 96 (2001): 751-57.

112. SM O'Brien, et al, "Cytokines: Abnormalities in Major Depression and Implications for Pharmacological Treatment," *Human Psychopharmacology* 19 (2004): 397-403.

113. BioHealth Diagnostics, "Chronic Stress Response™ Chart."

114. Ibid.

115. RC Lawrence, et al, "Estimates of the Prevalence of Arthritis and Other Rheumatic Conditions in the United States Part II," *Arthritis and Rheumatism* 58 (2008): 26-35.

116. W. Riedel, et al, "Secretory Patterns of GH, TSH, Thyroid Hormone, ACTH, cortisol, FSH, and LH in Patients With Fibromyalgia Syndrome Following Systemic Infection of the Relevant Hypothalamic-releasing Hormones," *Zeitschrift für Rheumatologie* 57 (1998): S81-87.

117. BS McEwan, "Sleep Deprivation as a Neurologic and Physiological Stressor: Allostasis and Allostatic Load," *Metabolism* 55 (2006): S520-523.

118. G. Addolorado, "Regional Cerebral Hypoperfusion in Patients With Celiac Disease," *American Journal of Medicine* 116 (2004): 312-7.

119. BioHealth Diagnostics, "Chronic Stress Response™ Chart."

120. O'Brien, "Cytokines," 397-403.

121. R. Ferguson, et al, "Coeliac Disease, Fertility, and Pregnancy," *Scandinavian Journal of Gastroenterology* 17 (1982): 65-8.

122. BioHealth Diagnostics, "Steroidal Hormone Principle Pathways."

123. Espelund Ulrick, et al, "Fasting Unmasks a Strong Inverse Association Between Ghrelin and Cortisol in Serum: Studies in Obese and Normal-weight Subjects," *The Journal of Clinical Endocrinology & Metabolism* 90 (2005): 741-746.

124. DF Swaab, et al, "The Stress System in the Human Brain in Depression and Neurodegeneration," *Ageing Research Reviews* 4 (2005): 141-194.

125. P. Collin, et al, "Coeliac Disease—Associated Disorders and Survival," *Gut* 35 (1994): 1215-8.

126. LM Sollid, "Coeliac Disease: Dissecting a Complex Inflammatory Disorder," *Nature Reviews Immunology* 2 (2002): 647-55.

127. Vodjani, "Medical Diagrams."

128. J. Cosnes, et al, "Incidence of Autoimmune Diseases in Celiac Disease: Protective Effect of the Gluten-free Diet," *Clinical Gastroenterology and Hepatology* 6 (2008): 753-8.

129. F. Cataldo, V. Marino, "Increased Prevalence of Autoimmune Diseases in First-degree Relatives of Patients With Celiac Disease," *Journal of Pediatric Gastroenterology and Nutrition* 36 (2003): 470-3.

130. RM Kline, "Correction of Celiac Disease After Allogeneic Hematopoietic Stem Cell Transplantation for Acute Myelogenous Leukemia," *Pediatrics* 120 (2007): e1120-2.

131. Cosnes, "Incidence of Autoimmune Diseases in Celiac Disease," 753-8.

132. Cataldo, "Increased Prevalence of Autoimmune Diseases," 470-3.

133. Collin, "Coeliac Disease—Associated Disorders and Survival," 1215-18.

134. SH Kim, et al, "Symptom Experience, Psychological Distress, and Quality of Life in Korean Patients With Liver Cirrhosis: A Cross-Sectional Survey," *International Journal of Nursing Studies* 43 (2006): 1047-56.

135. A. Carroccio, et al, "Screening for Celiac Disease in Non-Hodgkin's Lymphoma Patients: A Serum Anti-transglutaminase-based Approach," *Digestive Diseases and Sciences* 48 (2003): 1530-6.

136. Ibid.

137. Merck Staff, "Dermatitis Herpetiformis," *The Merck Manual of Medical Information—Second Home* Edition, http://www.merck.com/mmhe/print/sec18/ch209/ch209d.html (accessed April 2, 2008).

138. O. Karabudak, et al, "Dermatitis Herpetiformis and Vitiligo," *Journal of the Chinese Medical Association* 70 (2007): 504-6.

139. T. Reunala, P. Collin, "Diseases Associated With Dermatitis Herpetiformis," *British Journal of Dermatology* 150 (2004): 136-8.

140. P. Humbert, et al, "Gluten Intolerance and Skin Diseases," *European Journal of Dermatology* 16 (2006): 4-11.

141. Pruessner, "Detecting Celiac Disease in Your Patients."
142. Collin, "Coeliac Disease—Associated Disorders and Survival,"
     1215-8.
143. LM Luft, et al, "Autoantibodies to Tissue Transglutaminase in
     Sjögren's Syndrome and Related Rheumatic Diseases," *The
     Journal of Rheumatology* 30 (2003): 2613-9.
144. Vodjani, "The Immunology of Gluten Sensitivity Beyond the
     Intestinal Tract."
145. Ibid.
146. Hartl, Barbara, "The Facts About Fosamax, Boniva
     (Bisphosphonates), et al," Reverse Osteoporosis Naturally,
     http://my-bone- density.com/bisphosphonates.htm (accessed
     April 2, 2008).
147. HJ Tsai, et al, "The Association of Diet With Respiratory
     Symptoms and Asthma in Schoolchildren in Taipei, Taiwan,"
     The Journal of Asthma 44 (2007): 599-603.
148. L. Chatzi, et al, "Protective Effect of Fruits, Vegetables and the
     Mediterranean Diet on Asthma and Allergies Among Children
     in Crete," *Thorax* 62 (2007): 677-83.
149. S. Farchi, et al, "Dietary Factors Associated With Wheezing and
     Allergic Rhinitis in Children," *The European Respiratory Journal*
     22 (2003): 772-80.
150. Vojdani, "Infections, Toxic Chemicals and Dietary Peptides,"
     189-99.
151. W. Dickey, N. Kearney, "Overweight in Celiac Disease:
     Prevalence, Clinical Characteristics, and Effect of a Gluten-free
     Diet," *The American Journal of Gastroenterology* 101 (2006):
     2356-9.
152. Reunala, "Diseases Associated With Dermatitis Herpetiformis,"
     136-8.
153. Collin, "Coeliac Disease—Associated Disorders and Survival,"
     1215-18.
154. AC Spadaccino, et al, "Celiac Disease in North Italian Patients
     With Autoimmune Thyroid Diseases," *Autoimmunity* 41 (2008):
     116-21.

155. E. Flatau, et al, "Prevalence of Hypothyroidism and Diabetes Mellitus in Elderly Kibbutz Members," *European Journal of Epidemiology* 16 (2000): 43-6.

156. D. Villalta, et al, "High Prevalence of Celiac Disease in Autoimmune Hepatitis Detected by Anti-tissue Tranglutaminase Autoantibodies," *Journal of Clinical Laboratory Analysis* 19 (2005): 6-10.

157. Luft, "Autoantibodies to Tissue Transglutaminase," 2613-9.

158. Fasano, et al, "Prevalence of Celiac Disease in At-Risk and Not-At-Risk Groups in the United States," Arch Intern Med 163 (2003): 286-292.

159. Major, Ralph H., *Classic Descriptions of Disease* (Charles C Thomas Pub. Ltd., 1978), 600-1.

160. WF Caspary, "Celiac Disease/Sprue—100 Years Following the Initial Detailed Description by Samuel Gee," *Zeitschrift für Gastroenterologie* 27 (1989): 344-51.

161. Hadjivassiliou, "Gluten Sensitivity," 560-563.

162. David Nelsen, Jr., MD, "Gluten-sensitive Enteropathy (Celiac Disease): More Common Than You Think," *American Family Physician* 66 (2002), http://www.aafp.org/afp/20021215/2259.html.

163. C. Gregory, et al, "Delay in Diagnosis of Adult Coeliac Disease," *Digestion* 28 (1983): 201-4.

164. J. Murray, "The Widening Spectrum of Celiac Disease," *The American Journal of Clinical Nutrition* 69 (1999): 354–65.

165. Nelsen, Jr. "Gluten-Sensitive Enteropathy."

166. C. Loftus, J. Murray, "Celiac Disease: Diagnosis and Management," *Hospital Physician* May (2003): 45-55.

167. PHR Green, C. Cellier, "Celiac Disease," *The New England Journal of Medicine* 357 (2007): 1731-1743.

168. Nelsen, Jr., "Gluten-Sensitive Enteropathy."

169. Ibid.

170. Kamin, "The Iceberg Cometh," 359-361.

171. M. Verkasalo, "Undiagnosed Silent Celiac Disease: A Risk for Underachievement," *Scandinavian Journal of Gastroenterology* 40 (2005): 1407-1412.

172. Dickey, "Overweight in Celiac Disease," 2356-2359.

173. A. Ventura, "Duration of Exposure to Gluten and Risk of Autoimmune Disorders in Patients With Celiac Disease," *The American Journal of Gastroenterology* 117 (1999): 297-303.

174. Ulrike Peters, PhD, et al, "Causes of Death in Patients With Celiac Disease in a Population-based Swedish Cohort," *Archives of Internal Medicine* 163 (2003): 1566-72.

175. Nelsen, Jr., "Gluten-Sensitive Enteropathy."

176. Vodjani, "Medical Diagrams."

177. Citizens Commission on Human Rights, "Common Psychiatric Drugs and Their Effects," Citizen Commission on Human Rights, http://www.cchr.org/media/pdfs/Common_Psychiatric_Drugs_and_Their_Effects.pdf.

178. Ibid.

179. S. Karande, "Autism: A Review for Family Physicians," *Indian Journal of Medical Sciences* 60 (2006): 205-15.

180. National Institute of Mental Health, "Attention Deficit Hyperactivity Disorder," National Institute of Mental Health, http://www.nimh.nih.gov/health/publications/adhd/complete-publication.shtml (accessed April 28, 2008).

181. Citizens Commission on Human Rights, "Common Psychiatric Drugs," 1-18.

182. R. Muhle, et al, "The Genetics of Autism," *Pediatrics* 113 (2004): e472-86.

183. Mark Sircus, Dr. Alan Clark, "Thimerosol, Autism and Vaccines: What Eli Lilly Isn't Telling You," BabySnark, http://www.babysnark.com/health/thimerosol-vaccines-autism.asp (accessed April 28, 2008).

184. SC Bello, "Autism and Environmental Influences: Review and Commentary," *Reviews on Environmental Health* 22 (2007): 139-56.

185. Knivsberg, "A Randomized Controlled Study," 251-61.

186. The National Center on Physical Activity and Disability, "Health Promotion: Autism and Nutrition," The National Center

on Physical Activity and Disability,
http://www.ncpad.org/nutrition/fact_sheet.php?sheet=105&view
=all (accessed April 28, 2008).

187. MI Kawashti, et al, "Possible Immunological Disorders in
Autism: Concomitant Autoimmunity and Immune Tolerance,"
The Egyptian Journal of Immunology 13 (2006): 99-104.

188. A. Vojdani, et al, "Immune Response to Dietary Proteins,
Gliadin and Cerebellar Peptides in Children With Autism"
Nutritional Neuroscience 7 (2004): 151-61.

189. Citizens Commission on Human Rights, "Common Psychiatric
Drugs," 1-18.

190. Ibid.

191. J. Biederman, et al, "Family-genetic and Psychosocial Risk
Factors in DSM-III Attention Deficit Disorder," *Journal of the
American Academy of Child and Adolescent Psychiatry* 29 (1990):
526-533.

192. SV Faraone, et al, " Neurobiology of attention-deficit
hyperactivity disorder," *Biological Psychiatry* 44 (1998): 951-958.

193. Citizens Commission on Human Rights, "Common Psychiatric
Drugs," 1-18.

194. Zelnick, "Range of Neurologic Disorders," 1672-6.

195. H. Niederhofer, K. Pittschieler, "A Preliminary Investigation of
ADHD Symptoms in Persons With Celiac Disease," *Journal of
Attention Disorders* 10 (2006): 200-4.

196. Citizens Commission on Human Rights, "Common Psychiatric
Drugs," 1-18.

197. G. Harris, B. Careyt, "Researchers Fail to Reveal Drug Pay," *The
New York Times*, June 8, 2008.

198. Citizens Commission on Human Rights, "The Silent Death of
America's Children," Citizen Commission on Human Rights,
http://www.cchr.org/media/pdfs/The_Silent_Death_of_America
s_Children.pdf.

199. Citizens Commission on Human Rights, "Common Psychiatric
Drugs," 1-18.

200. Ibid.

201. Citizens Commission on Human Rights, "International Warnings on Psychiatric Drugs Since 2004," Citizen Commission on Human Rights, http://www.cchr.org/press_room/int_drug_warnings_since_200 4/ (accessed June 11, 2008).

202. National Alliance for the Mentally Ill, "Holland Court Rules ADHD Not a Disease," National Alliance for the Mentally Ill Santa Cruz County, http://www.namiscc.org/News/2002/Fall/ADHD-NotDisease.htm (accessed April 25, 2008).

203. S. Mackie, et al, "Cerebellar Development and Clinical Outcome in Attention Deficit Hyperactivity Disorder," *The American Journal of Psychiatry* 164 (200): 647-55.

204. Knivsberg, "A Randomized Controlled Study," 251-61.

205. National Center for Chronic Disease Prevention and Health Promotion, "Arthritis Types—Overview," Centers for Disease Control and Prevention, http://www.cdc.gov/arthritis/arthritis/generic.htm (accessed May 3, 2008).

206. Ibid.

207. HealthWise, "Sjogren's Syndrome—Topic Overview," WebMD, http://arthritis.webmd.com/tc/sjogrens-syndrome-topic-overview (accessed May 3, 2008).

208. Gregory Stacy, MD, "Osteoarthritis, Primary" eMedicine, http://www.emedicine.com/radio/topic492.htm (accessed May 3, 2008).

209. Ibid.

210. Ibid.

211. Mayo Clinic Staff, "Rheumatoid Arthritis," MayoClinic.com, http://www.mayoclinic.com/health/rheumatoid-arthritis/DS00020 (accessed May 3, 2008).

212. Ibid.

213. Ibid.

214. William C. Shiel, Jr., MD, FACP, FACR, "Sjogren's Syndrome," MedicineNet.com, http://www.medicinenet.com/sjogrens_syndrome/article.htm (accessed May 3, 2008).

215. Ibid.
216. E. Lubrano, et al, "The Arthritis of Coeliac Disease: Prevalence and Pattern in 200 Adult Patients," *British Journal of Rheumatology* 35(1996): 1314-8.
217. O. Slot, H. Locht, "Arthritis as Presenting Symptom in Silent Adult Coeliac Disease. Two Cases and Review of the Literature," *Scandinavian Journal of Rheumatology* 29 (2000): 260-3.
218. P. Carli, et al, "Inflammatory Rheumatism and Celiac Disease in Adults: Coincidence or Pathogenic Relationship?" *La Presse Médicale* 24 (1995): 606-10.
219. F. Falcini, et al, "Recurrent Monoarthritis in an 11-year-old Boy With Occult Coeliac Disease. Successful and Stable Remission After Gluten-free Diet," *Clinical and Experimental Rheumatology* 17 (1999): 509-11.
220. L. Paimela, et al, "Gliadin Immune Reactivity in Patients With Rheumatoid Arthritis," *Clinical and Experimental Rheumatology* 13 (1995): 603-7.
221. I. Hafström, et al, "A Vegan Diet Free of Gluten Improves the Signs and Symptoms of Rheumatoid Arthritis: The Effects on Arthritis Correlate With a Reduction in Antibodies to Food Antigens," *Rheumatology* 40 (2001): 1175-9.
222. AM Teppo, CP Maury, "Antibodies to Gliadin, Gluten and Reticulin Glycoprotein in Rheumatic Diseases: Elevated Levels in Sjögren's Syndrome," *Clinical and Experimental Immunology* 57 (1984): 73-8.
223. P. Szodoray, et al, "Coeliac Disease in Sjögren's Syndrome—a Study of 111 Hungarian Patients," *Rheumatology International* 24 (2004): 278-82.
224. M. Lidén, et al, "Gluten Sensitivity in Patients With Primary Sjögren's Syndrome," *Scandinavian Journal of Gastroenterology* 42 (2007): 962-7.
225. National Institutes of Health, "Diabetes Overview," National Diabetes Information Clearinghouse, http://diabetes.niddk. nih.gov/dm/pubs/overview/index.htm (accessed May 5, 2008).
226. Ibid.

227. Ibid.
228. DM Nathan, et al, "Intensive Diabetes Treatment and Cardiovascular Disease in Patients With Type 1 Diabetes," *The New England Journal of Medicine* 353 (2005): 2643-53.
229. National Institutes of Health, "Diabetes Overview."
230. Ibid.
231. Ibid.
232. Medina Y. Nóvoa, et al, "Impact of Diagnosis of Celiac Disease on Metabolic Control of Type 1 Diabetes," *Anales de Pediatría* 68 (2008): 13-7.
233. D. Hansen, et al, "Prevalence of Coeliac Disease (CD) in Children With Ttype 1 Diabetes (T1D)," *Ugeskrift for Laeger* 169 (2007): 2029-32.
234. M. My liwiec, et al, "Prognostic Factors of Celiac Disease Occurrence in Type 1 Diabetes Mellitus Children," *Endokrynologia, Diabetologia i Choroby Przemiany Materii Wieku Rozwojowego* 12 (2006): 281-5.
235. M. Barbato, et al, "Association Between Insulin Dependent Diabetes Mellitus and Coeliac Disease: A Study on 175 Diabetes Patients," *Minerva Gastroenterologica e Dietologica* 44 (1998): 1-5.
236. National Institutes of Health, "Diabetes Overview."
237. AG Ziegler, et al, "Early Infant Feeding and Risk of Developing Type 1 Diabetes-associated Autoantibodies," *JAMA* 290 (2003): 1721-8.
238. S. Verbeke, et al, "Risk Markers for Insulin-dependent Diabetes Mellitus and Duration of Exposure to Gluten in Celiac Patients," *Revista Médica de Chile* 132 (2004): 979-84.
239. G. Frisk, et al, "A Unifying Hypothesis on the Development of Type 1 Diabetes and Celiac Disease: Gluten Consumption May Be a Shared Causative Factor," *Medical Hypotheses* 70 (2008): 1207-9.
240. C. Poulain, et al, "Prevalence and Clinical Features of Celiac Disease in 950 Children With Type 1 Diabetes in France," *Diabetes & Metabolism* 33 (2007): 453-8.

241. C. Goh, K. Banerjee, "Prevalence of Coeliac Disease in Children and Adolescents With Type 1 Diabetes Mellitus in a Clinic Based Population," *Postgraduate Medical Journal* 83 (2007): 132-6.

242. My liwiec, "Prognostic Factors," 281-5.

243. MR Pastore, et al, "Six Months of Gluten-free Diet Do Not Influence Autoantibody Titers, but Iimprove Insulin Secretion in Subjects at High Risk for Type 1 Diabetes," *The Journal of Clinical Endocrinology and Metabolism* 88 (2003): 162-5.

244. M. Füchtenbusch, et al, "Elimination of Dietary Gluten and Development of Type 1 Diabetes in High Risk Subjects," *The Review of Diabetic Studies* 1 (2004): 39-41.

245. E. Valletta, et al, "Early Diagnosis and Treatment of Celiac Disease in Type 1 Diabetes. A Longitudinal, Case-control Study," *La Pediatria Medica e Chirurgica* 29 (2007): 99-104.

246. National Institutes of Health, "Diabetes Overview."

247. A. Franzese, et al, "Update on Coeliac Disease and Type 1 Diabetes Mellitus in Childhood," *Journal of Pediatric Endocrinology & Metabolism* 20 (2007): 1257-64.

248. JM Duggan, "Coeliac Disease: The Great Imitator," *The Medical Journal of Austraila* 17 (2004): 524-6.

249. National Institutes of Health, "Irritable Bowel Syndrome," National Digestive Diseases Information Clearinghouse, http://digestive. niddk.nih.gov/ddiseases/pubs/ibs/ (accessed May 7, 2008).

250. C. O'Leary, et al, "Celiac Disease and Irritable Bowel-type Symptoms," *The American Journal of Gastroenterology* 97 (2002): 1463-7.

251. P. Usai, et al, "Effect of Gluten-free Diet and Comorbidity of Irritable Bowel Syndrome-type Symptoms on Health-related Quality of Life in Adult Coeliac Patients," *Digestive and Liver Disease* 39 (2007): 824-8.

252. National Institutes of Health, "Irritable Bowel Syndrome."

253. Ibid.

254. Ibid.
255. B. Shahbazkhani, et al, "Coeliac Disease Presenting With Symptoms of Irritable Bowel Syndrome," *Alimentary Pharmacology & Therapeutics* 18 (2003): 231-5.
256. U. Wahnschaffe, et al, "Celiac Disease-like Abnormalities in a Subgroup of Patients With Irritable Bowel Syndrome," *Gastroenterology* 121 (2001): 1329-38.
257. BD Cash, et al, "The Utility of Diagnostic Tests in Irritable Bowel Syndrome Patients: A Systematic Review," *The American Journal of Gastroenterology* 97 (2002): 2812-9.
258. BM Spiegel, et al, "Testing for Celiac Sprue in Irritable Bowel Syndrome With Predominant Diarrhea: A Cost-effectiveness Analysis," *Gastroenterology* 126 (2004): 1721-32.
259. SM Mein, et al, "Serological Testing for Coeliac Disease in Patients With Symptoms of Irritable Bowel Syndrome: A Cost-effectiveness Analysis," *Alimentary Pharmacology & Therapeutics* 19 (2004): 1199-210.
260. O'Leary, "Celiac Disease and Irritable Bowel-type Symptoms," 1463-7.
261. SN Adler, et al, "Positive Coeliac Serology in Irritable Bowel Syndrome Patients With Normal Duodenal Biopsies: Video Capsule Endoscopy Findings and HLA-DQ Typing May Affect Clinical Management," *Journal of Gastrointestinal and Liver Diseases* 15 (2006): 221-5.
262. Mary Shomon, "Thyroid Disease Is Far More Widespread Than Originally Thought," Thyroid-Info, http://www.thyroid-info.com/ articles/thyroid-prevalence.htm (accessed May 10, 2008).
263. Mayo Clinic Staff, "Grave's Disease," MayoClinic.com, http://www.mayoclinic.com/health/graves-disease/DS00181 (accessed May 10, 2008).
264. Ibid.
265. Ibid.
266. Ibid.

267. Ibid.

268. Ibid.

269. Mayo Clinic Staff, "Hashimoto's Disease," MayoClinic.com, http://www.mayoclinic.com/health/hashimotos-disease/DS00567 (accessed May 10, 2008).

270. Ibid.

271. Ibid.

272. Ibid.

273. Ibid.

274. LM da Silva Kotze, et al, "Thyroid Disorders in Brazilian Patients With Celiac Disease," *Journal of Clinical Gastroenterology* 40 (2006): 33-6.

275. Spadaccino, "Celiac Disease in North Italian Patients," 116-21.

276. R. Iuorio, et al, "Prevalence of Celiac Disease in Ppatients With Autoimmune Thyroiditis," *Minerva Endocrinologica* 32 (2007): 239-43.

277. MN Akçay, G Akçay, "The Presence of the Antigliadin Antibodies in Autoimmune Thyroid Diseases," *Hepato-gastroenterology* (2003): 1-5.

278. FM Melo, et al, "Association Between Serum Markers for Celiac and Thyroid Autoimmune Diseases," *Arquivos Brasileiros de Endocrinologia e Metabologia* 49 (2005): 542-7.

279. L. Cuoco, et al, "Prevalence and Early Diagnosis of Coeliac Disease in Autoimmune Thyroid Disorders," *Ital Journal of Gastroenterology and Hepatology* 31 (1999): 283-7.

280. S. Faesch, et al, "Thyroiditis and Gluten Intolerance: Extrapancreatic Auto-immune Diseases Associated With Type 1 Diabetes," *Archives de Pédiatrie* 14 (2007): 24-30.

281. N. Ansaldi, et al, "Autoimmune Thyroid Disease and Celiac Disease in Children," *Journal of Pediatric Gastroenterology and Nutrition* 37 (2003): 63-6.

282. R. Valentino, et al, "Prevalence of Coeliac Disease in Patients With Thyroid Autoimmunity," *Hormone Research* 51 (1999): 124-7.

283. M. Buysschaert, "Coeliac Disease in Patients With Type 1

Diabetes Mellitus and Auto-immune Thyroid Disorders," *Acta Gastro-enterologica Belgica* 66 (2003): 237-40.

284. CL Ch'ng, et al, "Celiac Disease and Autoimmune Thyroid Disease," *Clinical Medicine & Research* 5 (2007): 184-92.

285. U. Volta, et al, "Coeliac Disease in Patients With Autoimmune Thyroiditis," *Digestion* 64 (2001): 61-5.

286. CL Ch'ng, et al, "Prospective Screening for Coeliac Disease in Patients With Graves' Hyperthyroidism Using Anti-gliadin and Tissue Transglutaminase Antibodies," *Clinical Endocrinology* 62 (2005): 303-6.

287. Joshua A. Hirsch, MD, "Osteopenia and Osteoporosis: Is There a Difference?" SpineUniverse, http://www.spineuniverse.com/displayarticle.php/article3148.html (accessed May 15, 2008).

288. Mayo Clinic Staff, "Osteoporosis," MayoClinic.com, http://www.mayoclinic.com/health/osteoporosis/DS00128 (accessed May15, 2008).

289. Hartl, "The Facts About Fosamax."

290. Mayo Clinic Staff, "Osteoporosis."

291. Ibid.

292. John J. Cannell, MD, Bruce W. Hollis, PhD, "Use of Vitamin D in Clinical Practice," *Alternative Medicine Review* 13 (2008): 6-20.

293. Mayo Clinic Staff, "Osteoporosis."

294. Ibid.

295. Ibid.

296. Ibid.

297. Hartl, "The Facts About Fosamax."

298. YA Gokhale, et al, "Celiac Disease in Osteoporotic Indians," *The Journal of the Association of Physicians of India* 51 (2003): 579-83.

299. US Kavak et al, "Bone Mineral Density in Children With Untreated and Treated Celiac Disease," *Journal of Pediatric Gastroenterology and Nutrition* 37 (2003): 434-6.

300. SE Meek, K Nix, "Hypocalcemia After Alendronate Therapy in a

Patient With Celiac Disease," *Endocrine Practice* 13 (2007): 403-7.

301. Cannell, "Use of Vitamin D," 6-20.

302. Ibid.

303. Vodjani, "The Immunology of Gluten Sensitivity Beyond the Intestinal Tract."

304. ML Bianchi ML, MT Bardella, "Bone and Celiac Disease," *Calcified Tissue International* 71 (2002): 465-71.

305. C. Hartman, et al, "Bone Quantitative Ultrasound and Bone Mineral Density in Children With Celiac Disease," *Journal of Pediatric Gastroenterology and Nutrition* 39 (2004): 504-10.

306. H. Vasquez, et al, "Risk of Fractures in Celiac Disease Patients: A Cross-sectional, Case-control Study," *The American Journal of Gastroenterology* 95 (2000): 183-9.

307. BioHealth Diagnostics, "Chronic Stress Response™ Chart."

308. BioHealth Diagnostics, "Steroidal Hormone Principle Pathways."

309. AV Stazi, B. Trinti, "Reproduction, Endocrine Disorders and Celiac Disease: Risk Factors of Osteoporosis," *Minerva Medica* 97 (2006): 191-203.

310. BioHealth Diagnostics, "Steroidal Hormone Principle Pathways."

311. C. Sategna-Guidetti, et al, "The Effects of 1-year Gluten Withdrawal on Bone Mass, Bone Metabolism and Nutritional Status in Newly-diagnosed Adult Coeliac Disease Patients," *Alimentary Pharmacology & Therapeutics* 14 (2000): 35-43.

312. Mayo Clinic Staff, "Osteoporosis."

313. S. Mora, et al, "Bone Density and Bone Metabolism Are Normal After Long-term Gluten-free Diet in Young Celiac Patients," *The American Journal of Gastroenterology* 94 (1999): 398-403.

314. Hartl, "The Facts About Fosamax."

315. Ibid.

316. Ibid.

317. Ibid.

318. WF Stenson, et al, "Increased Prevalence of Celiac Disease and Need for Routine Screening Among Patients With Osteoporosis," *Archives of Internal Medicine* 28 (2005): 393-9.
319. M. Szathmári, et al, "Bone Mineral Content and Density in Asymptomatic Children With Coeliac Disease on a Gluten-free Diet," *European Journal of Gastroenterology & Hepatology* (2001): 419-24.
320. T. Kemppainen, et al, "Osteoporosis in Adult Patients With Celiac Disease," *Bone* 24 (1999): 249-55.
321. Mayo Clinic Staff, "Autoimmune Hepatitis," MayoClinic.com, http://www.mayoclinic.com/health/autoimmune-hepatitis/DS00676 (accessed May 20, 2008).
322. S. Caprai, et al, "SIGENP Study Group for Autoimmune Liver Disorders in Celiac Disease. Autoimmune Liver Disease Associated With Celiac Disease in Childhood: A Multicenter Study," *Clinical Gastroenterology and Hepatology* 6 (2008): 803-6.
323. Mayo Clinic Staff, "Autoimmune Hepatitis."
324. Barbero Villares, et al, "Hepatic Involvement in Celiac Disease," *Gastroenterología y Hepatología* 31 (2008): 25-8.
325. FM Stevens, RM McLoughlin, "Is Coeliac Disease a Potentially Treatable Cause of Liver Failure?" *European Journal of Gastroenterology & Hepatology* 17 (2005): 1015-7.
326. A. Rubio-Tapia, et al, "Celiac Disease Autoantibodies in Severe Autoimmune Liver Disease and the Effect of Liver Transplantation," *Liver International* 28 (2008): 467-76.
327. Stevens, "Is Coeliac Disease a Potentially Treatable Cause," 1015-7.
328. Cantarero Vallejo, MD, et al, "Liver Damage and Celiac Disease," *Revista Española de Enfermedades Digestivas* 99 (2007): 648-52.
329. Caprai, "SIGENP Study Group for Autoimmune Liver Disorders," 803-6.
330. G. Maggiore, S. Caprai, "Liver Involvement in Celiac Disease," *Indian Journal of Pediatrics* 73 (2006): 809-11.

331. M. Pazo, et al, "Liver Abnormalities in Adult Celiac Disease. Clinicopathologic Characterization and Outcome After Therapy," *Gastroenterología y Hepatología* 29 (2006): 383-9.

332. Caprai, "SIGENP Study Group for Autoimmune Liver Disorders," 803-6.

333. Maggiore, "Liver Involvement in Celiac Disease," 809-11.

334. Mayo Clinic Staff, "Autoimmune Hepatitis."

335. Mayo Clinic Staff, "Depression," MayoClinic.com, http://www.mayoclinic.com/health/depression/DS00175 (accessed May 26, 2008).

336. Ibid.

337. GS Sachs, et al, "Effectiveness of Adjunctive Antidepressant Treatment for Bipolar Depression," *The New England Journal of Medicine* 356 (2007): 1711-22.

338. Mayo Clinic Staff, "Depression."

339. Ibid.

340. C. Hallert, J. Aström , "Psychic Disturbances in Adult Coeliac Disease. II. Psychological Findings," *Scandinavian Journal of Gastroenterology* 17 (1982): 21-4.

341. C. Hallert, T. Derefeldt, "Psychic Disturbances in Adult Coeliac Disease. I. Clinical Observations," *Scandinavian Journal of Gastroenterology* 17 (1982): 17-9.

342. WrongDiagnosis staff, "Prevalence and Incidence of Depression," WrongDiagnosis, http://www.wrongdiagnosis.com/d/depression/ prevalence.htm (accessed May 26, 2008).

343. Hallert, "Psychic Disturbances in Adult Coeliac Disease. I. Clinical Observations,"17-9.

344. PA Pynnönen, et al, "Mental Disorders in Adolescents With Celiac Disease," *Psychosomatics* 45 (2004): 325-35.

345. Pynnönen, "Gluten-free Diet May Alleviate Depressive and Behavioural Symptoms," 14.

346. P. Potocki, K. Hozyasz, "Psychiatric Symptoms and Coeliac Disease," *Psychiatria Polska* 36 (2002): 567-78.

347. Potocki, "Psychiatric Symptoms" 567-78.

348. M. Kieslich, et al, "Brain White-matter Lesions in Celiac Disease: A Prospective Study of 75 Diet-treated Patients," *Pediatrics* 108 (2001): E21.

349. Dickey, "Overweight in Celiac Disease," 2356-9.

350. National Center for Health Statistics, "Overweight," Centers for Disease Control and Prevention, http://www.cdc.gov/nchs/fastats/ overwt.htm (accessed May 29, 2008).

351. Mayo Clinic Staff, "Obesity," MayClinic.com, http://www. mayo clinic.com/health/obesity/DS00314 (accessed May 29, 2008).

352. Ibid.

353. Ibid.

354. Ibid.

355. Dickey, "Overweight in Celiac Disease," 2356-9.

356. P. Mariani, et al, "The Gluten-free Diet: A Nutritional Risk Factor for Adolescents With Celiac Disease?" *Journal of Pediatric Gastroenterology and Nutrition* 27 (1998): 519-23.

357. AG Nieuwenhuizen, F. Rutters, "The Hypothalamic-pituitary-adrenal-axis in the Regulation of Energy Balance," *Physiology & Behavior* 94 (2008): 169-77.

358. SL Teegarden, TL Bale, "Effects of Stress on Dietary Preference and Intake Are Dependent on Access and Stress Sensitivity," *Physiology & Behavior* 93 (2008): 713-23.

359. Nibali S. Conti, et al, "Obesity in a Child With Untreated Coeliac Disease," *Helvetica Paediatrica Acta* 42 (1987): 45-8.

360. O. Oso, NC Fraser, "A Boy With Coeliac Disease and Obesity," *Acta Paediatrica* 95 (2006): 618-9.

361. WrongDiagnosis Staff, "Prevalence and Incidence of Fibromyalgia," WrongDiagnosis, http://www.wrongdiagnosis.com/f/fibromyalgia /prevalence.htm (accessed June 2, 2008).

362. Mayo Clinic Staff, "Fibromyalgia," MayoClinic.com, http://www.mayoclinic.com/health/fibromyalgia/DS00079 (accessed June 2, 2008).

363. Ibid.

364. Ibid.
365. Ibid.
366. JD Smith, et al, "Relief of Fibromyalgia Symptoms Following Discontinuation of Dietary Excitotoxins," *The Annals of Pharmacotherapy* 35 (2001): 702-6.
367. K. Kaartinen, et al, "Vegan Diet Alleviates Fibromyalgia Symptoms," *Scandinavian Journal of Rheumatology* 29 (2000): 308-13.
368. KA Azad,,et al, "Vegetarian Diet in the Treatment of Fibromyalgia," *Bangladesh Medical Research Council Bulletin* 26 (2000): 41-7.
369. RD Zipser, et al, "Presentations of Adult Celiac Disease in a Nationwide Patient Support Group," *Digestive Diseases and Sciences* 48 (2003): 761-4.
370. G. Triadafilopoulos, et al, "Bowel Dysfunction in Fibromyalgia Syndrome," *Digestive Diseases and Sciences* 36 (1991): 59-64.
371. D. Veale, et al, "Primary Fibromyalgia and the Iirritable Bowel Syndrome: Different Expressions of a Common Pathogenetic Process," *British Journal of Rheumatology* 30 (1991): 220-2.
372. DJ Wallace, DS Hallegua, "Fibromyalgia: The Gastrointestinal Link," *Current Pain and Headache Reports* 8 (2004): 364-8.
373. WrongDiagnosis Staff, "Prevalence and Incidence of Dermatitis Herpetiformis," WrongDiagnosis, http://www.wrongdiagnosis.com/d/dermatitis_herpetiformis/prevalence.htm (accessed June 4, 2008).
374. P. Collin, T. Reunala, "Recognition and Management of the Cutaneous Manifestations of Celiac Disease: A Guide for Dermatologists," *American Journal of Clinical Dermatology* 4 (2003): 13-20.
375. H. Kraus, Jr., "Rashes/Skin Problems," Chronic Illness: Gluten and Celiac Disease Links and Notes, http://members.cox.net/harold.kraus/gluten/anno_symptoms_files/skin.htm (accessed June 3, 2008).

376. Merck Staff, "Dermatitis Herpetiformis," The Merck Manuals Online Medical Library, http://www.merck.com/mmhe/sec18/ch209/ch209d.html (accessed June 3, 2008).

377. SI Katz, et al, "Dermatitis Herpetiformis: The Skin and the Gut," *Annals of Internal Medicine* 93 (1980): 857-74.

378. Merck Staff, "Dermatitis Herpetiformis."

379. Katz, "Dermatitis Herpetiformis," 857-74.

380. M. Nino, et al, "A Long-term Gluten-free Diet as an Alternative Treatment in Severe Forms of Dermatitis Herpetiformis," *The Journal of Dermatological Treatment* 18 (2007): 10-12.

381. MO Eriksson, et al, "Palmoplantar Pustulosis: A Clinical and Immunohistological Study," *The British Journal of Dermatology* 138 (1998): 390-8.

382. Kraus, Jr., "Rashes/Skin Problems."

383. U. Lindqvist, et al, "IgA Antibodies to Gliadin and Coeliac Disease in Psoriatic Arthritis," *Rheumatology* 41 (2002): 31-7.

384. M. Seyhan, et al, "The Mucocutaneous Manifestations Associated With Celiac Disease in Childhood and Adolescence," *Pediatric Dermatology* 24 (2007): 28-33.

385. T. Reunala, "Dermatitis Herpetiformis: Coeliac Disease of the Skin," *Annals of Medicine* 30 (1998): 416-8.

386. S. Meyers, et al, "Cutaneous Vasculitis Complicating Coeliac Disease," *Gut* 22 (1981): 61-4.

387. WrongDiagnosis Staff, "Prevalence and Incidence of Alzheimer's Disease," WrongDiagnosis, http://www.wrongdiagnosis.com/a/alzheimersdisease/prevalenc e.htm (accessed June 5, 2008).

388. Mayo Clinic Staff, "Mild Cognitive Impairment," MayoClinic.com, http://www.mayoclinic.com/health/mild-cognitive-impairment/DS00553 (accessed June 5, 2008).

389. Ibid.

390. Ibid.

391. L. Luostarinen, et al, "Coeliac Disease Presenting With Neurological Disorders," *European Neurology* 42 (1999): 132-5.
392. MR Turner, et al, "A Case of Celiac Disease Mimicking Amyotrophic Lateral Sclerosis," *Nature Clinical Practice. Neurology* 3 (2007): 581-4.
393. E. Karakoç, et al, "Encephalopathy Due to Carnitine Deficiency in an Adult Patient With Gluten Enteropathy," *Clinical Neurology and Neurosurgery* 108 (2006): 794-7.
394. WT Hu, et al, "Cognitive Impairment and Celiac Disease," *Archives of Neurology* 63 (2006): 1440-6.
395. U. Volta, et al, "Clinical Findings and Anti-neuronal Antibodies in Coeliac Disease With·Neurological Disorders," *Scandinavian Journal of Gastroenterology* 37 (2002): 1276-81.
396. M. Hadjivassiliou, et al, "Autoantibody Targeting of Brain and Intestinal Transglutaminase in Gluten Ataxia," *Neurology* 66 (2006): 373-7.
397. Mayo Clinic Staff, "Mild Cognitive Impairment."
398. P. Usai et al, "Frontal Cortical Perfusion Abnormalities Related to Gluten Intake and Associated Autoimmune Disease in Adult Coeliac Disease. 99mTc-ECD Brain SPECT Study," *Digestive and Liver Disease* 36 (2004): 513-8.
399. G. Addolorato, et al, "Regional Cerebral Hypoperfusion in Patients with Celiac Disease," *The American Journal of Medicine* 116 (2004): 312-7
400. S. Helms, "Celiac Disease and Gluten-associated Diseases," *Alternative Medicine Review* 10 (2005): 172-92.
401. A. Fasano, "Clinical Presentation of Celiac Disease in the Pediatric Population," *Gastroenterology* 128 (2005): S68-73.
402. Helms, "Celiac Disease and Gluten-associated Diseases," 172-92.
403. B. Lebwohl, PH Green, "Screening for Celiac Disease," *The New England Journal of Medicine* 3 (2003): 1673-4.
404. A. Tursi, "Can Histologic Damage Influence the Severity of Coeliac Disease? An Unanswered Question," *Digestive and Liver Disease* 39 (2007): 30-2.
405. S. Rashtak, et al, "Comparative Usefulness of Deamidated

Gliadin Antibodies in the Diagnosis of Celiac Disease," *Clinical Gastroenterology and Hepatology* 6 (2008): 426-32.

406. Tursi, "Can Histologic Damage Influence," 30-2.

407. AD Hopper, et al, "What Is the Role of Serologic Testing in Celiac Disease? A Prospective, Biopsy-confirmed Study With Economic Analysis," *Clinical Gastroenterology and Hepatology* 6 (2008): 314-20.

408. Rahstak, "Comparative Usefulness," 426-32.

409. D. Villalta, et al, "Testing for IgG Class Antibodies in Celiac Disease Patients With Selective IgA Deficiency. A Comparison of the Diagnostic Accuracy of 9 IgG Anti-tissue Transglutaminase, 1 IgG Anti-gliadin and 1 IgG Anti-deaminated Gliadin Peptide Antibody Assays," *Clinica Chimica Acta* 382 (2007): 95-9.

410. Helms, "Celiac Disease and Gluten-associated Diseases," 172-92.

411. P. Patinen, et al, "Salivary and Serum IgA Antigliadin Antibodies in Dermatitis Herpetiformis," *European Journal of Oral Sciences* 103 (1995): 280-4.

412. AF Rodrigues, HR Jenkins, "Investigation and Management of Coeliac Disease," *Archives of Disease in Childhood* 93 (2008): 251-4.

413. Lebwohl, "Screening for Celiac Disease," 1673-4.

414. JA Abrams, et al, "Seronegative Celiac Disease: Increased Prevalence With Lesser Degrees of Villous Atrophy," *Digestive Diseases and Sciences* 49 (2004): 546-50.

415. D. Goldberg, et al, "Screening for Celiac Disease in Family Members: Is Follow-up Testing Necessary?" *Digestive Diseases and Sciences* 52 (2007): 1082-6.

416. Carlo Catassi, "A Prospective, Double-blind, Placebo-controlled Trial to Establish Safe Gluten Threshold for Patients With Celiac Disease," *American Journal of Clinical Nutrition* 185 (2007): 160-166.

417. Biagi Federico, "A Milligram of Gluten a Day Keeps the Mucosal Recovery Away: A Case Report," *Nutrition Reviews* 62 (2004): 360-63.

418. Hadjivassiliou, "Neuromuscular Disorder," 770-5.
419. Hallert, "Evidence of Poor Vitamin Status," 1333-9.
420. Hallert, "Evidence of Poor Vitamin Status," 1333-9.
421. A. Fasano, "Celiac Disease—How to Handle a Clinical Chameleon," *The New England Journal of Medicine* 348 (2003): 2568-70.
422. Green, "Celiac Disease," 1731-43.

GLOSSARY

ACTH (adrenocorticotrophic hormone): a hormone produced by the pituitary gland; an important player in how the brain and the adrenal glands interact.

Adrenal glands: two small glands that sit just above your kidneys. They are immediately adjacent to some of your major blood vessels so that they can release hormones into the bloodstream and respond to feedback from other hormones and chemicals. In this way, they control how other systems operate.

One of the primary roles of the adrenal glands is to help the body respond to physical, biochemical or emotional stress. They are also mainly involved in anabolic work—that is, repairing and anti-aging effects. Another of their roles is to keep the immune system properly functioning and, at the same time, to balance other bodily systems to promote optimal health.

Adrenaline (epinephrine): a hormone secreted by the adrenal glands.

Aldosterone: a hormone that balances our electrolytes, such as sodium and potassium, and our fluid balance

Allopathic medicine: conventional medicine which normally utilizes medications as its main treatment tool.

Alzheimer's disease: the seventh-leading cause of death. The disease results in memory loss caused by premature aging of the brain.

Amino acids: the building blocks of proteins; the subunits from which proteins are assembled.

Amyotrophic lateral sclerosis (Lou Gehrig's disease): a progressive, usually fatal disease of the nervous system caused by degeneration of the part of the nervous system that controls voluntary muscle movement.

Antibodies: substances your immune system makes to identify and destroy foreign objects.

Anti-endomysial antibodies (EM-Ab): antibodies that are made against proteins of the smooth muscle cells of the intestine; endomysial antibodies are produced and directed against your body's own tissue.

Antigens: any substance that causes the production of antibodies by the body's immune system. Common antigens include bacteria, viruses and pollen grains.

Anti-gliadin antibodies: antibodies that the immune system creates to identify and attack gliadin molecules (gluten protein).

Antioxidants: substances, such as vitamin C, vitamin E, vitamin A, beta carotene and selenium, which protect cells from damage that can later lead to health problems such as heart disease or cancer.

Anti-tissue transglutaminase antibodies (tTG Ab): antibodies directed against your own tissue, specifically against the enzyme transglutaminase. After gliadin crosses the intestinal lining, the enzyme, tissue transglutaminase, binds to gliadin and takes off a portion of the protein. tTG antibodies are produced and directed against this complex of gliadin attached to tissue transglutaminase.

Ataxia: poor coordination and balance.

Autoantibodies: antibodies made against your own body's tissues due to your immune system mistaking those tissues for foreigners.

Autoimmune disease: disorders that work against your own body tissue. Diseases such as arthritis, cancer, diabetes and others are known to have an autoimmune component. There are more than forty defined autoimmune disorders and, in total, these are among the top ten leading causes of death. Only one-third of those afflicted with autoimmune diseases are diagnosed.

Autoimmune polyglandular syndrome: a syndrome wherein gluten sensitivity, diabetes and thyroid disease are often linked together.

B cells: white blood cells that play a large role in your bloodstream's immune response. Their principal function is to make antibodies against antigens. B cells are made in the bone marrow.

Beta cells: the special cells of the pancreas that produce insulin in response to a rise of glucose in the bloodstream.

Body mass index (BMI): this index figures in your height and weight and then calculates a number for an assessment of weight category. A BMI of less than twenty-five is normal; a BMI from twenty-five to thirty is overweight; and a BMI greater than thirty is obese.

Calcitriol: a form of vitamin D that occurs in humans. It is a hormone made from cholesterol that acts to balance calcium and phosphorus in your body.

Calcitonin: a hormone produced by the thyroid that slows down bone loss. When it's deficient, bone destruction occurs.

Casein: a milk protein that can cause allergic reactions in affected people.

Catabolism: destructive metabolism resulting in the breakdown of body tissues.

Celiac disease: an intestinal disease that creates damage to the small intestine, thereby compromising absorption of nutrients. It is genetic in nature and predisposes the patient to other disease processes. The only treatment is lifelong avoidance of gluten.

Celiac hepatitis: liver damage seen in patients who have celiac disease or gluten sensitivity. Celiac patients are found to be resistant to the hepatitis B vaccine and such resistance can be a clue to untreated celiac disease.

Cellular mimicry: some molecules of one tissue can look very similar to molecules of another. This phenomenon is one way in which gluten triggers immune disorders throughout the body.

Central tolerance: early in the development of your body, cells of the immune system (called T cells and B cells) begin to seek and destroy other cells that would normally attack your own body. The first wave of this is called central tolerance.

Cerebellum: a part of your brain that helps coordinate perceptions with muscle movement so that you know where parts of your body are and motions are smooth and coordinated.

Cholecystokinin: a hormone that causes the gall bladder and pancreas to produce enzymes so that fat can be digested.

Cirrhosis: damage to the liver from chronic inflammation, which creates scarring.

Colitis: inflammation of the colon that affects the lining of the intestines. Colitis is an autoimmune disease.

Cortisol: commonly referred to as our "stress hormone." It increases blood pressure and sugar levels, and it decreases the function of the immune system.

CT scan (computed tomography): A scan that uses X-rays to provide a three-dimensional image of your body.

Deaminated gliadin: the result of the actions of the enzyme tissue transglutaminase once it breaks apart gliadin, removing a particular amino acid called glutamine. It's the beginning of gliadin's digestion.

Deaminated gliadin antibodies: the specific antibodies that the immune system makes against deaminated gliadin. These are different antibodies as compared to those made against an intact gliadin protein.

Dermatitis herpetiformis (DH): one of the more common autoimmune disorders associated with gluten sensitivity. This disorder is selectively associated with gluten sensitivity and can be the major presenting symptom. It consists of small blisters that often develop over the buttocks, lower back, knees, elbows and back of the head. Usually, itching and burning of the skin are significant.

DEXA scans (dual energy X-ray absortiometry): an X-ray test to measure the density of bones.

DHEA (dehydroepiandosterone): a precursor hormone of our sex hormones (estrogen, testosterone and progesterone).

DNA: molecules that contain the genetic instructions for how an organism will develop and function. DNA is found in all living organisms.

Eczema: characterized by redness, swelling, itching, dryness, crusting and flaking.

Enzymes: proteins that facilitate the rates of reactions in the body, such as digesting food.

Excitotoxins: found in today's prepackaged, preservative-rich foods. They can be particularly detrimental to the intestinal lining. They include artificial sweeteners, MSG and nitrites.

Fatty acids: fats that are required for cells to function normally. The body cannot make them on its own. Therefore they must be made available through the diet. Vegetable oils are rich in omega 6, while fish oil is rich in omega 3. The current Western diet consists of way too much omega 6 and not enough omega 3. Ideally your diet should reflect a ratio of 1.5:1 (omega 6 :omega 3). Currently it averages 20:1 in our diets!

Fibromyalgia: a disorder of fatigue, joint aches and muscle aches. Other symptoms include fatigue with poor sleep digestive complaints, headaches, depression, tingling, numbness and brain fog.

Folic acid: an important nutrient for the development of a fetus; its deficiency can cause miscarriages and birth defects so it's important that women planning to become pregnant have adequate amounts.

Gastrin: a hormone that causes the secretion of gastric acid (hydrochloric acid) by the stomach.

Ghrelin: a hormone produced in the digestive tract that is directly affected by cortisol levels. Ghrelin stimulates appetite and appears to be related to growth hormone release.

Gliadin: one of the major proteins in gluten, along with glutenin. They are present in equal, fifty-fifty portions for the most part. Gliadin gives wheat its ability to be stretched, known as extensibility. Glutenin gives wheat its ability to return to its shape when stretched, known as elasticity. Both are needed to make good breads. Gliadin is the protein that creates the immune response in gluten sensitivity.

Glutamine: gliadin contains two problematic amino acids—proline and glutamine—that create digestive problems for the body.

Gluten: the main protein in wheat, representing eighty-five percent of all wheat proteins present.

Glutenin: one of the major proteins in gluten, along with gliadin. They are present in equal, fifty-fifty portions for the most part. Gliadin gives wheat its ability to be stretched, known as extensibility. Glutenin gives wheat its ability to return to its shape when stretched, known as elasticity. Both are needed to make good breads

Gluteomorphins: have effects on morphine-like receptors in our brains and create cravings. As with glucose, there are believed to be other physiological cravings that develop when wheat becomes a regular component of our diet.

Gluten sensitivity: a condition in which gluten is the underlying cause of a variety of health problems. For individuals who are gluten-sensitive, removal of gluten completely from the diet generally results in improved health along many of the body's systems.

Goiter: an enlargement of the thyroid gland.

Grave's disease: results in high thyroid function, or hyperthyroidism.

Hashimoto's thyroiditis: results in low thyroid function or hypothyroidism.

HealthNOW Method: distinguished from the common, allopathic view by addressing the root of the problem and not simply symptom relief. The body is looked at as a whole and diagnostic procedures, along with dietary and lifestyle changes, are implemented to restore optimal body function. Learn more at www.healthnowmedical.com.

H. pylori: a bacterium in the stomach that can cause stomach ulcers and stomach cancer when severe.

Hepatitis: injury to the liver resulting in inflammation of the organ. It can heal on its own or progress to scarring of the liver.

HLA genes: a group of genes that carry the blueprints for our immune systems. In people who are gluten-sensitive, a group of specific blueprints surface on these genes. These have been labeled HLA-DQ2 and HLA-DQ8. Our immune cells that carry these patterns affect our ability to see gluten as a "safe" dietary protein. The result is that the immune system begins attacking the gluten molecules.

HLA-DQ2 (see "HLA genes," above): approximately ninety-five percent of patients with celiac disease have the HLA-DQ2 gene while close to five percent have the HLA-DQ8 gene (see below). Twenty-five to forty percent of the United States population has either DQ2 or DQ8.

HLA-DQ8 (see "HLA genes," above): approximately ninety-five percent of patients with celiac disease have the HLA-DQ2 gene while close to five percent have the HLA-DQ8 gene. Twenty-five to forty percent of the United States population has either DQ2 or DQ8.

Hormones: chemical messengers that transport signals from one cell to another. Hormones are released by cells that then affect cells in other parts of the body.

HP axis (Hypothalamic-Pituitary Axis): The HP axis represents a key interface between the brain and nervous systems and is divided into two parts: the hypothalamus and the pituitary gland (both of which are located in the brain). The hypothalamus responds to many signals generated by the brain as well as by other hormone glands. In response to these signals, the hypothalamus releases hormones or molecules that stimulate or suppress the pituitary gland. The pituitary gland produces a hormone called ACTH and is an important player in how the brain and the adrenal glands interact.

Hypothyroid: refers to a low-functioning thyroid gland that fails to produce enough thyroid hormone.

IBS (irritable bowel syndrome): an uncomfortable syndrome resulting in abdominal complaints such as cramping, bloating, constipation and diarrhea.

IgA (immunoglobulin A): the chief antibody found in the digestive tract. IgA is primarily produced along the intestinal lining and represents an important part of our bodies' defense systems against foreign bacteria, viruses and parasites that may come from our diets. If someone is sensitive to gluten, the immune system works overtime to attack gluten as it attempts to enter the bloodstream from the intestines. IgA antibodies are produced in high numbers in the intestinal lining as a defense barrier.

IgG (immunoglobulin G): a chief antibody found in the blood. IgG levels don't tend to get depleted and therefore are a more accurate test of gluten intolerance in people with low IgA levels.

Immune system: the system that protects against disease by identifying and eradicating disease-causing agents and cancer cells. It can detect a wide variety of hostile agents and, in order to function properly, needs to distinguish those hostile agents from the organism's own healthy tissues.

Insulin: a hormone that allows the cells of your body to absorb glucose so that your blood sugar reduces.

Insulin resistance: a condition in which the cells of the body become resistant to the effects of insulin. As a result, higher levels of insulin are needed in order for it to be effective. Insulin resistance is associated with obesity, fatty liver, type 2 diabetes, heart disease and polycystic ovary disease.

Intestinal biopsy: while a patient is lightly sedated a surgeon inserts a small camera down the esophagus and into the stomach and upper portion of the small intestine. The surgeon then uses small pinchers to take little pieces of tissue that can be examined later under a microscope. Specifically, in gluten disorders, findings sought include villous atrophy and inflammation of the wall of the small intestine.

Latent gluten sensitivity: called "silent" or "latent" because the patients do not yet have symptoms, despite having gluten reactivity occurring within their bodies, or because the inflammation cannot yet be detected.

Leaky gut: the tight junctions between the lining cells of the intestine become disrupted due to inflammation, allowing gluten and other substances to bypass the lining cells and gain access directly to the bloodstream.

Leukemia: cancer of the blood or bone marrow.

Neuropathy: altered function of the nerves resulting in a variety of symptoms including pain, weakness or numbness.

Lupus (systemic lupus erythematosis): an autoimmune disease that can involve the skin alone or the skin and the heart, lungs, kidneys, joints and nervous system. When it involves multiple systems it's called "systemic lupus"; when it only involves the skin it's called "discoid lupus."

Lymphoma: a cancer that is usually diagnosed due to lymph node enlargement. The cancer starts in the white blood cells, called lymphocytes.

Malabsorption: decreased ability to absorb nutrients from the diet.

Metabolites: substances produced by metabolism or breakdown.

Metabolic pathways: trace reactions within a cell that occur for the cell to maintain itself and its functioning within your body. For example, a cell produces energy as a result of a metabolic pathway.

Metabolism: chemical reactions that occur in your body in order to maintain life. Such reactions allow you to grow, reproduce, maintain your body's structure and respond to the environment.

Modified elimination diet (MED): a hypoallergenic diet, followed for ten days, that eliminates gluten and other common food allergens such as cow's milk, corn and soy products while invoking a good balance of healthy foods such as lean protein, good quality fat, vegetables and fruits.

MRI (magnetic resonance imaging): a medical imaging technique used to visualize the structure and function of the body. It's especially useful for visualizing soft tissue as opposed to bone.

Mucosa: moist tissue that lines the inside of your body, including your nose, mouth, lungs and gastrointestinal tract.

Myocarditis: an autoimmune attack causing inflammation of the heart.

Non-Hodgkin's lymphoma: a cancer that develops from lymphocytes, a type of white blood cell. Your white bloods cells are part of your immune system.

Oral tolerance: Normally, as infants and children are gradually exposed to foods, including wheat and gluten, the immune system catalogs these as "safe" and normal. In this way, when the gluten and gliadin process through our digestive system, there is no immune attack triggered. Because the immune system learned early in life that these are beneficial to our nutrition and cause no harm to our health, it tolerates these substances.

Opiate receptors: areas of the brain which, when activated, cause symptoms such as diminished alertness, concentration and memory.

Osteoarthritis: also known as degenerative joint disease. Accounts for more than half of all cases of arthritis. Weight-bearing joints such as the hips, knees and spine are typically affected as well as the hands.

Osteopenia: means "a deficiency of bone" and is considered a predecessor to osteoporosis.

Osteoporosis: means "porous bone." If bone density is moderate to severely reduced, it is defined as osteoporosis.

Paleolithic: pertaining to cultures from the Stone Age.

Palmoplantar pustulosis: a type of psoriasis appearing on the palms of the hands and the soles of the feet.

Pathology: a disease process.

Peripheral tolerance: the phase of the immune system's development that occurs in the tissues and bloodstream. Peripheral tolerance is handled mostly by special T cells called "regulatory T cells." They continue to identify immune cells that are targeting self tissues and suppress them or make them inactive

Phytonutrients: substances that come from edible plants and are rich in nutrients.

Pituitary gland: located at the base of the brain. It secretes hormones regulating body function and produces hormones that cause other glands to secrete their own hormones. For example, the thyroid stimulating hormone produced by the pituitary stimulates the thyroid to secrete its hormones.

Pregnenelone: often called the "mother hormone" as it is a precursor to DHEA and progesterone. It is the basic building block not only of cortisol but also of DHEA, progesterone (a female sex hormone) and aldosterone (a hormone that causes the retention of sodium and water in the body).

Probiotic: nutritional supplements containing healthy, beneficial bacteria that improve the function of your immune system.

Proline: gliadin contains two problematic amino acids, proline and glutamine, that create digestive problems for the body.

Proteus: a bacteria responsible for many urinary tract infections.

Psoriasis: a common skin disease that affects the life cycle of skin cells, increasing it from a month to only days. As a result, cells build up rapidly, forming thick, silvery scales and itchy, dry, red patches that can be painful.

Purkinje cells: These cells are found in your brain and are the main components of your balancing center and coordination.

Regulatory T cells: special cells that render ineffective any cells that would attack your own tissues (called autoimmune cells). This process starts while you are an embryo and continues throughout your life.[38] There is a constant monitoring process by these regulatory T cells, which watch out for autoimmune cells.

Rheumatoid arthritis: an inflammatory form of arthritis that causes joint pain, swelling and eventually deformity. It is an autoimmune arthritic disorder that is three times more common in women than men, commonly occurring between the ages of forty and sixty. Its juvenile form is the most common arthritis in childhood.

Rotavirus: a virus that carries proteins within it that look very similar to the gliadin or deaminated gliadin particles. In this way, not only does it cause a disrupted intestinal lining when a child contracts it, but it can also directly trigger the same immune attack as gliadin due to its similar composition.

Secretin: a hormone that regulates the pH of the stomach.

Serotonin: a neurotransmitter that affects mood, sleep and appetite in addition to other factors.

Silent gluten sensitivity: a patient is considered to be in a silent" or "latent" category when they do not yet have symptoms despite having gluten reactivity occur within their bodies, or when the inflammation cannot yet be detected.

Sjogren's syndrome: an autoimmune disease that can involve the joints and can occur secondarily to other forms of arthritis, like rheumatoid arthritis or lupus. It attacks the tear ducts and salivary glands, resulting in dry eyes and a dry mouth. It is nine times more common in women than men.

Steroid: important compounds such as cholesterol, the sex hormones (testosterone and estrogen) and adrenal hormones are all steroids.

Stressors: stress can come in many different varieties, other than from our diets. Some examples are sleep deprivation, pain, emotional stress, infections, toxins and injuries.

T4: a pre-hormone produced by the thyroid that does very little until activated by an enzyme that turns it into T3, the active thyroid hormone.

T3: the active form of the body's thyroid hormone.

T cells: belong to a group of white blood cells (known as lymphocytes) and play an important role in your cell's immune response. They are called "T cells" because the thymus gland is responsible for their production.

Tetracycline: made from certain microorganisms (Streptomyces) and used as a broad-spectrum antibiotic.

Thymus gland: located behind the top of the breastbone, it serves as the site of T cell production. The thymus increases gradually in size and activity until puberty and then shrinks, becoming mostly inactive.

Thyroid stimulating hormone (TSH): stimulates the thyroid gland to make thyroid hormone, which is important for your metabolism (how quickly and efficiently you burn your food to create energy).

Thyroxin: a thyroid hormone.

Tight junctions: the structures that hold the lining cells of the intestine together along their sides.

Tissue transglutaminase (tTG): a special enzyme that breaks down gliadin in the small intestine. tTG can be the focus of an immune attack once it's attached to the gluten proteins.

Toxins: poisons that can damage tissues of the body.

Transaminase: any of a group of enzymes that cause the removal of a part of an amino acid and its transfer to another amino acid. The enzymes are important in protein metabolism.

Tryptophan: an amino acid needed to make serotonin.

Villi: the lining of the small intestine is normally covered with finger-like projections, called villi, that serve to help absorb nutrients. These villi greatly increase the surface area of the intestines (imagine the size of a tennis court), allowing a large area from which nutrients can enter your body.

Vasculitis: inflammation of the body's blood vessels.

Villous atrophy: the villi of the small intestine are damaged and diminish in size.

Vitiligo: a skin disorder wherein there is a loss of the natural pigment, resulting in white patches on the body.

INDEX

RESOURCES

HealthNOW Medical Center—home of the HealthNOW Method
www.healthnowmedical.com
www.healthnowmethod.blogspot.com
1309 S. Mary Ave., Suite 100
Sunnyvale, CA 94087
408-733-0400

Institute of Functional Medicine
www.functionalmedicine.org
You can refer to their list of doctors around the country
  to find a practitioner close to where you live.

Labs

Genova Diagnostics: www.genovadiagnostics.com
Biohealth Diagnostics: www.biodia.com
Metametrix: http://www.metametrix.com
Entero Lab: https://www.enterolab.com
Prometheus Laboratories: www.prometheuslabs.com
Kimball Genetics: www.kimballgenetics.com
Neuroimmunology Labs: www.neurorelief.com

Books

Celiac Disease: A Hidden Epidemic by Peter H.R. Green, M.D., and Rory Jones
Dangerous Grains by James Braly, M.D., and Ron Hoggan, M.A.
Going Against the Grain by Melissa Diane Smith
The Gluten-Free Bible by Jax Peters Lowell
The Schwarzbein Principle by Diana Schwarzbein, M.D., and Nancy Deville
Ultrametabolism by Mark Hyman, M.D.
Digestive Wellness by Elizabeth Lipski, Ph.D., C.C.N.
Digestive Wellness for Children by Elizabeth Lipski, Ph.D., C.C.N.
Leaky Gut Syndrome by Elizabeth Lipski, M.S., C.C.N.
The Metabolic Typing Diet by William Wolcott and Trish Fahey
Genetic Nutritioneering by Jeffrey S. Bland, Ph.D.
The Gut Flush Plan by Ann Louise Gittleman, Ph.D., C.N.S.

Magazines
Living Without
Gluten-Free Living

Web Sites and Blogs
Celiac Disease and Gluten-free Diet Information: www.celiac.com
Celiac Sprue Association: www.csaceliacs.org
Simply…Gluten-Free (cooking blog):
    www.simplygluten-free.blogspot.com
The Gluten Doctors: www.glutendoctors.blogspot.com
Gluten Intolerance Group® of North America: www.gluten.net
The Gluten Syndrome (patient perspectives on gluten grain
    intolerances and sensitivities): www.glutensensitivity.net
National Foundation for Celiac Awareness: www.celiaccentral.org